RESEARCH

SUCCESSFUL APPROACHES

RESEARCH

SUCCESSFUL APPROACHES

Elaine R. Monsen, PhD, RD, Editor

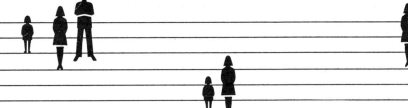

THE AMERICAN DIETETIC ASSOCIATION

Library of Congress Cataloging-in-Publication Data

Research: Successful Approaches/Elaine R. Monsen, editor.
   p.   cm.
   Includes bibliographical references and index.
   ISBN 0-88091-092-5
   1. Nutrition — Research.   2. Dietetics — Research.   I. Monsen, Elaine R.   II. American
Dietetic Association.
TX367.R46 1991   91-31303
363.8′072 — dc20   CIP

The views expressed in this publication are those of the authors and do not necessarily reflect policies and/or official positions of The American Dietetic Association. Mention of product names in this publication does not constitute endorsement by the authors or The American Dietetic Association. The American Dietetic Association disclaims responsibility for the application of the information contained herein.

Printed in Mexico.

CONTRIBUTORS

Editor

Elaine R. Monsen, PhD, RD
Editor, *Journal of The American
    Dietetic Association*
Professor of Nutrition and
Medicine
University of Washington
Seattle, Washington

Authors

Cheryl L. Achterberg, PhD
Associate Professor, Nutrition
    Department
The Pennsylvania State University
University Park, Pennsylvania

Carol J. Boushey, MPH, RD
Research Assistant, Nutritional
    Sciences
University of Washington
Seattle, Washington

Jean C. Burge, PhD, RD
Assistant Professor, Medical
    Dietetics Division
The Ohio State University
Columbus, Ohio

Carrie L. Cheney, PhD, RD
Research Associate
Fred Hutchinson Cancer Research
    Center
Seattle, Washington

Ronni Chernoff, PhD, RD
Associate Director, Geriatric
    Research Education and
    Clinical Center
John L. McClellan Memorial
    Veterans Hospital
Professor of Nutrition and Dietetics
University of Arkansas for Medical
    Sciences
Little Rock, Arkansas

Anne M. Dattilo, PhD, RD
Assistant Professor, Foods and
    Nutrition
The University of Georgia
Athens, Georgia

Barbara H. Dennis, PhD, RD
Research Associate Professor,
    Department of Nutrition
School of Public Health
University of North Carolina
Chapel Hill, North Carolina

Doris D. Disbrow, DrPH, RD
Field Faculty/Adjunct Lecturer
Director, Dietetic Internship
Public Health Nutrition Program
University of California, Berkeley
Berkeley, California

Rebecca A. Dowling, PhD, RD
Director, Department of Food and
    Nutrition Service
Rush–Presbyterian–St. Luke's
    Medical Center
Chicago, Illinois

Judith A. Ernst, DMSc, RD
Associate Professor of Nutrition
    and Dietetics
Pediatric–Neonatal Dietitian
Indiana University School of
    Medicine
J. W. Riley Hospital for Children
Indianapolis, Indiana

Judith A. Gilbride, PhD, RD
Associate Professor, Department of
    Nutrition, Food and Hotel
    Management
New York University
New York, New York

Mary B. Gregoire, PhD, RD
Associate Professor, Department of
    Hotel, Restaurant, Institution
    Management and Dietetics
Kansas State University
Manhattan, Kansas

Jean H. Hankin, DrPH, RD
Research Nutritionist
Professor of Public Health
Cancer Research Center
University of Hawaii
Honolulu, Hawaii

P. M. Kris-Etherton, PhD, RD
Professor, Nutrition Program
College of Human Development
The Pennsylvania State University
University Park, Pennsylvania

M. Eileen Matthews, PhD, RD
Professor, Foodservice
    Administration Program
Department of Food Science
University of Wisconsin–Madison
Madison, Wisconsin

David J. Mela, PhD
Head of Food Acceptance Section
Consumer Sciences Department
Agricultural and Food Research
    Council
Institute of Food Research
Reading, United Kingdom

Judy L. Miller, PhD, RD
Professor and Head, Department of
    Hotel, Restaurant, Institution
    Management and Dietetics
Kansas State University
Manhattan, Kansas

Denise Ouellet, MBA, DtP
Foodservice Administration
    Program
Department of Food Science
University of Wisconsin–Madison
Madison, Wisconsin

Sara C. Parks, MBA, RD
Dean and Associate Professor,
    College of Health and Human
    Development and School of
    Hotel, Restaurant, and
    Institutional Management
The Pennsylvania State University
University Park, Pennsylvania

Jean A. T. Pennington, PhD, RD
Associate Director for Dietary
    Surveillance
Division of Nutrition
Center for Food Safety and Applied
    Nutrition
Food and Drug Administration
Department of Health and Human
    Services
Washington, DC

Judy Perkin, DrPH, RD
Program Manager, University of
    Florida Shands Cancer Center
Shands Hospital
Gainesville, Florida

M. Rosita Schiller, PhD, RD
Professor and Director, Medical
    Dietetics Division
The Ohio State University
Columbus, Ohio

Sandra K. Shepherd, PhD, RD
Assistant Professor, Department of
    Clinical Nutrition
Rush University
Rush–Presbyterian–St. Luke's
    Medical Center
Chicago, Illinois

Bettylou Sherry, PhD, RD
Assistant Professor, Maternal and
    Child Health
School of Public Health
University of Washington
Seattle, Washington

Margaret D. Simko, PhD, RD
Clinical Professor
University of Medicine and
    Dentistry of New Jersey
Robert Wood Johnson Medical
    School
Department of Family Medicine
New Brunswick, New Jersey

Carol West Suitor, DSc, RD
Study Director, Food and
    Nutrition Board
Institute of Medicine
National Academy of Sciences
Washington, DC

Faye L. Wong, MPH, RD
Branch Chief, Center for Chronic
    Disease Prevention and Health
    Promotion
Centers for Disease Control
US Department of Health and
    Human Services
Atlanta, Georgia

Catherine E. Woteki, PhD, RD
Director, Food and Nutrition Board
Institute of Medicine
National Academy of Sciences
Washington, DC

CONTENTS

FOREWORD

Few people remember or even know that it was a group of research dietitians who were among the first to organize themselves as a special interest group within The American Dietetic Association. Six energetic and enthusiastic research dietitians from around the country, representing clinical research centers of the National Institutes of Health, met during the 47th Annual Meeting of The American Dietetic Association in Portland, Oregon. On July 29, 1964, at that same meeting, the Research Dietitians Group, as it was then called, was established.

In 1977, dietetic practice groups as we now know them were officially incorporated as distinct units within The American Dietetic Association. Today there are more than 20 dietetic practice groups representing a wide range of specialties within the profession of dietetics and nutrition. All dietetic practice groups have a defined working environment and area of interest. The Nutrition Research Dietetic Practice Group is unique, however, in that the research process, our underlying specialty and common thread, is a fundamental building block and part of all dietetic practice. Consequently, our membership works in many different arenas. Whether these job settings are in education, government agencies, the community, foodservice, private industry, private practice, clinical settings, or the laboratory, it is research that provides the new knowledge to stimulate growth, change, and progress.

As dietitians, we recognize that it is the understanding and application of scientific methodology that will give us the skills to interpret data and make decisions that will lead to growth within our individual careers and our profession.

Elaine Monsen is a strong advocate of the importance of research to the practitioner, the profession, and the Association. As Editor of the *Journal of The American Dietetic Association*, she sees the broad spectrum and application of research to all areas of nutrition and dietetics. From her vast experience, insight, and expertise this book has evolved. The contributing authors she invited are experts in their own fields, and contributors to all areas of nutrition research application.

The Nutrition Research Dietetic Practice Group views this text as a valuable resource for all dietetic practitioners: as a guide to independent creativity, to the interpretation of new knowledge for future growth, and to the development of new avenues of opportunity.

Janis Swain, MS, RD, 1990–1991 Chairman
Gail Frank, DrPH, RD, 1989–1990 Chairman
Deborah Golden, MS, RD, 1991–1992 Chairman
Nutrition Research Dietetic Practice Group

INTRODUCTION

This monograph describing the why, what and how of research is targeted toward the nutrition, dietetics, and allied health professional. The Editor, Dr. Elaine Monsen, and several of the contributors are current or past members of the Council on Research. The authors represent successful researchers in the field. Thus, we can learn and be motivated by their cumulative experience and practical examples. The Council on Research hopes this monograph will stimulate research relevant to the field of dietetics and encourage members to get involved in the research process.

Research has been recognized as the "backbone" of our profession. It is the supporting framework from which our body of knowledge and activities evolve. It is necessarily integrated into the matrix of all Association activities. As such, research must be properly formed, well nourished, and practically functional. It must be supported by new research to remain healthy and enduring.

We cannot let our profession fall behind in the quest for new information. Each of us must assume the responsibility and challenge to contribute to the development and future of our profession. The opportunity to build from within and develop our skills so we can successfully position ourselves in the demanding marketplace is critical to our overall professional viability.

Research must become an integral part of all levels of dietetic practice. Research can range from a simple systematic gathering of facts to answer a question; a problem-solving technique; the evolution of a new method or product; comparisons of product, interventions, or delivery systems; or analysis of an important phenomenon. The decision is yours to be creative, practical, and correct in your methods. The information presented in this monograph will support you in these efforts.

Research is becoming a necessity, rather than a luxury, for every one of us. The purpose of this monograph is to present the basic components of applied research in our profession, to describe methods, and to present perspectives that will be directly applicable to practicing dietitians. It is enthusiastically supported by the Council on Research and ADA's Department of Research, and it will be used extensively in future workshops and programs of the Association. We look forward to significant contributions in research from our members and other health professionals who use this publication.

Sachiko T. St. Jeor, PhD, RD, 1990–1991 Chairman
Ronnie Chernoff, PhD, RD, 1991–1992 Chairman
Janet R. Hunt, PhD, RD, 1992–1993 Chairman
Council on Research

PART 1
RESEARCH METHODS: DESIGN, DATA ANALYSIS, AND PRESENTATION

The chapters collected here present insights and guidance from experts in diverse areas of nutrition and dietetics research. I was impressed that the authors' excitement and satisfaction in research is evident throughout their discussions of the challenges and rigor of research. The practical observations provided by these experienced investigators will make research accessible to all readers.

The book, organized in eight parts, begins with an overview of research design, analysis, and presentation. The following part, on the research environment, discusses ethical issues that pertain to conducting and presenting research, and it supplies useful information about preparing research proposals and funding applications. The core middle parts provide clear discussions of descriptive and analytical research, major techniques used in research, and statistical analyses. The final two parts highlight effective processes in presenting research and beneficial interactions of practice and research. A detailed index completes the book.

Chapter 1, the impetus for the book, presents a paradigm of research issues in which research is categorized by its purpose, that is, either to describe or to analyze. Descriptive research generates data, both qualitative and quantitative, that define the state of nature at a point in time. Assessments of selected populations, well-constructed surveys, accumulated vital statistics, and observations and interviews of individuals or groups are among the methods used frequently to secure descriptive data (see also chapters 4 through 7). Often the objective is to obtain baseline data for use in decision making or in monitoring changes over time. Descriptive research offers effective ways by which associations may be established and hypotheses generated; however, descriptive research can neither assess hypotheses nor ascertain cause and effect.

Analytical research techniques, through observational or experimental designs, allow the evaluation of hypotheses and the determination of causal relationships. Case-control and cohort studies are two types of observational analytical studies (see also chapter 8). Experimental research designs in which intervention is carefully controlled by the researcher permit verification of causal relationships. Clinical trials are designed to evaluate clearly defined treatment group(s) in which the investigator manipulates the variable(s) of interest and compares resulting data from the study group(s) with those from a control group (see also chapters 8 and 9).

As the initial effort, chapter 1 was pivotal. Thus, it deserved and received the valued review and input of more than 40 experts in nutrition and dietetics research. Many of those whose comments were solicited actively participate on the Board of Editors of the *Journal of The American Dietetic Association,* the ADA Publications Committee, the ADA Council on Research, and the Nutrition Research Dietetic Practice Group. Their assistance is greatly appreciated.

Each of the 24 chapters that follow chapter 1 has also benefited from the capable review and expertise of individuals in each specialized area. The mammoth task of reviewing the entire 25 chapters was accomplished by Idamarie LaQuatra, PhD, RD, and Martha T. Conklin, PhD, RD. Final reviewers were Susan Laramee, MS, RD, chairman of the ADA Publications Committee, and Mary Carey, PhD, RD, member of the ADA Board of Directors and liaison to the ADA Publications Committee.

The exceptional chapters of the 28 contributing authors have been transformed into this monograph through the diligence and gusto of Carol J. Boushey, MPH, RD, the publishing expertise of Karen Izui and Roberta Cooper-Meyer, RD, and the unflagging support and encouragement of Deborah L. McBride. That the book has become a reality is a tribute to all.

ERM, Editor

1. RESEARCH DESIGN, ANALYSIS, AND PRESENTATION

Elaine R. Monsen, PhD, RD, and Carrie L. Cheney, PhD, RD

Research is the backbone of nutrition and dietetics. It supports practice and offers new directions. Research allows objective measurement of complex environments and tangible evaluation of the outcomes of procedures and treatments. Through research, associations can be observed, hypotheses tested, programs compared, and protocols evaluated. Research procedures can be used to document practice, to monitor activities, to assure quality, and to assess cost-effectiveness. The strength of a discipline, whether in health sciences or management, is associated closely with its research base. Strong research supports a strong profession.

Dietitians are assuming an increasingly major role in research, both as leaders and as collaborators. Research has an impact on all areas of dietetics. Dietetic and nutrition education are guided and updated by research findings. Practice-related research will continue to drive the future of dietetic professionals.

The ten sections on research methods in nutrition and dietetics presented in this chapter are guides for design and interpretation of research. The chapter is an overview and includes the major types of research designs. As a guide for research, the chapter addresses principal issues and points out potential problems of various research designs.

Research may be broadly classified according to purpose as descriptive or analytical. Descriptive studies include qualitative research (section 2.0), case reports and case series (section 3.0), and survey research (section 4.0). Those designs describe the state of nature at a point in time. They are useful for generating hypotheses regarding the determinants of a condition or disease or the characteristic of interest. The studies provide baseline data and can monitor change over time, eg, nutritional status of the nation. Descriptive studies can establish associations among factors but do not allow causal relationships to be determined.

Analytical research includes both experimental designs (section 5.0), such as clinical trials, and observational research designs, such as cohort or follow-up studies (section 7.0) and case-control studies (section 8.0). Analytical studies are designed to test hypotheses concerning the effects of specific factors of interest and allow causal associations to be detected. Only experimental studies in which intervention is designed by the researchers provide proof of cause and effect. Partially controlled or quasi-experimental designs (section 6.0) are less rigorous than analytical research and thus less definitive. The last sections survey a variety of tests used in statistical analyses (section 9.0) and discuss application of research data, conclusions that the data can support, and the ensuing research project (section 10.0).

This chapter originally appeared, in a slightly different form, in *J Am Diet Assoc.* 1988;88:1047-1065. Used by permission.

The choice of research design depends upon the nature of the research question, the setting in which the study is to take place, and available resources.

Each section and subsection is numbered for easy referral and reference. Subsections of particular interest are ethics in research (section 1.6); human subject review and confidentiality (sections 3.2 and 5.1); subject selection (sections 3.3, 4.3, 5.4, 7.3, 8.3, and 8.4); validity, accuracy, reliability, and precision (section 4.5); sensitivity and specificity (section 4.6); and statistical analysis and interpretation (sections 3.5, 4.7, 5.9, 7.7, 8.6, 9.0).

Examples of research in clinical dietetics, foodservice, dietetic education, and nutrition are given throughout the chapter to illustrate the various research designs. The examples are abstracted from published research, elaborations and expansions of published research, or, for the most part, fabricated for illustration.

1.0 THE RESEARCH QUESTION

1.1 Select the Research Topic

The research process is a problem-solving, decision-making procedure involving a series of interrelated decisions. When one focuses on one decision at a time, the research process becomes manageable. Each option can be considered, and the most appropriate option can be selected. Research projects should be meaningful; they should expand current knowledge and practice of the profession.

Initially, select issues important to your practice and, thereby, important to the field of dietetics. In selecting specific areas, researchers develop and extend their own areas of expertise. Research questions evolve from many sources, including ideas to improve patient health, suggestions to increase effectiveness of services and products, untested concepts in published literature, application of business research methods,[1,2] and uncharted boundaries in basic research of all areas of advanced study. In selecting the research topic, observe and thoughtfully consider the needs of your own practice. Then, in addressing the overall topic, break the problem down into its component parts and select a component that is feasible to study in your setting. Start with a simple question. Data generated in response to the initial question will lead to many other questions and aspects of the problem that subsequent studies can address.

1.2 Prepare for the Project

It is necessary to review the published research literature related to your topic. In your review, emphasize both current scientific literature and seminal classic articles. Computerized literature search can speed and facilitate your review. A critical review of previous work in the field can be the base upon which to build solid new research projects. Shortcomings can be improved and suggested new areas developed. Contact people who are interested and/or experienced in the field. Discuss the problem with them personally by telephone or by electronic communication. Actively seek out information that may be useful to you from colleagues in related fields.

Available resources and personnel need to be assessed, eg, patient population, laboratory and library facilities, foodservice equipment, nutrient databases, data processing capabilities, computer facilities, personnel resources, statistical consultants, other consultants, and collaborative opportunities. Team efforts permit quality research that provides major benefits to the profession. Practicing dietitians can demonstrate leadership in research by directing such team efforts.

Direct and indirect costs to perform the research need to be estimated. If a study is well designed and carefully developed, it may be accomplished with existing personnel and facilities. If it is necessary to obtain funds, consider a variety of funding sources.[3,4] As you prepare for the project, you should be formulating the research question and evaluating its feasibility.

1.3 State Clearly the Question To Be Researched

A concise, simple, straightforward statement of the research question focuses the research design process. Clearly define the question and strive to keep it uncomplicated. Use objective, measurable, operational terms, such as *identify, compare, differentiate,* and *describe.*

Components of the research question are:
- *Who (Which):* The subjects or units being assessed need to be defined in broad terms, eg, patients with diabetes, dietetics students, food items, tray lines, foodservice costs.
- *What:* The factor of interest needs to be stated specifically, eg, body weight, knowledge, iron intake, tray error, labor costs.
- *How assessed:* The outcome to be assessed needs to be stated specifically, eg, disease incidence, change in knowledge, alterations in food selection, tray errors per meal, labor costs per patient day.

When the research question has been stated clearly, the research project can be designed more easily. Consider several research designs to see which is best suited to the research question and the setting. Among items to consider are (a) the variables, ie, characteristics or attributes of the persons or objects that vary within the study population (eg, fiber intake, serum cholesterol); (b) the dependent variables, ie, the outcome variables of interest (eg, serum cholesterol); and (c) the independent variable, ie, the variable that is thought to influence the dependent variable and is manipulated in experimental designs (eg, fiber intake).

Other study design characteristics relate to time and direction of data collection and include (a) cross-sectional studies, ie, a study based on data collected from a group of subjects at a single point in time; (b) longitudinal studies, ie, a study based on data collected at more than one point in time; (c) prospective studies, ie, a study that begins with examination of presumed causes (eg, fiber intake) and goes forward in time to observed presumed effects (eg, cardiovascular disease); and (d) retrospective studies, ie, a study that begins with manifestations of an outcome (eg, cardiovascular disease) and goes back in time to uncover relationships with presumed causes (eg, fiber intake).

1.4 Prepare Research Protocol

Research protocols are useful to concentrate research efforts and to provide needed information to key parties. Components to include in the research protocol are first, the research question, focused and concisely stated; second, a literature review; third, importance and potential value of the research; and fourth, the research design, which presents a clear outline of who, what, and how assessed. The research design component should be composed of manageable subsections, including methods, data analysis, and appropriate statistical analysis.

When research funding is sought, research proposals need to conform with the funding agency's guidelines. Many private and public agencies model their guidelines after those of the National Institutes of Health (NIH). The initial section of an NIH grant application is composed of a title page, an abstract of the research plan, a table of contents, biographical sketches of investigators and other key project personnel, other existing or pending sources of support, and an assessment of the availability of needed resources and the appropriateness of the environment in which the research will be conducted.

The second section of an NIH grant application is composed of eight subsections. First, the specific aims and objectives of the research project are to be summarized succinctly. Second, the significance of the research is to be presented to support the practical and theoretical relevance of the project, including a critical concise review of the literature. Third, published and unpublished preliminary studies done by the investigators, including pilot studies, are to be discussed.

Fourth, the research design and methods to be employed are given in detail. Within this subsection, it is customary to present the research question; methods of sample selection, including statements about selection bias; justification of sample size estimates; experimental intervention if planned; instrumentation and the reliability and validity of planned measuring instruments; data collection procedures, including where and how; plans for analysis of data; and a project schedule or work plan.

Fifth, human subject approval procedures to assure protection of subjects' rights and to disclose the potential risks undertaken are outlined. Prior approval obtained from the local institutional review board can be included to support the research grant application. Sixth, if vertebrate animals are to be used in the research project, justification as to their need in the research and their welfare during the research must be provided.

Seventh, if consultants are to be used during the project, letters confirming their willingness to participate must be provided. Eighth, the literature cited within the application is listed.

1.5 Conduct a Pilot Study

A trial or pilot study is strongly advised. The pilot study will provide experience prior to conducting the full research project. Many refinements in methods and measuring instruments may be suggested to the researcher. Although it is tempting to design an instrument and immediately use it in collecting data, time is more effectively used if the instrument is tested before it is used in the major study. Making adjustments before instigating the major study can make data collection easier and more successful. In some cases, a researcher will wish to redraft the research question as well as the research protocol. Think through what data you need and what you will do with them statistically. If you do not know what you will do with the data, then you should ask yourself whether you need to collect them. Data and experience generated from the pilot study can be used to gain support and funding for the major project.

1.6 Assure Ethics in Research

In preparing for research activities, researchers need to adhere to ethical procedures in all aspects of design and conduct of the research.[5,6] Ethics are important in the choice of topics, the samples selected, the interventions designed, and the data collection procedures. After data are collected, ethics are of great importance in the analysis and reporting of data.[7]

2.0 QUALITATIVE RESEARCH

A qualitative study often precedes other research designs. Its primary purpose is to explore the phenomenon of interest as a prelude to theory development.[8] The design is necessarily flexible so that the researcher can discover ideas, gain insight, and, ultimately, formulate the problem for further investigation. Kidder and Judd[9] refer to qualitative studies as formulative or exploratory studies, characterized by the receptive, seeking attitude of the investigator and an intense study of the individuals or groups. One approach is grounded theory research, where data "grounded" in real-life observations are collected and analyzed with the purpose of developing theoretical propositions.

Example. Grounded theory research may be used to explore and describe the major attributes of effective practitioners, such as foodservice administrators, dietetic technicians, or clinical dietitians. The question "What specific dimensions are associated with an effective nutrition counselor?" can be addressed initially by developing a set of criteria for selecting effective clinical dietitians. The criteria are based on existing research, role delineation studies, peer evaluation, student evaluation, recommendation by supervisors, peer recognition, and award. Data are collected through systematic focused interviews and direct observations during daily activities in clinical settings. Individuals who interact closely with the selected clinical dietitians are interviewed: patients, students, peers, and supervisors. All data are treated confidentially. Commonalities and differences in patterns of behavior, and cognitive and affective domains will emerge. From results of the grounded theory research, prior theories can be refined and new hypotheses, to be tested quantitatively in future research, can be generated.

Subjects are selected according to their experience with the phenomenon being explored. Thus, they have special characteristics and are not considered to be typical or representative of the population. Data are collected by such methods as observation, interviews, and questionnaires. The interview format may range from structured—restricting the range of responses—to less structured—permitting an unlimited range of responses. The less structured or unstructured interview may be focused on a particular topic or experience (a focused interview) or may have minimal direction (a nondirective interview).[9]

If a group of respondents is assembled together to answer questions on a specific topic, the term *focus group* is applicable. The Delphi technique utilizes a panel of experts who may answer separately; their judgments are collated and circulated to the panel members, who may then be requestioned two or three times until a general consensus is reached. The process results in the reduction of the variability of judgments among panelists. The Delphi technique is useful in developing solutions to problems, planning, and forecasting.

Example. Priorities in nutrition and dietetics research will be examined using the Delphi technique with three cycles of question, analysis, feedback, and response. Panel members recognized for their interest and expertise in research will be identified by dietetic practice groups. The first questionnaire will request each panel member to identify seven research areas of highest priority. Responses will be analyzed, and the areas most frequently identified will be sent back to the panel members, along with a questionnaire requesting that the areas be ranked as to importance and potential impact on the field. Responses will be summarized and sent with the last questionnaire requesting further comment on areas in which the panelists disagree. Final results will be sent to all panelists.

3.0 CASE SERIES

3.1 Uses

A case series is a report of observations on one subject (a case report) or more than one subject (a case series) that may be used in administrative as well as educational and clinical settings. The purpose of this design is to describe quantitatively the experience of a series of cases with a disease or condition in common. Investigators using this design attempt to identify the variables that are important to the etiology, care, or outcome of subjects with a particular condition.

A carefully prepared case series report helps to generate hypotheses for future studies. The information gathered can provide evidence for an association between the disease or condition and a suspected etiological or therapeutic factor. It also provides the data necessary to justify the need for future studies and can help determine the methods to be used in such studies. Results from case series research cannot be generalized unless the cases are selected with the rigor required to be representative of the target populations. (See section 4.3.)

3.2 Institutional Approval and Confidentiality

Most research involving human subjects requires prior approval by an institutional review board. (See section 5.1.) Check with administrative authorities about local review procedures of both the research site and the researcher's affiliated institution.

The privacy of the information gathered must be protected during all phases of the study, including record keeping, data storage, data retrieval, follow-up, computing, reporting, and procedures. Procedures to assure confidentiality are those that prevent the identification of the individual subjects. Code numbers are used as identifiers rather than names. Other steps to protect confidentiality should be planned in advance.

In studies in which non-routine tests or measures are collected, informed written consent must be obtained from each subject. Even when routine tests are used, informed consent may be necessary so that the data can be used. (See section 5.1.)

3.3 Features and Subject Selection

A case series is an expansion of the case report, in which observations of a single or a few cases are reported. The series is composed of all cases of a specific disease or condition occurring or presenting to a particular clinic or locality during a specified period of time. For example, the series may consist of patients with gastric cancer who were referred to the nutrition support service for consultation during a 6-month period. This method of subject selection yields a convenience sample that cannot be considered representative of all gastric cancer patients (section 3.5); therefore, the results cannot be generalized to larger groups.

Example. A case report will be generated through evaluating opportunities for cost saving through private consultation in the operation of a single, long-term-care facility. Permission for quality assurance review will be obtained from the administrator of the facility. Two areas will be emphasized: first, food production with observation of sanitation procedures and the use of standardized recipes; second, overview of the nutritional needs of the residents as observed by chart review of residents with decubiti, insulin-dependent diabetes, renal failure requiring dialysis, or severe or chronic weight loss. Medical records will be reviewed for charting of height, weight, and caloric intake. If residents are receiving parenteral or enteral feeding, records will be reviewed for charting of energy, protein, and fluid requirements and intake.

3.4 Data Collection

Most commonly, existing records provide the data; however, data generated concurrently may be collected. The advantage of concurrent data collection is the opportunity to obtain complete information in a standardized way, although that may also be possible with existing data.

Example. A concurrent case series determined labor minutes per meal equivalent and percentage of time spent in direct work, indirect work, delay time, and total time. A preliminary study identified 14 areas in which employees worked most frequently in the foodservice department, the average number of employees per work area, and an estimate of the required number of readings needed for the projected study on labor time. Data were collected from activity sampling studies of foodservice workers in the same community hospital for 7 days (Monday to Sunday) during the second week of February for 12 consecutive years. The longitudinal study provided an opportunity to assess trends in the distribution of labor time, examine patterns among work and delay activities, and identify factors in the foodservice environment that may have an impact on labor productivity.[10]

Data concerning relevant factors are collected by chart or record review, questionnaire, interview, or examination. A combination of collection methods may be used. The data usually cover a broad range of factors in-depth, forming a detailed description of the cases. The variety and depth allow a number of factors to be considered but of necessity limit the number of subjects or objects under study.

Example. A case series was generated from all reports of foodborne illness received over the past 5 years by the regional public health department. Reports selected for review had to include microbiological analysis of suspected foods. Descriptive analysis of the data will allow patterns related to food type and geographic distribution to emerge.

3.5 Statistical Analysis and Interpretation

Simple descriptive statistics—such as means, medians, standard deviations, ranges, and frequencies—are appropriate. Alternatively, the actual data for each subject may be presented for the most important variables, especially if the size of the series, eg, the number of subjects, is small. Regardless of sample size, statistical tests for inference are usually not appropriate because hypotheses are not investigated in that type of study.

When the researchers interpret results of a case series report, they must acknowledge that the sample is not representative of a larger population of cases. The series of cases is selected by the investigators according to certain conditions and may consist of cases unique in certain characteristics. It remains to be shown in further study whether the results can be generalized beyond the individuals chosen for the study.

Example. A series was generated from a chart review of all acute-care patients who were given albumin infusions during hospitalization, in an effort to identify factors related to the use of albumin and to describe the outcome of its use. The requisite for selection was the existence of records that included complete daily intake and output records and laboratory reports and could be evaluated. Many important cases were omitted because records were incomplete. Some of the factors that resulted in an incomplete record were known, such as interruptions because of emergency procedures and incontinence in patients not catheterized. The number of patients omitted was listed along with the known factors. But the investigators suspected other unidentified reasons existed because most of the omitted patients were on the gastrointestinal surgical service. These patients were likely to be different in other ways from those selected for study. Those differences may have related in some way to albumin use or outcome. The investigators were careful to describe the study patients thoroughly and resisted generalizing the results.

4.0 SURVEY

A survey is research designed to describe and quantify characteristics of a defined population. A survey lacks a specific hypothesis, although the investigator may suspect that certain relationships exist. The purpose of a survey is to obtain a statistical profile of the population.[11] A survey, for example, may be designed to assess nutrient content of the food supply.

Example. To determine the variation in nutrient composition of fast-food fried chicken, a preliminary study was conducted to determine the design for a nationwide sampling for a descriptive study, ie, a survey. From each selected city and vendor, five breast-wing and five thigh-leg units were purchased. Each sample was deboned, homogenized, coded, and frozen prior to analysis. Replicate samples were analyzed for fat, protein, moisture, and vitamin content, utilizing appropriate chemical and microbiological methods. Control samples were prepared by identical procedures and analyzed along with each laboratory run.[12]

4.1 Uses

A survey may be useful for establishing associations among variables or factors and often provides clues for further study. Surveys can also provide baseline data about the prevalence of a condition or factor of interest in the population. A major use of the survey method is for planning health services.

Example. The clinical dietitian for a large prepaid health plan wants to know what proportion of the plan's enrollees are interested in weight reduction. The dietitian hopes to plan a weight reduction clinic and needs the estimated participation rates for budget purposes. A random sample of enrollees will be selected to receive a pilot-tested questionnaire regarding their interests. The results will be used to tailor the clinic to the participants' needs; thus, questions about what help enrollees want for weight reduction will be asked.

Most aspects of dietary services can be investigated in this way through careful survey research.

Example. A patient survey will be designed for quality assurance. Randomly selected patients will be questioned with regard to their satisfaction with tray presentation. Assessment will be made on cold food, hot food, time of delivery, and tray appearance. The random survey will be repeated periodically so that tray service can be monitored, trends can be observed, and actions can be taken to improve service.

4.2 Features

As it is usually not feasible to measure the entire population, a sample is selected based on a probability design. The individuals who consent to participate in the sample are then questioned or examined for the disease or characteristic of interest and other relevant variables.

Example. Foodservice managers in health care and educational institutions that applied computer technology to their operations were surveyed to examine the extent to which computers were applied to management and client service functions. The research questionnaire was designed to collect data on the characteristics of the institution, the types of computers in use, the applications for which computers were being used, and the reasons for not using computers. The questionnaire was pretested by a panel of experts using the Delphi technique. The expert panel was composed of specialists in foodservice management, computer systems, and survey research methods. The experts were asked a series of questions, the answers to which were used by the researcher to devise the final questionnaire upon which the panel agreed. Questionnaires were mailed to 2064 persons randomly selected from the membership listings of several professional organizations related to foodservice management.[13]

4.3 Subject Selection

Results of a survey can be generalized with confidence only if the sample is representative of the target population. This means the target population must be defined and enumerated; then a sample is drawn at random from it. A probability sample scheme is devised by which all the individuals in the target population have a known chance of being included in the sample; that is, the chances of being selected are specified in the sampling scheme. A probability sampling method allows the sampling errors to be calculated and increases the likelihood that the study is representative of the target population. A high rate of participation (response rate) increases the chances that the results are representative, as it is never certain that responders and non-responders are similar.

Possible sampling schemes range from the simple random method to complex methods utilizing varying selection probabilities among subgroups (strata) of the population. Elwood[14] discusses the rationale for probability sampling in nutrition research, and Williams[15] provides details on methodology.

The appropriate sample size for a survey depends upon many factors, including how precisely the sample should estimate the population parameters. Methods for calculating sample size requirements are given by Cohen.[16]

A survey based on an accidental or convenience sampling scheme is of limited value because its results cannot be generalized. The reference population is undefined or is defined by the conscious or unconscious selection biases of the investigator. Further, the selection itself may be influenced by the condition or factor under study.

Example. A survey was conducted to identify factors related to noncompliance to diet among patients treated for hypertension with medication plus diet. The study included a convenience sample of patients who returned for follow-up at the hypertension clinic. Unfortunately, this scheme selected those patients who were likely to be more compliant to the diet simply because they returned for follow-up. Despite the purpose of the study, no information on the patients who did not comply with follow-up visits was generated.

4.4 Data Collection

Data are collected most frequently by using a questionnaire or interview but may also be generated by physical examination, for example, anthropometric measurement, laboratory evaluation of specimens, such as blood analysis for hemoglobin levels, or direct observation, such as employee productivity.

One of the most difficult aspects of survey methodology is designing the questionnaire.[17] Given the research objectives, standard or tested instruments can be used, if available. If questions must be developed, they need to be unambiguous yet concise and tactful. The length of the questionnaire, its format, and how it is to be administered are also important considerations. Rimm et al[18] and Polit and Hungler[19] present guidelines and suggestions for questionnaire development.

Consider how the questionnaire will be analyzed in the design phase. Once constructed, a pilot study of the instrument helps to detect problems. Subjects in the pilot test should be individuals similar to those eligible to participate in the formal study.

Questions can be administered by personal interview or telephone interview or by computer-assisted or self-administered questionnaire. Interviews allow questions to be clarified and more detailed information to be collected. The interviewers must be highly trained and objective and adhere to a set questioning routine to minimize their influence on the subject's responses.

Information about physical traits or symptoms can be collected by observation in some settings, particularly institutional or clinical settings. Criteria and definitions by which observations are made must be specific to improve accuracy. The observation technique should be standardized and each observer carefully trained to minimize intra- and inter-observer variation. Verify that laboratory methods are reliable and standardized and their accuracy is quantified. If laboratory analyses are to be done out of the researcher's laboratory, select laboratories that are certified by a recognized agency, such as the College of Medical Pathologists. For any assessment that is dependent to some degree upon the judgment of the observer, eg, self-reports of appetite, assessment of a more objective, "hard" variable, eg, measured caloric intake, is helpful. It is also an aid to establishing validity of a subject's self-report.

Example. To examine the entry-level role responsibilities in community dietetics, questionnaires were sent to randomly selected subjects consisting of 152 Plan IV representatives, 82 internship directors, and 740 dietetic interns. Postage-paid return envelopes were enclosed. A follow-up postcard was mailed 2 weeks later. Questionnaires were color-coded according to the seven geographic areas used by the ADA House of Delegates; all materials were otherwise anonymous. Data collected from dietetic interns were self-reports of perceived competence at two points in time, one being the current moment and the other being at the start of the dietetic internship experience. Data collected from internship directors used the same scale, but ratings were opinions as to the perceived degree of competence that students should possess at the completion of their academic work.[20]

4.5 Validity, Accuracy, Reliability, and Precision

Four measurement qualities critical to all research are discussed here; they relate to all research projects and data interpretation. Any instrument devised needs to be pilot tested, revised, and retested to assure its validity and reliability.

The validity of a test or instrument refers to its ability to measure the phenomenon it intends to measure. Validity of an instrument can be readily assessed when the true state of the phenomenon can be measured. Unfortunately, if such a method exists, it is often costly and time-consuming.

A quantitative measure of the validity of an instrument is accuracy. The accuracy of an instrument is the measure of the systematic error in measurement.[18] The difference between the measured and the true values expresses the accuracy of the instrument. Observer subjectivity also affects the accuracy of the instrument. For example, observers may be more likely to report even values when reporting the terminal digit of a caliper reading. An average of repeated readings may help to minimize the error in accuracy. Questionnaires requiring recall of diet or other events are particularly subject to inaccuracy. Supplementing responses with other types of information may help to establish validity. (See section 4.4.)

The reliability of a test or an instrument is determined by its consistency of results when applied to the same specimen repeatedly, administered by either the same or different persons. The reliability of clinical tests can be determined by repeated assays of aliquots taken from the same specimen. The reliability of observational reports or physical examinations can be assessed by comparing the data from the same subjects gathered by two or more observers. Follow-up questionnaires can be administered to a subset of the sample to determine whether the instrument elicits the same responses.

A quantitative measure of the reliability of an instrument is precision. The precision of an instrument is described by the amount of variation that occurs randomly, a measure of its random error.[18] The dispersion (variation) of measurements around the true value expresses the precision. Less random variation results in greater precision in the measurement and greater reliability.

4.6 Sensitivity and Specificity

If a survey or other research protocol involves screening for a particular condition, there is a need to address both sensitivity and specificity. For example, the intent of a survey may be to determine the prevalence of a certain condition or diagnosis, such as folate deficiency in pregnant women. Tests or observations are used to classify subjects as to the presence or absence of folate deficiency as defined by a cut-off value of 6 nmol/L (3 ng/mL).[21] How well the cut-off criteria categorize the population is quantified by two measures: sensitivity and specificity.

The sensitivity of a test or criterion is the proportion of afflicted individuals who test positive, ie, the proportion of those individuals with folate deficiency whose serum folate is less than 6 nmol/L (3 ng/mL). Likewise, the specificity of a test or criterion is the proportion of non-afflicted individuals who are identified as non-afflicted, ie, who test negative. Griner et al[22] review the principles of test interpretation, including calculating sensitivity and specificity. Begg[23] describes the sources of bias in diagnostic tests and critiques the measures of test efficacy, sensitivity, and specificity.

The choice of a single cut-off value to categorize individuals may not be clear when the test yields a continuous scale of values. A cut-off value chosen to maximize sensitivity will unavoidably cause the test to be less specific.[24] The selection of an appropriate cut-off point is aided by use of a graph plotting true-positive against false-positive ratios, known as a "ROC curve" (receiver-operating-characteristic curve). Several authors discuss constructing and using a ROC curve.[24-26]

4.7 Statistical Analysis and Interpretation

Results of surveys can be described using simple descriptive statistics, such as means, medians, standard deviations, and frequency distributions. Plot the frequency distributions of important variables to determine skewness, or departure from the normal bell-shaped curve. If skewness is present and the mean and median differ substantially, more information about the distribution must be presented, such as a histogram of the distribution. Relationships between variables are best presented as scatter diagrams,[18] and subsequently defined by mathematical models, such as correlation coefficients. Prevalence rates can also be calculated.[18]

The National Health and Nutrition Examination Surveys (NHANES) provide examples of positive or right skewed data. The mean intake of vitamin C for females, aged 6 months to 74 years, as assessed for 10 339 subjects in NHANES II, was 93 mg/day[27]; the median intake was 63 mg/day. With such strong positive skewness, presenting the median intake with high and low percentiles, such as 10th and 90th (11 and 209 mg), provides a clearer picture of the intake of the study population than does the mean with either its standard deviation (163 mg) or its standard error (1.6 mg). (See sections 9.1 and 9.3.)

When survey results are interpreted, limitations inherent in the study methodology should be considered. Major among them is a low response rate, since nonrespondents may differ in important ways from respondents. The response rate affects the confidence given the results and limits the degree to which the results can be generalized. Efforts should be vigorous to follow up on nonrespondents and increase the response rate. A low response rate can seriously damage an otherwise well-designed study, as it increases the sampling error (error due to sampling only the responsive portion of the target population).

A second major limitation occurs because measurements are taken at one point in time. Since all variables are measured simultaneously, the temporal relationship between factors and the condition or disease of interest is not known. It is not clear that exposure to a suspected causal agent preceded the onset of the disease. For the same reason, it is not possible to distinguish between a risk factor and a prognostic factor.

Use discretion in applying inferential statistical tests to data from survey research. Because survey studies are designed to be descriptive rather than analytical, formal tests of hypotheses are undertaken after the data are viewed, and the test result is likely to be biased toward a spurious statistically significant result. (See section 4.8.) Such inferential tests are to be regarded as exploratory, useful in generating questions for future analytical studies.

4.8 Ex Post Facto Analysis

Analysis "after the fact," or ex post facto, should be used with caution. In ex post facto research, variations in the variable of interest have not been manipulated by the researcher but rather have occurred at various times prior to data collection in the natural course of events. Subjects have not been assigned randomly into treatment groups, and no control or comparison group has been studied.

While providing information regarding associations of variables, ex post facto analysis cannot yield satisfactory answers regarding causal relationships for the reasons outlined in section 4.7. The preferable approach in testing causal relationships would be to devise an analytical study, such as an experimental design (section 5.0), an observational analytical study, eg, a cohort (follow-up) study (section 7.0), or a case-control study (section 8.0). If it is not possible to design an analytical research project, then ex post facto analysis may be considered, but the results should be viewed as exploratory and must not be interpreted falsely as causal. Instead, ex post facto analysis serves as the springboard for future analytical designs.

Example. Cross-sectional data on food consumption, supplement usage, and bone density could be obtained from 1000 postmenopausal women randomly selected from the Midwest region. If ex post facto analysis of the data showed a statistically significant positive association between dietary calcium intake and bone density and between supplementary calcium intake and bone density, analytical studies could be designed to test the hypothesis that calcium intake affects bone density of postmenopausal women.

An observational analytical study using a case-control design (section 8.0) could be developed from the existing survey data by identifying cases and controls and obtaining retrospective data from existing records, personal interview, and questionnaire.

A different analytical research study could be devised using an experimental design in which a subset of postmenopausal women with low bone density was randomly assigned to one of four treatment groups: placebo plus diet counseling to increase calcium intake, calcium supplementation plus diet counseling to increase calcium intake, placebo alone, and calcium supplement alone. Bone density of the subjects would be followed by dual photon absorptiometry at the initiation of the study and at 6 months and 1 year. The experimental design outlined is a double-blind (section 5.5), placebo-controlled randomized clinical trial (section 5.2) that conforms to a 2×2 factorial design (section 5.10).

5.0 EXPERIMENTAL DESIGN

Experimental design is the gold standard of analytic research because in that design all factors are held constant save those manipulated by the investigator. Certain observational designs, such as cohort (follow-up) studies (see section 7.0) and case-control studies (see section 8.0) are analytical but not experimental. The intent of analytic research is to test a hypothesis concerning causal relationships, perhaps a hypothesis generated from an earlier descriptive study.

Example. The variation in nutrient composition of fast-food fried chicken described in a nationwide survey (section 4.1) may lead to further research to test the effects on fat content of two different frying techniques.

5.1 Human Subjects Review and Informed Consent

Investigations involving human subjects must meet ethical guidelines to protect the rights, privacy, and welfare of individuals. The Declaration of Helsinki, drafted in 1964 by the World Medical Association, serves as the basis for the ethical guidelines that are now detailed regulations issued by governmental agencies, such as the NIH. A local institutional review board has the task of reviewing all investigations using human subjects to assure ethical conduct and to evaluate potential risks and benefits.

Key among the principles for ethical conduct is the investigator's responsibility to explain to the potential subject the nature of the study, including the possible risks and discomforts he or she may experience. Following the full verbal and written description, the subject is invited to participate in the study. If he or she accepts, the subject must sign a written consent. Confidentiality of all data is mandated by all review boards. (See section 3.2.) Specific elements to be included in the informed consent procedure are designated by the local review board.

5.2 Randomized Clinical Trial: Uses

The experimental design in medical research, referred to as a clinical trial, is the most powerful design for evaluating practices and medical treatments. It is used to prove the feasibility and safety of a treatment. After safety has been established, a clinical trial may be designed to determine the optimal regimen to obtain the desired effect. Most commonly, a clinical trial is employed to compare the efficacy of two or more treatments or practices.

5.3 Features

There are four general features of the randomized clinical trial. First, subjects are informed about the study purposes and risks and asked to participate. (See section 5.1.) Those consenting to participate are assigned randomly to one of two or more treatment or intervention groups. The group receiving the standard treatment (or treatments) constitutes the control group. The third feature is random assignment, ie, chance determines treatment assignment. Finally, subjects are observed for the occurrence of particular outcomes or end points following or concurrent with intervention or treatment.

Example. By randomly assigning dietetics students to a group that received a short curriculum in death education or to a group that did not, the effectiveness of the curriculum could be assessed. This analytical research is a logical extension of a prior quasi-experiment (section 6.0) that utilized a pretest/post-test format for a single group of students who received the curriculum in death education.[28] The prior study provides baseline data and testing of the evaluation instruments that measured the students' change in knowledge of the grief process, personality traits of empathy and dogmatism, fear of death, fear of interacting with the dying, and attitudes toward working with seriously terminally ill clients. Clinical performance of empathic counseling was assessed by direct observations.

5.4 Selection of Subjects

The degree to which the study group is representative of a reference population determines whether the results can be generalized. This must be reconciled with the equally important requirement that, with a high degree of probability, the treatment effect can be seen. In general, select subjects who are relatively homogeneous in major characteristics (eg, diagnosis and nutritional status) so that extraneous sources of variation are eliminated. Other factors to consider when selecting subjects are subject compliance, ease of follow-up, and cost of enrolling and monitoring.[29]

Compliance may be enhanced by offering appropriate incentives to all participants, such as special information or health care. Assessment of compliance prior to the start of the study may be helpful. This can be done by planning a pre-study requirement for all potential subjects. Repeated 24-hour urine collections or several days of dietary intake records are useful requirements for judging compliance. Subjects who are unable to complete the pre-study tasks are less likely to comply with study demands and are excluded from the study before it begins. The resulting sample is necessarily biased, composed as it is of persons selected for their compliant behavior.

The ease of follow-up is related, in part, to the study setting. Follow-up is facilitated in highly restrictive settings or those in which the subject can be readily observed, such as in hospital settings. Unless the research question is relevant in such restricted settings, however, imposing severe restrictions on subjects can impair the study's ability to correspond to a natural setting and can decrease its usefulness.

The cost of enrolling and monitoring subjects influences the number of subjects in the study. (See section 5.7.) In many cases, facilities and resources are available and information is collected routinely, thus lowering the costs per subject.

5.5 Choice of Intervention or Treatment

As with subject selection, the choice of intervention is made to maximize the likelihood that an effect can be detected. The more the treatment of the intervention group differs from the treatment of the comparison or control group, within the range of safe or acceptable levels, the more likely measurable differences will be seen. The comparison or control treatment should have, insofar as possible, a reasonable expectation of benefit at least equal to that of the experimental treatment.[29] An untreated group as control is valid if there is no recognized treatment. Otherwise, the control group should receive the standard or an accepted treatment for the disease or condition of interest.

If there is no recognized treatment and it is thought that a psychological effect or observer bias is likely, a placebo is recommended.[30] The result is a blind study in which the subjects are unaware of the treatment assignment. The placebo, or sham treatment, must be inert and identical to the experimental treatment in appearance and mode of administration. The blinding efficacy should be evaluated before and during the trial to assure that blinding is maintained.[31] If both subjects and investigators are unaware of the treatment assignment, the trial is a double-blind clinical trial, a powerful design because it eliminates expectation bias on the part of the subject and the investigative staff. The effect of expectation cannot be underestimated, as illustrated in the following example.

Example. The NIH conducted a double-blind (neither subject nor investigator was informed as to which treatment group the subject was assigned) randomized controlled trial of the effectiveness of ascorbic acid on reducing the frequency and severity of the common cold.[32] A lactose capsule placebo that could be easily distinguished from the vitamin C tablet by taste was used, although the investigators gave little thought to the possibility that their subjects might actually bite into the capsules.

Early in the study, the investigators learned that their volunteers were quite curious and many had bitten into the capsules; a significant number of subjects knew which medication they were receiving. Although the study was no longer a double-blind study, it did illustrate an association between severity and duration of symptoms and knowledge of the medication taken. Among those subjects who tasted their capsules, those receiving vitamin C had shorter, milder colds, while the converse was true for the placebo group. Among those subjects who remained blind to their treatment, no effect of vitamin C was seen.

5.6 Assignment to Treatment Groups

A random method of treatment assignment is essential. The random method eliminates the selection bias that can occur if the subject or the investigator selects the treatment. It also mitigates nonintentional bias, or the chance formation of groups that are not comparable because of differences in factors that affect the response to treatment, such as age and gender. The random method does not guarantee comparable groups, however, and a chance imbalance between groups is possible, especially if the sample size is less than 200.[33] Restricted randomization is a method of randomization that ensures that groups are equal or similar in numbers of subjects with certain characteristics, such as age and gender.

A crossover design uses subjects as their own controls rather than using a separate control group. This design requires fewer subjects because the within-subject variation is less than between-subject variation. It is useful when the study involves conditions that are chronic and the treatment effects, if present, are not long lasting. In a crossover design, the subjects are randomly assigned to two groups differing in the sequence of treatments. This assures that an effect due to order of treatment is eliminated from the observed treatment effect.[34]

Although seemingly simple and appealing, the crossover design is difficult to justify in most circumstances. That is because the validity of the comparison rests upon the assumption that the subject enters each time period—treatment and control—in an identical state. There can be no carry-over effects of the treatment and no appreciable change in the subject's condition. The crossover design is not appropriate when the treatment acts systemically[35] or when the physical condition of the subjects is unstable over the period of the trial.[36] The relevant issues are discussed by Hills and Armitage[34] and by Louis et al.[37]

Instead of randomizing patients to a control group, it is often tempting to use a historical control group composed of subjects, usually patients, who were treated in some manner recognized as standard in the past. Unfortunately, it is difficult to establish the validity of historical controls. The biases present in such a series of patients are rarely completely identifiable and may irretrievably weight the outcome of the comparison in favor of the new treatment.[38] It is not possible to assure comparability between current and previous patients and the treatments used. A suggested alternative is to use both historical and concurrent randomized controls but only when certain conditions are met as outlined by Pocock.[39]

Some clinical questions cannot be addressed by a randomized controlled trial because a comparison group of internal controls cannot be formed for ethical or logistic reasons. Other comparison groups—external controls—are necessary. If those controls are well chosen, the studies can make valuable contributions. General advice on the proper use and interpretation of studies using external controls is offered by Bailar et al.[40]

5.7 Size of the Sample

The ability of a clinical trial to detect a difference between treatment and control groups depends, in part, on the sample size. Determining the sample size is an estimate only and is based on several assumptions and judgments about circumstances of the study. The procedures for estimating the size of a study are detailed by Lachin.[41] Briefly, the procedure involves six steps:
1. Choose the main end point of interest and its method of measurement. The main end point selected should be the most important variable amenable to measurement of the variables studied.
2. Choose the statistical test to be applied to the data.
3. Specify the magnitude of the difference that is meaningful to detect. A smaller difference requires a larger sample size. The amount of difference specified should be one that is meaningful, ie, is significant in practice.
4. Estimate the expected variability using published research or results from pilot studies. Sometimes data are not available, and a "best guess" must be made.
5. Specify the acceptable chances of being wrong. Formally, these are the probability levels of type I and type II errors.[41] A type I error (α error) is the probability that a difference will be detected when in truth there is no difference. A type II error (β error) is the probability that a true difference will not be detected. The power of a study, which is the probability that a difference in specified size will be detected successfully, is determined by the formula $1 - \beta$.
6. Apply the appropriate calculations.

If the resulting number is larger than is reasonable with available resources, a second question should be asked: Given the available resources and the sample size feasible to accrue, what is the chance that a meaningful difference can be detected (ie, what is the power of the study)? This can be calculated by the same methods but solving for power instead of sample size. A study may not be worth doing if there is a low probability of detecting a relevant difference. If, in the final analysis, sufficient resources cannot be obtained, the project should be redesigned in such a fashion as to require fewer assets.

5.8 End Points and Data Collection

The end point of a study is the variable by which the treatments are compared. The choice of a meaningful end point is often clear from the nature of the research question. However, the preferred end point for some research questions is not measurable for a variety of reasons, such as the length of time required for the end point to occur or the sophisticated equipment necessary to measure the end point. In such cases, a surrogate for the end point is chosen, often an antecedent to the end point. The surrogate or antecedent condition must be highly predictive of the end point for it to serve as a valid answer to the study question.[29] Collecting more than a single surrogate may be advisable to help corroborate findings.

Example. In a study comparing two parenteral solutions differing in amino acid composition, the end point of interest was lean body mass (LBM) and the comparison was efficacy of sparing LBM. Because the study was done in an acute-care setting, it was not possible to use the more accurate estimates of LBM given by neutron activation analysis or isotope dilution techniques. The investigators decided to measure urine creatinine excretion to estimate muscle catabolism and changes in muscle mass. This surrogate yields an acceptable answer, to the extent that other factors bearing on creatinine excretion, such as renal function or creatinine intake, were measured and considered in the analysis of the data. Nitrogen balance was also measured. Neither urine creatinine excretion nor nitrogen balance is a direct measure of lean body mass, but the two measures did offer useful information in the absence of the true end point.

As Weiss cautions, the possibility exists that the treatment affects only the antecedent or surrogate and not the end point of interest.[29] In choosing the surrogate, consider all available information to help prevent that from occurring.

The choice of end point may be between "hard" (objective) and "soft" (subjective) evidence. The terms "hard" and "soft" have been applied to data, referring to the degree of subjectivity in observing or measuring data. Serum cholesterol and body weight are hard data; degree of headache pain and severity of flu symptoms are soft data. The more objective, hard variables are preferred because they are more reliable and easier to measure. Relevant soft variables should not be dismissed, however, since they are frequently the most interesting and important outcomes and can be useful in interpreting hard data. A combination of a few carefully chosen hard and soft variables provides a useful approach.

The assessment and measurement procedures should be standardized and applied to all subjects equally and in the same manner. To minimize observer biases in evaluating the end point, the person who evaluates the end point should be unaware of the treatment assignment (blind evaluation). This is especially important if the observation requires a subjective assessment.

Variation between observers is also a potential problem when the assessment method involves making a judgment. Suggestions to reduce between-observer variation are given by Gore.[42]

Variables in addition to the end point should be measured. Collect data on variables that help characterize the subjects or that are relevant to the study end point. Such variables have the potential to distort the treatment comparison if they differ in frequency or magnitude between groups. Randomization does not assure that the groups are balanced in all factors, and some adjustment or stratification in the analysis may be necessary.

Example. A study was conducted to compare the nitrogen-sparing efficacy of two levels of parenterally administered solutions containing different concentrations of branched-chain amino acids in patients undergoing intensive and prolonged cancer treatment.[43] Since it is known that physiological stress exacerbates nitrogen loss, the investigators collected information on the severity of stress the patients experienced during the study. Neither the investigators nor the patients were aware of the amino acid solution given, so that there was little chance that one group would be scrutinized to a greater degree than another or that symptoms would be more likely to be reported in one group. At the end of the study, one group had indeed experienced a greater frequency of severe stress than had the other group. The investigators were able to account for this difference in the analysis by stratifying the severity of stress, thus controlling (to some degree) the influence of stress on the outcome measure. If that had not been done, the estimate of the treatment effect would have been distorted by group differences in stress.

When measuring a numeric variable with the intent to categorize the levels, such as low and high serum cholesterol levels, retain the value intact in data collection, eg, 5.95 mmol cholesterol per liter serum (230 mg/dL). This provides more information and can be used with greater flexibility than a single dimension or category.

5.9 Statistical Analysis and Interpretation

Several excellent references describe statistical procedures for testing hypotheses in experiments.[18,44-46] A general review of selected tests follows (section 9). Among the major problems frequently encountered when one is analyzing and interpreting results of clinical trials are noncompliance and loss of subjects.

Even with the best efforts to maintain strict adherence to the treatment protocol, noncompliance often occurs. Adherence to treatment should be monitored to learn of practical aspects of the treatment. All subjects should be followed to the same extent, regardless of their compliance with treatment. At the time of analysis, retain subjects in the originally assigned treatment group whether or not they actually received it. This comparison reflects how the treatments perform in practice.[44] A selection bias is introduced if the subjects are excluded or analyzed in groups other than the group to which they were randomly assigned. A secondary analysis could evaluate the outcomes of the treatments actually received, but that analysis is not given more weight or relevance.

Withdrawal of subjects presents another opportunity for selection bias to occur. Subjects who are withdrawn from the study should be followed in the same manner as study subjects if possible.[47] As in the problem of noncompliance, these subjects should be analyzed as part of the original treatment group. Report reasons for withdrawal and compare them among groups. One treatment may favor withdrawal because it is less acceptable or has unexpected side effects.

Reporting side effects will aid in evaluating the practicality of the treatment and in planning future studies. If follow-up is not possible and the outcome is not known, compare the known characteristics of the subjects withdrawn with the characteristics of the subjects who complete the study. This may help determine the nature of the bias introduced into the results by the subjects' withdrawal. As an additional step in estimating the effect of removing the subjects, a secondary analysis could be done assuming an unfavorable outcome for those subjects. Compare this "worst outcome" result with that obtained with known end points.

Experimental design is an appropriate analytical research method, regardless of whether the subjects are human beings, experimental animals, or inanimate objects. In each case, criteria for subject selection need to be established, appropriate sample size needs to be estimated, the treatment(s) must be clearly defined, and end points must be established. After a preliminary study has been conducted and the experiment has been designed, data need to be collected and analyzed suitably (section 9.0) to permit appropriate interpretation and application.

5.10 Factorial Design

The study designs previously described (sections 5.4 to 5.9) consider only one study question and investigate only one factor. Their simplicity makes them preferred designs in most settings. If the facilities allow, however, it may be useful and efficient to study more than one factor in a single study using a factorial design. A factorial design includes study groups for all combinations of levels of each factor under study. For example, a two-factor factorial design with two levels per factor would have four treatment groups (*Figure 1.1*).

Figure 1.1
An example of a 2^p factorial design in which two factors are at two levels each. The effects of Factor A (cells 1 and 3 vs cells 2 and 4), Factor B (cells 1 and 2 vs cells 3 and 4), and the interaction of $A \times B$ may be calculated using two-way analysis of variance.

		FACTOR A		
		YES	NO	
FACTOR B	YES	Cell 1 Yes–Yes	Cell 2 Yes–No	1 + 2
	NO	Cell 3 No–Yes	Cell 4 No–No	3 + 4
		1 + 3	2 + 4	$A \times B$

The comparison of levels of factor A is achieved by comparing groups with factor A (cells 1 and 3) to groups without factor A (cells 2 and 4); the comparison of levels of factor B is achieved by comparing groups with factor B (cells 1 and 2) with groups without factor B (cells 3 and 4). These comparisons are made using two-way analysis of variance. This design also allows a synergistic effect (interaction) to be detected.[44] Snedecor and Cochran[48] provide details for design and analysis of factorial experiments.

Example. The impact of incentive programs on effectiveness of employee training will be assessed in a 2×2 factorial design in which a monetary bonus is compared with bonus points. All employees will be enrolled in a course on customer service, and each will be given an audiocassette and a self-paced workbook. Employees will be randomly divided into one of four groups receiving bonus points only, monetary bonus only, both bonus points and monetary bonus, or no bonus. Outcomes to be measured are knowledge and attitude scores pretest and post-test, reported customer satisfaction, and job performance evaluations before and 3 months after the course.

6.0 PARTIALLY CONTROLLED OR QUASI-EXPERIMENTAL DESIGNS

All research involves a balance of the ideal with the feasible. Certain situations exist in which randomized treatment assignment or assembly of an appropriate control group is impossible. (See also section 5.6.) Other study design options are available, although each has limitations, and none is as convincing as the randomized controlled trial. Zelen[49] describes two principal types of nonrandomized trials. Other research options to consider are the observational analytic study designs, ie, cohort and case-control studies.

7.0 COHORT (FOLLOW-UP) STUDY

Cohort (follow-up) studies are observational analytic studies that are designed to mimic the randomized clinical trial. A cohort study does not involve investigator manipulation and, thus, is not categorized as experimental, but it does test a hypothesis of a causal relationship and, thus, is analytical in approach.

A cohort is a group of persons, followed over time, having a common characteristic or factor of interest. A cohort or group is assembled on the basis of factors thought to relate to the development of the end point under study. This allows investigation of a hypothesis concerning the etiology of the outcome of interest. The study involves following the group or cohort forward in time to observe its experience. The outcome studied most commonly is a disease; for convenience, the following discussion refers to the studied outcome as *disease*. This design is by no means limited to the study of diseases, however. Many other conditions can be studied in the same manner. The possible causal factors under investigation, referred to as *exposures,* may cover a wide range of environmental and life-style characteristics.

7.1 Uses

A cohort design is useful to determine the frequency of a newly developed disease or a health-related event and to assess the exposure-disease relationship. In the cohort design, exposure to a suspected risk factor is identified when individuals are free of detectable disease, ie, the cohort is identified on the basis of exposure to certain factors thought to affect risk but without the presence of disease. Exposure to the factor of interest clearly precedes the detection of disease. Because it helps establish the temporal sequence of risk factor and end point, the cohort design is appealing for the study of causes of disease. A drawback is that sufficient time must elapse between assessing the exposure and detecting the outcome, causing a typical cohort study to be long. Cohort studies are most useful when the time between exposure and detection of the end point is thought to be relatively short.

Unless the disease studied is extremely common in the population to be studied, most individuals in a cohort will not develop it. Therefore, a large number of subjects is required in order to compare incidence between exposure groups. This design is more feasible for conditions that are relatively common in the population studied.

Example. The association between raw food intake and the incidence of infection was investigated in a cohort study of hospitalized patients who were severely immunocompromised due to chemoradiotherapy for cancer, a population in which infection is common. Daily food intake was recorded, as were microbiologically confirmed cases of bacteremia, septicemia, and enteritis. The incidence rates of infection were compared among groups differing in exposure to raw foods.

7.2 Features

The subjects in a cohort are apparently free of the disease under study and are selected on the basis of the presence or absence of a factor of interest, termed an *exposure*. Subjects are then followed forward in time to determine the occurrence of the disease or of a specific end point serving as an indicator of the disease. The monitoring process can be concurrent or nonconcurrent. The direction of the study is always prospective because the exposure is identified before the disease is detected. However, the follow-up period may be concurrent or nonconcurrent. Follow-up may proceed at the same time as the study is conducted (concurrent follow-up); current records generate data on disease occurrence. Alternatively, follow-up may have occurred earlier in time (nonconcurrent follow-up); existing records yield data on disease occurrence. Clearly, the latter scheme alleviates the need to wait for the cohort to go through time.

7.3 Selection of Subjects

The subjects making up the cohort must be at risk for developing the disease or outcome of interest but free of the disease at the start of the study. The subjects may be members of a single cohort and classified according to their exposure to the factor of interest, or the subjects may be members of different cohorts, selected from special exposure groups so that the cohort exposed can be compared with the one not exposed. The validity of the comparison between cohorts depends upon the assumption that the cohorts are comparable in all relevant factors other than the exposure.

7.4 Sample Size

The size of cohort required for study is related to the frequency that the end point of interest occurs. A low frequency requires a large sample size. Most cohort studies involve hundreds to thousands of individuals. Several authors address the issues and procedures of estimating sample size.[50-53] The basic concepts for estimating sample size for cohort studies are similar to those discussed in section 5.7.

7.5 Assessing Exposure Status

Exposure to the factor of interest is observed or measured for each subject at the start of the study. The technique of assessment should be standardized to improve reliability. (See sections 4.4 and 5.8.) Information relating to exposure and other important characteristics can be collected from existing records, personal interviews, and questionnaires.

Assessing dietary intake poses special problems. Dietary intake methodology is the subject of continuing investigation, as no single method has been shown to be reliable and valid for all types of research. When selecting the method for collecting dietary data, one needs to review three issues thoroughly: first, the limitations and use of available dietary intake collection methods, eg, an in-depth food history, a 3-day food record, or a 24-hour dietary recall[54]; second, the uses to which the data are to be addressed, eg, comparisons of an individual subject's nutrient intake and laboratory values; and third, the specific research goals, eg, estimating intakes of individuals or of groups.[55-61]

A difficulty of cohort studies is that a change in exposure status may occur during the follow-up period. A change in exposure status may dilute the study's ability to detect a difference in risk between exposed and unexposed groups. If possible, measure the factor again during the follow-up period.[62]

7.6 Assessing End Point, Disease

The end point should be defined in detail to be an unambiguous and reliable definition. The method and type of follow-up should be identical for all subjects, regardless of exposure status. This is facilitated by making the evaluators unaware of the subjects' exposure status, ie, blind assessment. Blinding assures that the efforts for follow-up and assessment methods used will be applied equally and will not be biased by the investigators' expectations.

The end-point events are counted as they occur during the follow-up period. However, end points occurring immediately after assessment of the exposure status cannot be counted in circumstances in which it is not clear that the exposure preceded the end point. This decision depends upon what is known or believed to be true about the length of the induction or latent period for the disease or end point in question.

It is often useful to supplement the information about the end point. Record the date of detection of the end point as well as its occurrence, depending upon the nature of the factor under study.

Complete follow-up on all members of the cohort is vitally important. Loss of subjects can seriously distort the results. Make vigorous efforts to assess the outcome of each subject at the end of the follow-up period.

The length of follow-up depends on the hypothesis and related knowledge of the latency period or the mechanisms of action of the risk factor. The longer the period, the more difficult the follow-up becomes because of changes of residence, death from other causes, changes in exposure status, and the added expense of staff for monitoring subjects and collecting data. Those considerations must be balanced with the need to allow sufficient time for the proposed effect to become manifest.

7.7 Statistical Analysis and Interpretation

Baseline characteristics of the cohort are described using descriptive statistics. The usual inferential comparative analysis of cohort studies involves determining incidence of disease and estimating the incidence ratio for exposed vs unexposed subjects. The incidence ratio is known as the relative risk and measures the strength of the association between the exposure factor and the disease. Rimm et al[18] discuss the rationale and provide methods for calculating the statistics. Often it is necessary to adjust for the effects of confounding variables by stratification[45]; a more complex analysis is indicated if several variables must be adjusted simultaneously.[63] Readers unfamiliar with the techniques are advised to seek statistical consultation.

The weakness in this observational design is that a relationship is not clearly causal. All factors are not held constant as in an experiment. Factors other than the exposure of interest may have a bearing on the outcome, and those factors may not be measured or known. The population may experience changes in environment or life-style that modify exposures and responses, yet such changes cannot be controlled by the investigators. Further, the end point may be related to the factors that determine the exposure status rather than to the exposure itself. The results are interpreted in light of other known evidence. The criteria for examining factors associated with disease risk are outlined by Hill.[64]

8.0 CASE-CONTROL STUDY

Case-control studies are observational analytical designs that investigate hypotheses of causal relationship. These designs are retrospective, historically oriented studies, also known as case-referent or case-comparison studies. Because case-control designs do not involve intervention by the investigators, they are not experimental but do adhere to as many principles of experimental design as possible.

8.1 Uses

A case-control design is used to explore etiology by comparing the prevalence of the exposure to factors of interest in persons who have a disease with that of a group without disease. It is useful in studies of rare diseases or end points. In general, case-control studies are less expensive to conduct and require less time than cohort studies. The use and methods of the case-control design are the subjects of an entire issue of the *Journal of Chronic Diseases.*[65]

8.2 Features

The case-control study design assesses exposure status after disease status is known and thus is retrospective. The comparison groups are formed on the basis of disease or outcome status, either with disease diagnosis (cases) or without disease diagnosis (controls). Subjects are then investigated for the current presence of or previous exposure to a factor or factors of interest. The prevalence of the factor is compared between cases and controls.

8.3 Selection of Cases

The goal in selection of cases is to obtain a sample that is representative of cases arising from a defined target population. This goal is difficult or impossible to attain in most circumstances. The ideal compromise is to select all incident (newly developed or detected) cases arising in a defined population over some specified period. Selecting incident cases rather than existing (prevalent) cases is preferred because factors related to survival, and, thus, to selection for the study, may differ from causal factors but cannot be distinguished when prevalent cases are used.

The definition of a case should be specific and objective to minimize the bias of personal judgment.

Example. To investigate the hypothesis that a low dietary fiber intake contributes to the risk of developing cholelithiasis, a case-control study was planned in a pre-paid health care setting. During a 2-year period, all newly diagnosed patients with cholelithiasis were asked to participate. The control group was randomly selected from the health care enrollee population and frequency-matched for age group and gender. Those agreeing to participate were interviewed in their homes for their usual intake of dietary fiber using a food frequency questionnaire administered by trained interviewers who did not know whether the subject was a case or a control. The reported fiber consumption (both quantity and type) was compared between cases and controls.

8.4 Selection of Controls

Selection of an appropriate comparison group depends largely upon the hypothesis. The goal in selecting the control subjects is that controls should be representative of the population from which the cases arose. A random probability sample (see sections 4.3 and 5.4) is ideal and is feasible if information is available on the sampling units (or community). A random probability sample is also feasible if the population is a closed one, such as a prepaid health plan or institution. Samples of convenience are often used, but the validity of the study rests upon the assumption that the subjects are similar to the reference or target population with regard to the factors of interest; this may or may not be a reasonable assumption.

Considerations in choosing a control group are cost, response rate, and interview setting. Compromises may have to be made to reduce the cost of accessing a control subject while maximizing the response rate. (See section 5.4.) The interview setting should be, insofar as possible, comparable with that for cases. Much of the information elicited is by recall and self-report, and factors bearing on those methods should be as identical as is feasible between the groups.

A selection bias in controls is undesirable but highly possible. Minimize bias by planning a structured selection system with established criteria for selecting control subjects. The criteria should be applied without the investigators' knowledge of the individuals' exposure status. Other sources of bias, such as age, gender, or socioeconomic status, may be eliminated by matching in the selection or by stratification in the analysis. How to select appropriate controls is not always clear; several authors review problems and give suggestions.[66-69]

8.5 Assessing Exposure

The historical information, including the exposure to the factor of interest, is obtained from existing records, examination, direct measurements, and personal interview or questionnaire. Schlesselman[67] provides guidelines for developing the research instrument, noting that the starting point for developing any data-gathering tool is a list of all pertinent variables, including the extent of detail needed. The methods for assessing past diet in case-control studies have been studied in a variety of settings. Investigators should review the literature before choosing the intake method.[70-73]

Regardless of the instrument used, the procedure for gathering information should be the same for cases and controls. The comparability of the procedure is increased if the interviewer or evaluator does not know whether the subject is a case or control. That may not be possible in a personal interview but may be feasible for a person gathering other objective data.

Sample size considerations include those discussed. (See section 5.7.) A detailed discussion is provided by Schlesselman.[67]

8.6 Statistical Analysis and Interpretation

The frequencies of the exposure of interest are presented for cases and controls. The association between the exposure and the disease is expressed by estimating the odds ratio, a statistical comparison of the prevalence of exposure between cases and controls. Rimm et al[18] present a brief overview of the basic methods of calculating the odds ratio. A typical analysis proceeds from the simple to the complex, involving stratification and possibly multivariate methods.[74] Detailed presentations are given by Schlesselman[67] and Breslow and Day.[66]

The observational method and retrospective nature of the case-control study present limitations that should be kept in mind when the results are interpreted. Sackett[75] reviews the possible biases and their effect on the interpretation of case-control studies. There are always alternatives to a causal explanation for an association.[67] Chief among them are the following three:
1. In a case-control study, it may be unclear whether the factor preceded the disease or resulted from it.
2. Recall bias is likely to be present; the self-report is influenced by the presence of the disease, especially if the subject is aware of the hypothesis being tested. If present, the observed association will overestimate the actual association.
3. The comparability of cases and controls may be questionable. The choice of control group is crucial to a valid study.

9.0 STATISTICAL ANALYSIS AND PRESENTATION OF RESULTS

An acquaintance with statistics at the introductory or basic level provides the basis for understanding the statistical aspects of research literature[76] but does not assure the expertise necessary for undertaking all research projects. Professional statistical assistance should be obtained during the planning stage of the research effort and thereafter as necessary. Familiarization with important statistical issues, which this section offers, will facilitate communication with a statistician.

Before beginning the analysis, review the hypothesis for the study. What is the question of interest and how is the study designed to answer it? Resist the temptation to answer all possible questions with the data or to suggest unrealistic applications. (See sections 3.5, 4.5, 4.6, 4.7, 5.9, 7.7, and 8.6.)

9.1 Steps in Analysis—Description and Inference

The two major purposes of analysis are description and inference (estimation). The sample is first described; then characteristics about the population (parameters) are estimated. Finally, probability may be determined as to whether these estimates are due to chance rather than to experimental variables.

Describe characteristics of the sample and values of important variables by plotting first, usually by use of a frequency histogram. Such plots usually allow errors to be detected. Nominal and ordinal variables, such as gender and anthropometric percentiles, can be presented simply in this manner or tabulated as proportions within categories or ranks. Continuous variables, such as age and weight, are customarily presented by summary statistics describing the frequency distribution. The choice of statistics depends on the symmetry of the plotted frequency histogram. The mean and standard deviation may be used when the distribution is relatively symmetrical. The median and a percentile range, such as the 25th and 75th percentiles, are preferable when the distribution is asymmetrical.[77] (See section 4.7.)

After the data are described, the hypotheses are evaluated by statistical inference, which involves estimation and significance testing. Conceptually, this is a technique for comparing the expected distribution with the observed distribution. The expected distribution is defined by the "null hypothesis" that there is no association or no effect of the factors under study. The null hypothesis specifies values for parameters which describe the underlying distribution. For most of the common tests, this is the Normal distribution, and the parameters are the mean and the variance. The sample is used to estimate these parameters for the population. The question then is: How likely is it to observe the mean and standard deviation given by the sample if the null hypothesis is true?

Many of the frequently used statistical tests are presented in *Table 1.1*. Refer to a basic statistical text, such as Rimm et al,[18] before applying any test in order to review the assumptions and constraints for its use.

Table 1.1
Statistical Tests Appropriate for Data Analysis

Relationship Among Samples	Type of Data	Normal Distribution	Statistical Test Two Samples	> Two Samples
Independent	Binary/classification	—	χ^2	χ^2
	Ordinal/ranked	—	Wilcoxon rank sum	Kruskal-Wallis
	Continuous/measured	Yes	t-test	One-way analysis of variance
		No	Wilcoxon rank sum	Kruskal-Wallis
Related	Binary/classification	—	χ^2	
Paired, repeated measures, replicate measures	Ordinal/ranked	—	Sign test Signed rank test	Friedman's test
	Continuous/measured	Yes	Paired t-test	Two(N)-way analysis of variance
		No	Signed rank test	Repeated measures analysis of variance Friedman's test

The validity of most standard tests depends upon the assumptions that (a) the data are from a Normal distribution and (b) the variability within groups (if these are compared) is similar. Tests of this type are termed *parametric* and are to some degree sensitive to violations of those assumptions. Other options should be considered if the conditions are not met. Data may be transformed (eg, logarithmically) to reduce skewness and minimize variation across groups.[78] Alternatively, *non-parametric* or distribution-free tests, which do not depend on the Normal distribution, can be used.[79] Non-parametric tests are also useful for data collected in categorical or interval form. Relative to their parametric counterparts, non-parametric tests have the advantage of ease but the disadvantage of less statistical power.

9.2 One-sided and Two-sided Significance Tests

A two-sided significance test (two-tailed) evaluates departures in either direction from the mean, while a one-sided test (one-tailed) is sensitive to differences in only one direction. For most situations, a two-sided test of significance is appropriate. The one-sided test is justified only in those rare situations in which the difference is expected to be in a specified direction and a difference in the opposite direction is of no interest. One-sided tests are less rigorous and thus are suspect if conclusions would change when a two-sided test is applied.

9.3 Standard Deviation and Standard Error

The standard deviation (SD) is descriptive and is used to describe the characteristics of the sample. The standard error (SE) is inferential and is used to indicate confidence in the population estimates. The SD indicates the distance from the center or mean, and describes the "spread" or variation around the sample mean. The SE describes the variation relative to the sample size, that is, the SE is the standard deviation of a sampling distribution. SE is a measure of the precision of the sampling estimate of a population parameter. Researchers should present the most appropriate statistic, not the smallest one. (See section 4.7.)

9.4 Confidence Intervals

Results of statistical analyses should be presented in detail. Important among the details are the test statistic (eg, $t=2.45$; $\chi^2=14.7$), the degrees of freedom, and the P value. The estimate of the parameter (such as the mean difference or relative risk) should be given as a point estimate and confidence interval.

The two products of any statistical test are (a) an estimate of the quantity of interest (eg, mean difference) and (b) the probability that this estimate is a chance occurrence. The two are usually presented as a mean difference and a P value. That provides only a single value to describe the difference, along with a single value describing its likelihood. An estimate of the population parameter is more meaningfully presented as a range of values within which the true value probably exists: a confidence interval. The confidence interval is the range from the smallest to the largest value that is plausible for the true population value, with a certain degree of confidence—usually 95%. It is calculated using the estimated value and its standard error.

Besides describing the possible magnitude of the value, the confidence interval provides information about the certainty in the estimate (precision). Gardner and Altman[80] present the rationale and methods for calculating the confidence interval for a number of statistical tests.

9.5 Repeated and Replicated Measurements

It is common to repeat measurements of a variable at several points in time. The simple approach for analysis is to calculate the mean and SD for each period and present them graphically by a line joining the means. Differences among the means are usually tested by several t-tests. However, these are not the most satisfactory methods for analysis of serial measurements.[77] The mean curve may not accurately summarize the data, especially if substantial individual variability is present. Further, multiple significance tests are likely to yield false positive results. (See section 9.6.) Likewise, regression and correlation analyses are not appropriate because the observations are related rather than independent.

A more useful analysis would be to evaluate some characteristic of individual curves, such as the time required to attain a specified level.[77] A Repeated Measures Analysis of Variance, using time as a main factor, can be used to determine whether groups differ in their responses over time. If there are missing values during the period, some adjustment is necessary to account for different amounts of information per subject. Statistical advice is recommended.

Replicate measurements, or several measures taken without regard to time, are also related observations, and the analysis must account for the fact that they were obtained from a single subject.

Analysis of variance can be used for replicate measurements of a continuous variable, provided the number of measurements is the same for each subject. If the number of observations varies among subjects, the analysis is more complex.[77,81] Statistical advice should be obtained.

9.6 Multiple Significance Tests

A common problem in nutrition literature is multiple significance testing,[82] as often occurs in studies of nutrient intakes when results from many subgroups are compared or many variables analyzed. The chances of finding a spurious significant result increase as the number of tests increases. The significance tests relating to the hypothesis serving as the basis for the study carry the greatest weight; other tests should be considered only as exploratory.[77] If those tests are done, the chances for false-positive results can be minimized by adjusting the criterion of statistical significance (ie, α, usually 0.05) downward, using a procedure such as the Bonferroni procedure.[18,83]

It is often necessary to compare the means of several groups. If multiple t-tests are used, the multiple comparison problem arises. Other methods to consider are analysis of variance and multiple-comparison methods specially designed to make several pairwise comparisons, such as the Least Significant Difference Method, the Scheffe Procedure, and the Walker-Duncan Procedure.[84]

9.7 Outliers

Outliers are extreme observations that are not consistent with the other observations. These cannot be excluded from the analysis unless there are other reasons to question their credibility.[62] Analyze the data with and without outliers to assess their effect on conclusions.

9.8 Missing Values

There is no single way to analyze data if there are missing values; consultation with a statistician is recommended. Missing values can have a pronounced impact on the results. They may be unavoidable, but they must not be ignored. The sample sizes of groups at each measurement period should be clearly presented, and the reasons for missing these observations given by group. The discussion should include an evaluation of how the missing values might affect the conclusions.

9.9 Regression and Correlation Analysis

The relationship between continuous variables is often expressed by a mathematical model describing a straight line, known as simple linear regression analysis. Regression analysis is commonly used to determine the association between two variables and to make predictions based on the linear relationship.

Results of regression analyses that may be presented include the fitted regression equation, variances of the slope and intercept coefficients, the variance of the residuals, and the proportion of the variation in the dependent variable explained by the regression equation.[85] When a plot is used to describe the relationship, include the regression line and the confidence interval curves on both sides of the line.

Correlation analysis and regression analysis differ in purpose, although they are related in technique. In correlation analysis, linear regression is used to yield only a measure of the strength of the association between the independent and dependent variables, the correlation coefficient. The presentation need not include the regression equation and associated variances but can present the correlation coefficient alone, along with the probability that the coefficient occurred by chance.

9.10 Complex Statistical Methods: Brief Descriptions

9.10a Cluster analysis. Cluster analysis refers to several multivariate statistical techniques used to classify into groups a set of previously unclassified objects or subjects.[86]

9.10b Factor analysis. Factor analysis constructs new independent factors to explain the relationships among several related variables. These new factors are then used in other analyses instead of the several related variables.[87]

9.10c Discriminant analysis. Discriminant analysis provides a mathematical model that discriminates between two populations on the basis of several independent variables. The populations are classified previously, such as those persons with and without cardiovascular disease. The method uses a linear model to describe the relationship between several independent variables and one nominal dependent variable.[87]

9.10d Multiple regression analysis. Multiple regression is used to describe the relationship between several independent variables considered simultaneously and a single dependent variable.[87]

9.10e Logistic regression analysis. Logistic regression adapts the multiple regression model for a binary response variable, such as mortality or the presence/absence of disease. This analysis yields estimates of relative risk while adjusting for covariates and is useful in cohort and case-control designs.[88]

9.10f Survival analysis. Survival analysis techniques determine the distribution of survival times (ie, death or other dichotomous event) for a cohort. From the survival distribution, the probability of survival (or death) for each specific period can be derived. Survival analysis methods include the life table (actuarial) method for grouped data and the Kaplan-Meier method for ungrouped exact times of death.[18,44]

9.10g Path analysis. Path analysis extends multiple regression analysis to examine a limited number of causal hypotheses or to build theoretical explanations for the observations.[46]

9.10h Meta-analysis. Recently developed, meta-analysis combines and analyzes the results of previous reports. Such analysis is particularly useful when several small studies but no larger studies of the hypothesis of interest are available and none of the small studies is acceptably large or acceptable with regard to α and β errors. The product has both quantitative and qualitative aspects and allows conclusions to be drawn and new studies to be planned. To assure quality meta-analysis, great care must be exercised in study design, choice of previous studies to combine, control of bias, statistical analysis, sensitivity analysis, and application of results.[89]

10.0 CONCLUSIONS FROM AND APPLICATION OF RESEARCH RESULTS

10.1 So What?

At that exciting moment when the research data have been collected and analyzed, the researcher is ready to present the data to and interpret the data for the scientific and professional community.[90] This is a thoughtful time of introspection, hope, concern, and truthfulness.

When drawing conclusions from research data, one needs to recognize the limitations of the study design and its execution. Among factors to consider are violations of the research protocol, sources of bias, subject selection, sample size, response rate, compliance, subjects lost to follow-up, and missing values. These limitations determine how clearly the research data answer the research question and, of great importance, whether and to what extent the answer can be generalized to populations beyond the study population.

The data can have great practical use when applied to the study population or used to document the investigator's practice even if extension to other populations is inappropriate. If the integrity of the study was maintained, if the study population was representative of the general population, if the sample size was sufficient, if response rate and compliance were high, if few subjects were lost to follow-up, if few values were missing, and if the differences observed were both statistically significant and of significance in practice, then the results can be applied with confidence to the larger population.

The last point, the distinction between statistically significant differences and differences of practical significance, is of substantial importance. A change in serum cholesterol of 0.05 mmol/L serum (2 mg/dL) may be highly statistically significant, but, for an individual or subgroup of the population, such a change may be of little import. It is only from differences that make a practical difference that meaningful recommendations may be made.

Studies that yield statistically nonsignificant results, or "negative studies," may be important to report. This is especially true if the negative study is of sufficient statistical power that a relevant difference could have been detected, suggesting that the true difference may be of impractical magnitude. At the least, negative studies provide valuable suggestions and show errors to avoid in future research.

Overall conclusions and recommendations drawn from the research data need to be only those that can be supported by the data. Further research may be needed before more global and more diverse recommendations can be supported, and thus, offered.

10.2 Now What?

With the successful completion of the research project, many ideas and questions appear. The researcher at this point will see new avenues of research ahead. It is a time to evaluate thoughtfully the completed research project and consider ways to make the next project more facile in execution. As the completed research project was devised after viewing the original research topic as a composite of its many component parts (section 1.1), the opportunities for future research are obvious. The advantage now is that the researcher can use the recent research project as a guide for the next.

References

1. Emory CW. *Business Research Methods.* Rev ed. Homewood, Ill: Richard D Irwin; 1980.
2. Blank SC. *Practical Business Research Methods.* Westport, Conn: AVI Publishing Co; 1984.
3. Moragne L, ed. *Nutrition Funding Report.* Washington, DC: Nutrition Legislation Services; 1986;1, monthly to date.
4. *The Foundation Directory.* 11th ed. New York, NY: Foundation Center; 1987.
5. Code of ethics for the profession of dietetics. *J Am Diet Assoc.* 1988; 88:1592–1596.
6. *Honor in Science.* New Haven, Conn: Sigma Xi, Scientific Research Society; 1986.
7. Angell M, Relman AS. Fraud in biomedical research. *N Engl J Med.* 1988; 318:1462.
8. Kerlinger FN. *Foundations of Behavioral Research.* 2nd ed. New York, NY: Holt Rinehart and Winston; 1973.
9. Kidder L, Judd CM. *Research Methods in Social Relations.* 5th ed. New York, NY: Holt, Rinehart and Winston; 1986.
10. Matthews ME, Zardain MV, Mahaffey MJ. Labor time spent in foodservice activities in one hospital: a 12-year profile. *J Am Diet Assoc.* 1986; 86:636.
11. Ferber R, Sheatsley P, Turner A, Wakesberg J. *What Is a Survey?* Washington, DC: American Statistical Association; 1980.
12. Bowers JA, Craig JA, Tucker TJ, Holden JM, Posati LP. Vitamin and proximate composition of fast-food fried chicken. *J Am Diet Assoc.* 1987; 87:736.
13. McCool AC, Garand MM. Computer technology in institutional foodservice. *J Am Diet Assoc.* 1986; 86:48.
14. Elwood PC. Epidemiology for nutritionists: 2. sampling. *Hum Nutr Appl Nutr.* 1983; 37A:265.
15. Williams WH. *A Sampler on Sampling.* New York, NY: John Wiley and Sons; 1978.
16. Cohen J. *Statistical Power Analysis for the Behavioral Sciences.* New York, NY: Academic Press; 1977.
17. Dillman DA. *Mail and Telephone Surveys: The Total Design Method.* New York, NY: John Wiley and Sons; 1978.
18. Rimm AA, Hartz AJ, Kalbfleisch JH, Anderson AJ, Hoffman RG. *Basic Biostatistics in Medicine and Epidemiology.* New York, NY: Appleton-Century-Crofts; 1980.
19. Polit DF, Hungler BP. *Essentials of Nursing Research: Methods and Applications.* Philadelphia, Pa: JB Lippincott Co; 1985.
20. Fruin MF, Lawler MR. Perceptions of competency attainment in community dietetics: Academic Plan IV vs. dietetic internship. *J Am Diet Assoc.* 1987; 87:1025.
21. Huber AM, Wallins LL, DeRusso A. Folate nutriture in pregnancy. *J Am Diet Assoc.* 1988; 88:791.
22. Griner PF, Mayewski RJ, Mushlin AI, Greenland P. Selection and interpretation of diagnostic tests and procedures. *Ann Intern Med.* 1981; 94:553.
23. Begg CB. Biases in the assessment of diagnostic tests. *Stat Med.* 1987; 6:411.
24. McNeil BJ, Keeler E, Adelstein SJ. Primer on certain elements of medical decision making. *N Engl J Med.* 1975; 293:211.
25. Hanley JA, McNeil BJ. The meaning and use of the area under a receiver operating characteristic (ROC) curve. *Radiology.* 1982; 143:29.

26. Department of Clinical Epidemiology and Biostatistics, McMaster University. Interpretation of diagnostic data: 4. How to do it with a more complex table. *Can Med Assoc J.* 1983; 129:832.
27. *Dietary Intake Source Data: United States, 1976-80.* Washington, DC: US Government Printing Office; 1983. DHHS publication PHS 83-1681.
28. Oakland MJ. The effectiveness of a short curriculum unit in death education for dietetic students. *J Am Diet Assoc.* 1988; 88:26.
29. Weiss NS. *Clinical Epidemiology: The Study of the Outcome of Illness.* New York, NY: Oxford University Press; 1986.
30. Gore SM. Assessing clinical trials—trial discipline. *Br Med J.* 1981; 283:211.
31. Farr BM, Gwaltney JM Jr. The problems of taste in placebo matching: an evaluation of zinc gluconate for the common cold. *J Chron Dis.* 1987; 40:875.
32. Karlowski TR, Chalmers TC, Frenkel LD, Kapidian AZ, Lewis TL, Lynch JM. Ascorbic acid for the common cold: a prophylactic and therapeutic trial. *JAMA.* 1975; 231:1038.
33. Gore SM. Assessing clinical trials—why randomize? *Br Med J.* 1981; 282:1958.
34. Hills M, Armitage P. The two-period cross-over clinical trial. *Br J Clin Pharmacol.* 1979; 8:7.
35. Gore SM. Assessing clinical trials—design I. *Br Med J.* 1981; 282:1780.
36. Willian AR, Pater JL. Using baseline measurements in the two-period crossover clinical trial. *Controlled Clin Trials.* 1986; 7:282.
37. Louis TA, Lavori PW, Bailer JC, Polansky M. Crossover and self-controlled designs in clinical research. *N Engl J Med.* 1984; 310:24.
38. Sacks H, Chalmers TC, Smith H. Randomized versus historical controls for clinical trials. *Am J Med.* 1982; 72:233.
39. Pocock SJ. The combination of randomized and historical controls in clinical trials. *J Chron Dis.* 1975; 29:175.
40. Bailar JC, Louis TA, Lavori PW, Polansky M. Studies without internal controls. *N Engl J Med.* 1984; 311:156.
41. Lachin JM. Introduction to sample size determination and power analysis for clinical trials. *Controlled Clin Trials.* 1981; 2:93.
42. Gore SM. Assessing clinical trials—between-observer variation. *Br Med J.* 1981; 283:40.
43. Lenssen P, Cheney CL, Aker SN, et al. Intravenous branched chain amino acid trial in marrow transplant recipients. *JPEN J Parenter Enteral Nutr.* 1987; 11:112.
44. Matthews DE, Farewell V. *Using and Understanding Medical Statistics.* New York, NY: Karger; 1985.
45. Fleiss JL. *Statistical Methods for Rates and Proportions.* 2nd ed. New York, NY: John Wiley and Sons; 1981.
46. Loether HJ, McTavish DG. *Descriptive and Inferential Statistics: An Introduction.* Boston, Mass: Allyn and Bacon; 1988.
47. Gore SM: Assessing clinical trials—rash adventures. *Br Med J.* 1981; 283:426.
48. Snedecor GW, Cochran WG. *Statistical Methods.* 7th ed. Ames, Iowa: Iowa State University Press; 1980.
49. Zelen M. Statistical options in clinical trials. *Semin Oncol.* 1977; 4:441.
50. Fleiss JL, Tytun A, Ury HK. A simple approximation for calculating sample sizes for comparing independent proportions. *Biometrics.* 1980; 36:343.
51. Greenland S. Power, sample size and smallest detectable effect determination for multivariate studies. *Stat Med.* 1985; 4:117.
52. Munoz A, Rosner B. Power and sample size for a collection of 2×2 tables. *Biometrics.* 1984; 40:995.
53. Palta M, McHugh R. Planning the size of a cohort study in the presence of both losses to follow-up and non-compliance. *J Chronic Dis.* 1980; 33:501.
54. Algert S, Stumbo P. *Validity and Reliability in Dietary Methodology—an Annotated Bibliography.* Chicago, Ill: Research Dietetic Practice Group; 1986.
55. Block G. A review of validations of dietary assessment methods. *Am J Epidemiol.* 1982; 115:492.
56. Byers T, Marshall J, Fiedler R, Zielezny M, Graham S. Assessing nutrient intake with an abbreviated dietary interview. *Am J Epidemiol.* 1985; 122:41.
57. Willett WC, Sampson L, Stampfer MJ, et al. Reproducibility and validity of a semiquantitative food frequency questionnaire. *Am J Epidemiol.* 1985; 122:51.
58. Jain M, Howe GR, Johnson KC, Miller AB. Evaluation of a diet history questionnaire for epidemiologic studies. *Am J Epidemiol.* 1980; 111:212.
59. Rider AA, Calkins BM, Arther RS, Nair PP. Concordance of nutrient information obtained by different methods. *Am J Clin Nutr.* 1984; 40:906.

60. Freudenheim JL, Johnson NE, Wardrop RL. Misclassification of nutrient intake of individuals and groups using one-, two-, three-, and seven-day food records. *Am J Epidemiol.* 1987; 126:703.
61. Morgan KJ, Johnson SR, Rizek RL, Reese R, Stampley GL. Collection of food intake data: an evaluation of methods. *J Am Diet Assoc.* 1987; 87:888.
62. Van Beresteyn ECH, van'T Hof MA, van der Heiden-Winkeldermaat HJ, ten Have-Witjes A, Neeter R. Evaluation of the usefulness of the cross-check dietary history method in longitudinal studies. *J Chron Dis.* 1987; 40:1051.
63. Breslow NE. Elementary methods of cohort analysis. *Int J Epidemiol.* 1984; 13:112.
64. Hill AB. *Principles of Medical Statistics.* 9th ed. London, England: Oxford University Press; 1971.
65. *J Chron Dis.* 1979; 32:1-144.
66. Breslow NE, Day NE. *Statistical Methods in Cancer Research. The Analysis of Case-Control Studies.* Lyons, France: International Agency for Research on Cancer; 1980;1.
67. Schlesselman JJ. *Case-Control Studies: Design, Conduct, and Analysis.* New York, NY: Oxford University Press; 1982.
68. Hayden GF, Kramer MS, Horwitz RI. The case-control study: a practical review for the clinician. *JAMA.* 1982; 247:326.
69. Horwitz, RI, Feinstein AR. Methodologic standards and contradictory results in case-control research. *Am J Med.* 1979; 66:556.
70. McKeown-Eyssen GE, Yeung KS, Bright-See E. Assessment of past diet in epidemiologic studies. *Am J Epidemiol.* 1986; 124:94.
71. Hankin JH, Nomura AMY, Lee J, Hirohata T, Kolonel LN. Reproducibility of a diet history questionnaire in a case-control study of breast cancer. *Am J Clin Nutr.* 1983; 37:981.
72. Jensen OM, Wahrendorf J, Rosenqvist A, Geser A. The reliability of questionnaire-derived historical dietary information and temporal stability of food habits in individuals. *Am J Epidemiol.* 1984; 120:281.
73. Willett WC, Sampson L, Browne ML, et al. The use of a self-administered questionnaire to assess diet from years in the past. *Am J Epidemiol.* 1988; 127:188.
74. Rothman KJ, Boice JD Jr. *Epidemiologic Analysis with a Programmable Calculator.* 2nd ed. Chestnut Hill, Mass: Epidemiology Resources; 1982.
75. Sackett DL. Bias in analytic research. *J Chron Dis.* 1979; 32:51.
76. Cheney CL. Presenting and discussing statistics. In: Chernoff R, ed. *Communicating as Professionals.* Chicago, Ill: The American Dietetic Association; 1986.
77. Altman DG, Gore SM, Gardner MJ, Pocock SJ. Statistical guidelines for contributors to medical journals. *Br Med J.* 1983; 286:1489.
78. Gore SM. Assessing methods—transforming the data. *Br Med J.* 1983; 283:1489.
79. Marascuilo LA, McSweeney M. *Nonparametric and Distribution-free Methods for Social Sciences.* Monterey, Calif: Brooks/Cole; 1977.
80. Gardner MJ, Altman DG. Confidence intervals rather than p values: estimation rather than hypothesis testing. *Br Med J.* 1986; 292:746.
81. Kleinbaum DG, Kupper LL. *Applied Regression Analysis and Other Multivariable Methods.* North Scituate, Mass: Duxbury Press; 1978.
82. Reid M, Hall JC. Multiple statistical comparisons in nutritional research. *Am J Clin Nutr.* 1984; 40:183.
83. Rimm AA, Tukey JW. Some thoughts on clinical trials, especially problems of multiplicity. *Science.* 1977; 198:679.
84. Godfrey K. Comparing the means of several groups. *N Engl J Med.* 1985; 313:1450.
85. Godfrey K. Simple linear regression in medical research. *N Engl J Med.* 1985; 313:1629.
86. Everitt B. *Cluster Analysis.* 2nd ed. New York, NY: Halsted Press; 1980.
87. Kleinbaum DG, Kupper LL. *Applied Regression Analysis and Other Multivariable Methods.* Boston, Mass: PWS Publishers; 1987.
88. Kleinbaum DG, Kupper LL, Morgenstern H. *Epidemiologic Research: Principles and Quantitative Methods.* New York, NY: Van Nostrand Reinhold Co; 1982.
89. Sacks HS, Berrier J, Reitman D, Ancona-Berk VA, Chalmers TC. Meta-analysis of randomized controlled trials. *N Engl J Med.* 1987; 316:450.
90. Monsen ER. On communicating effectively. In: Chernoff R, ed. *Communicating as Professionals.* Chicago, Ill: The American Dietetic Association; 1986.

PART 2
THE RESEARCH ENVIRONMENT

Preparing for research is an exciting, creative time, a time of opportunity. During planning, one focuses on the research question and looks forward to the answers and applications. The two chapters that follow are designed to help create a productive environment that is conducive to research.

The chapter on ethics considers two interrelated topics: human error and research errors. Human error may be the consequence of inadvertent actions, negligence, or fraud. Professionals circumvent human error through responsible, truthful behavior. Research errors may result from inappropriate sampling, nonresponse, measurement error, or improper representation of oneself, one's research design, or one's data. Through careful research design, conduct, statistical analysis, and presentation, research errors may be prevented. "Data-dredging" and fragmentation of reports—ie, "LPUs"—are two easily avoidable problems.

Strategies to minimize research errors are of considerable import and are discussed not only in chapter 2, but throughout the volume as well. For example, sampling strategies are also discussed in chapters 8, 9, and 12. The use of human subjects and the need for appropriate consent forms is considered in chapter 9. Reduction of measurement error is detailed in the various chapters of parts 3, 4, and 5. Appropriate uses of statistical analyses are described in chapter 21. Strategies to enhance presentation of research findings are considered in chapters 22, 23, and 24. Issues of authorship are incorporated into chapter 24.

Chapter 3 guides the reader in writing research proposals and securing funding for research projects. Devising research questions, reviewing the literature, identifying collaborators and advisers, and locating funding sources are thoughtfully discussed. The sections on preparation of the proposal, the timeline, the budget, and the budget justification give much needed detail and pertinent checklists.

First-time investigators and experienced researchers alike will want to read this chapter once for an overview of the topic and again for the specific points presented. It is a road map, complete with encouragement and instructions, for commencing and continuing the adventure of research.

ERM, Editor

2. THE ETHICS OF CONDUCTING AND PRESENTING RESEARCH

Elaine R. Monsen, PhD, RD

All knowledge attains its ethical value and its human significance only by the human sense in which it is employed.

—Hermann Nothnagel

Ethics encompasses the principles of conduct governing an individual or a group, and as such, it pervades all aspects of personal and professional life. As have other responsible professional groups, The American Dietetic Association has adopted a voluntary, enforceable code of ethics. The current version of the code, which became effective in 1989, delineates 19 principles to guide dietetics professionals in their conduct, commitments, and obligations to "self, client, society, and the profession."[1] According to the code of conduct, practitioners act with objectivity and respect for the unique needs and values of individuals; avoid discrimination; maintain confidentiality; base practices on scientific principles and current information; conduct professional affairs with honesty, integrity, and fairness; and remain free of conflict of interests.

Not all judgments are ethical judgments; many evaluations and decisions are based on considerations of practicality, aesthetics, or professional values. Furthermore, diversity exists within ethical deliberations.[2] Ethical judgments reflect divergent opinions. Each case can be evaluated on an individual basis; indeed, case analysis is a major pillar of moral reasoning.[3] Nonetheless, despite this disparity, people of all cultures and eras are found to agree on the actions that are basically constructive—or destructive—to human interaction. Ethical conduct underscores behavior that supports positive relationships between persons.

At each step of research, ethical issues arise. Designing, conducting, reporting, and interpreting research all involve decisions in which professional ethics are pivotal. Whenever human subjects are involved in research, the bioethics of the research must be recognized and carefully considered. Bioethics, a major component of professional ethics, is associated with the much-debated issues of nutrition and hydration of the terminally ill, [4,5] but it also includes the ethics of human experimentation.[6] Issues related to authorship and to conflict of interests are also of critical import in research ethics. These various ethical issues will be addressed in this chapter; additionally, the key errors in research design and presentation—and practical strategies—are discussed.

RESEARCH ERROR, HUMAN ERROR, AND FRAUD

Whether they are consequences of flawed design, improper conduct of research, or unintentional or intentional human error, scientific errors can seriously deflect scientific progress. Repercussions of error are manifold. Time and finances can be lost in pursuing blind alleys, misapplication can be damaging to society, and scientific careers can be severely thwarted. Tainted literature, like an ocean blackened by an oil spill, requires time to be cleansed.[7] Poor and inadequate supervision is not acceptable in scientific enterprises. It is critical that researchers assume responsibility and enable investigation if misconduct is charged in any research projects in which they have participated.

Researchers need to, and generally can, circumvent research errors: those of design, execution, and presentation. Research errors may be categorized into six types: sampling error, noncoverage error, nonresponse error, measurement error, error of data distortion and overgeneralization, and errors of misrepresentation to human subjects, in authorship, and in conflict of interests. Quality research demands that research errors be minimized; moreover, allowing such errors may cause major ethical dilemmas in the future. This chapter discusses the six research errors and proposes strategies to avert them.

Human errors are a different class of error. Generally, they are more hidden and less readily detected than research errors. Human errors are an unfortunate—and one hopes infrequent—occurrence in research.

Three sources of human error need to be differentiated: *inadvertent behavior, negligence,* and *intentional actions.* As scientists are fallible, inadvertent errors can occur. An honest mistake is tolerable to the scientific community and the public if it is promptly and properly handled when uncovered. However, preventable mistakes attributable to carelessness or negligence are not tolerable to either science or society; sloppy science is a form of intentional error.

Fraud, or intentional deception, destroys science by eroding trust and integrity. The scientific method is built upon hypotheses and honest observation; deception is anathema to science. Fraud comes in varying degrees, including concealing data not supportive of a hypothesis and presenting only supportive data (ie, "selective" reporting or "cooking" data), revising observed data to conform to a hypothesis (ie, "trimming" data), and blatant fabrication of data. Each is an intentional deception, though the extent of misconduct differs dramatically. Falsifying and fabricating data occur rarely, but their calamitous impact can annihilate laboratories and brutally cripple participating institutions. Plagiarism is a further category of intentional fraud. Its damaging effects are felt keenly by the offended parties, and the perpetrator is subject to severe criticism from the scientific community and the alert public.

ETHICS IN RESEARCH INVOLVING HUMANS

Nuremberg Code and Declaration of Helsinki

Current guidelines and regulations regarding human experimentation have evolved over the last half century in reaction to public and scientific outcry over a few individual cases of gross human injustice. One of the first to receive public scrutiny was the heinous behavior of physicians toward the inmates of Nazi concentration camps in Germany during World War II. Following the war, 20 doctors were tried in Nuremberg before an international tribunal for war crimes and crimes against humanity. The resulting Nuremberg Code of 1947 established ten principles that must be followed in human experimentation to satisfy moral, ethical and legal concepts.[8] These principles, for the first time, established as essential informed voluntary consent of human subjects.

The second major international code of ethics was the Declaration of Helsinki adopted by the World Medical Association in 1964, with a proviso that the text be reviewed periodically. The basic principles in the Declaration of Helsinki were extended by the 29th World Medical Assembly in Tokyo in 1975, and further revised in 1983.[9] The 12 basic principles delineated the concept of submitting experimental protocols to an independent committee for consideration, comment, and guidance. This was the genesis of the future institutional review board, which has become a major force in ensuring the rights of human subjects. The Helsinki Declaration also counseled researchers to exercise caution in conducting research that could affect the environment and to respect the welfare of animals used for research.

Belmont Report

A third important document supporting the rights of human subjects is the 1978 Belmont Report issued by the National Commission for the Protection of Human Subjects of Biomedical and Behavioral Research.[10] This President's Commission was formed in 1974 in rapid response to disclosure of two scandalous research studies of the 1930s.[11] One, a study of the immune response, involved the injection of live, malignant cells into several aged patients in a chronic disease hospital without the patients' prior consent. The second study concerned long-term observation of the "natural" course of syphilis in men who were recruited into the study without informed consent. More despicably, these men were observed for several decades but did not receive penicillin, the efficacy of which in the treatment of syphilis was established several years after the initiation of the study.

The Belmont Report addresses ethical conduct of research involving human subjects and argues for balancing society's interests in protecting the rights of subjects with its interests in furthering knowledge that can benefit society as a whole. To assess benefit and risk of any research protocol, three basic principles are evoked: *respect for persons, beneficence,* and *justice.*

The Belmont Report argues that "respect for persons" incorporates at least two basic ethical convictions (or assurances): that individuals be treated as autonomous agents and that individuals in need of protection because of diminished autonomy are entitled to protection. Beneficence is understood to encompass acts of kindness and charity that go beyond strict obligation. The duality of beneficent actions extends from doing no harm to maximizing possible benefits and minimizing possible harms. Justice, the third principle, demands that each person be treated fairly. Justice requires that burdens and benefits are shared with equity. Those who may reap the benefits of the research are those who should shoulder the risk.

The reports issued by the National Commission established recommendations for the protection of special categories of human subjects, including the human fetus, children, prisoners, and people institutionalized as mentally infirm. To protect the rights of subjects, institutional review boards were empowered through federal regulations.

In all aspects of human experimentation, it is critical that researchers avoid misrepresentation to human subjects. The paramount strategy to avoid this research error relies on the three ethical principles of respect, beneficence, and justice. These principles affirm full and comprehensible disclosure to subjects, noncoercive consent, autonomous right of free choice, including the right to terminate participation without penalty, confidentiality, protection of privacy, and equity in subject selection. A research project should be terminated if, at any point, the data warrant such action.

ETHICS IN DESIGNING, CONDUCTING, AND ANALYZING RESEARCH

The scientific method is the basis for research design.[12] Initially, the existing body of scientific knowledge is carefully assessed. Questions of import to science and society are formulated, and in response to the research questions a vigorous and rigorous research design is crafted. Ethical scientific conduct includes accurate recording of data in such a way that they are readily available and understandable to current and future colleagues. To ensure appropriate data accessibility, the data need to be recorded at the time they are generated both correctly and in the detail necessary for ready comprehension. Original data books need to be retained and made available if requested.

Throughout the research process, careful attention needs to be paid to details of subject selection, method choice, and execution. If critical details are disregarded, if sloppy science is allowed, ethical predicaments may develop. This becomes of great concern when results are generalized.

Dillman,[13] who is recognized for his research on survey methodology, outlined four potential research errors that invalidate research: *sampling error, noncoverage error, nonresponse error,* and *measurement error.* The impact of such errors extends beyond survey design to other descriptive research techniques and to analytical research as well. By minimizing and, one hopes, eliminating these sources of error, one's research will gain substantially greater utility.

Sampling Error

Errors of sampling result from the differences between the study sample and the actual population. To have a true probability sample, each individual in the study population must have an equal chance of being selected as a subject. Sampling errors may be random; that is, they may occur by chance as samples from the same populations are drawn. Ensuring that each individual within the study population has the same likelihood of participating will minimize random sample error.

Another key element in minimizing sampling error is ensuring that the sample size is appropriate to the goals of the research (see chapter 20). Random sampling errors generally decrease as the sample size increases. A rule of thumb is that random sampling error will be reduced by one-half if the sample size is quadrupled.[13]

Noncoverage Error

Noncoverage error results from a sampling format that excludes some individuals within the study population from being selected as subjects. Noncoverage errors are, in general, systematic and difficult to overcome.[13] They are caused by bias in specifying or selecting the study sample.[4] For example, the subjects may be selected from outdated lists that exclude recent additions; from published telephone listings that exclude people with unlisted numbers; or from a group of people who are able to attend lectures in the evening, excluding those who work at that time. Bias generally occurs when samples of convenience are selected, eg, members of a group, volunteers responding to advertisements, or people from different health care institutions in whom a specific disease is diagnosed. Such biases impinge on the degree to which the data generated may represent the population at large. Issues of biases are of concern in both qualitative and quantitative research. When bias cannot be eliminated, it is particularly important to recognize it and declare it to those who are considering the results of the study.

Other examples of sampling bias[4] are:
- differences in geographical, temporal, or economic access to diagnostic procedures
- differences in treatment modalities that are standard for specific localities
- differences resulting from the fact that people with specific disorders or exposures gravitate toward certain health care facilities
- different diagnostic labels or treatment plans for the same condition at different points in space or time (secular changes in definitions, exposures, diagnoses, and treatments may make noncontemporaneous controls noncomparable)
- differences in exposure or outcome between "early comers," volunteers, or respondents (who tend to be "healthier") and "late comers," nonvolunteers, or nonrespondents
- membership in certain groups (employed, college graduates, or bicyclists), which may imply a degree of health or health awareness that systematically differs from that of the general population
- previous history that, if not reported and taken into account, may bias outcome because of the impact of prior diagnostic or treatment tactics

Noncoverage error, as does any systematic sampling error, distorts results. Because the bias of systematic errors is usually difficult to assess, the findings from the study become clouded. One cannot assume that the data collected from the faulted sample adequately represent the entire population. Thus, generalizations of the results to either the study population or other populations must be limited by the constraints of the actual subjects sampled.

Nonresponse Error

The third category of error is that of nonresponse. In surveys, the response rate is the percentage of those who actually answer the survey queries.[13] A low response rate raises serious questions as to whether the observed data accurately represent the study population: whether the nonresponders differ significantly from the responders. In many studies, researchers strive to improve response rate by devising various strategies to motivate, remind, and cajole subjects to respond.

Unfortunately, researchers may pay little attention to a modest response rate unless there is a marked disparity between projected and actual observations. One way to quiet some of the concern over a low response rate is to evaluate demographic and other available data of nonresponders and responders to ascertain whether important differences exist between the two groups. A further dilemma results when responders provide incomplete data sets, eg, omitted or partial responses to some questions in a survey. Among the ways to decrease inadequate responses to survey questions are to evaluate and pilot test the survey carefully, assuring clarity of the questions and ease of reply.

A corollary of nonresponse in clinical trials is error resulting from loss of subjects to follow-up. To minimize such loss, researchers make valiant efforts to complete the data sets. For example, to secure 25 years of follow-up data, some researchers have commissioned private detectives to investigate the whereabouts and life or death status of cohorts. Other examples are missing data for some laboratory values or anthropometric measurements or incomplete food intake records. In each case, the complete and incomplete data sets must be evaluated to ascertain whether the missing data skew the apparent results.

Unless one can be confident that inclusion of incomplete data does not misguide, the complete and incomplete data sets should be handled separately, rather than as single, blended data.

Faulty Measurement Error

Measurement error is the fourth type of research error. Whereas the first three types of error result from nonobservation, measurement error is one of observation.[13] As such, errors in conducting or executing the research are akin to measurement error. For example, if a question is worded in such a way that it cannot be answered accurately or if the questionnaire is structured so that unequal emphasis is placed on certain questions, measurement error will result. Impact of the placement of questions is influenced by whether the respondent receives the questions verbally or visually. In all cases, it is critical to recognize that biased questions and biased organization produce biased answers.

Characteristics of the subjects may also produce measurement error. Other biases[4] in executing research projects need to be avoided. One frequent error results when the experimental group and control group are treated differently in ways beyond what is designated by the specified intervention, as in giving additional attention or care to the experimental group. When the control group does not receive care and attention in amounts equal to what the experimental group receives, differences in outcome may be inaccurately attributed to the intervention.

Another type of bias occurs when issues of efficacy become confounded with those of compliance, as may occur when the experimental design requires patients to adhere to specified therapies. For example, some subjects may have a low rate of attendance at the education sessions of a program being evaluated. As suggested in the section on nonresponse error, the researcher can compare the complete data sets with the incomplete data sets to determine whether the data can be merged. Similarly, subjects who either withdraw or are withdrawn from an experiment may differ systematically from those who remain, causing withdrawal bias. Furthermore, preconception bias is likely to occur unless the experimental design is masked, or blinded, striving to allow the investigation to proceed and data to be collected without influence or bias from either subject or investigator.

Well-Crafted Design

The well-crafted research design minimizes research errors. All people in the population one wishes to observe have an equal probability of being subjects, avoiding noncoverage error. Individual subjects within that population are randomly selected, and the number selected is sufficiently large to provide the desired precision, minimizing sampling error. Every subject selected responds and is not lost to follow-up, avoiding response error. The techniques for estimating response are precise, accurate, reproducible, and equally valid for each subject; each subject complies fully to the assigned regimen, limiting measurement error; and all data are truthfully and fully recorded.

Thoughtful and adequate supervision of all research projects is essential to ensure that the data are properly collected. Each person in a research team must assume responsibility for all aspects of the research in his or her domain and maintain awareness of the project in its entirety. The sense of team involves

ETHICAL PRESENTATION AND INTERPRETATION OF RESEARCH

graduate students, research assistants, intradisciplinary and interdisciplinary professionals, and faculty. Although the chief supervisor must assume ultimate accountability, responsibility for ethical conduct falls on everyone's shoulders.

Honesty, truthfulness, and full disclosure are requisite in presenting research. It is the researcher's obligation to publish valid data, to analyze the data objectively and dispassionately, and to present a fair and unbiased interpretation to readers.[14] Inference must be supportable by the data. Authors must recognize the power of inference and avoid misleading the reader.

As a parallel, readers are obligated to use data ethically, without distortion. The Council of Biology Editors contends that equal care must be exercised by researchers and authors as to the message they send and by readers as to the message they receive and use.[14]

The Whole Truth, and Nothing but the Truth

The ethical investigator truthfully reports and fully discloses research data and the methods whereby the data were generated. Limitations of the study design, eg, subject bias, should be clearly stated. The ethical investigator objectively evaluates the data and provides a fair interpretation. To do more or less is ethically unsupportable. At all times, scientific proof must be rigorous and without bias.

Several practices in handling data are considered unethical and may be considered *errors of data distortion*: data-dredging, selective reporting of findings, fragmentation of reports, redundant publication, and inappropriate statistical tests.[14] Data-dredging is the process of combing through a large pool of data to pick up "significant findings" from research that was not designed to produce those results. Data-dredging is particularly noxious when only "positive" results are reported and "negative" results are ignored, thus making the former appear to be of substantial import, rather than merely significant by chance. Because the accepted level of statistical significance is a probability of 0.05 or less, the chance that a relationship would be considered significant is 1 in 20. Thus, if the number of comparisons are many, as could occur if data collected from ten laboratory values and the dietary intake of ten nutrients were compared, the 100 potential comparisons would undoubtedly yield several (perhaps five) "significant relationships," most of which would be by chance and lacking relevance.

The relationships that are appropriate to evaluate are those decreed by the original research design, driven by the research question and hypothesis. Chance observations may encourage further research, and if the new research question results in data that replicate the earlier "positive" results, publication of the findings would be justified.

Selective reporting of research findings is a form of advertent fraud, often motivated by efforts to support a hypothesis when the data do not clearly provide adequate support. Such actions as concealing data, presenting solely favorable data, or in any other way shaping or trimming data to accommodate the hypothesis disregards scientific and ethical principles. Such conscious acts are ignoble, premeditated actions to distort data and to mislead one's colleagues and the public.

Research findings that are fragmented and published in multiple small units are a disservice to readers. The whole picture is not visible, and interrelationships are lost. Scientific editors discourage submission of "least publishable units," commonly called LPUs, and refer to such fragmentation as "salami science." A similar wasteful practice is duplicate or redundant publication: presentation of essentially the same study with little if any modification.

Statistics to Interpret Data

Statistics is the art and science of interpreting quantitative data. It includes framing questions that are answerable, designing the study, exercising quality control of the data to reduce both variance and bias, drawing inferences from data, and generalizing results to other situations.[14]

Fienberg[15] suggests that the following eight points be addressed in a statistical review of a submitted manuscript. The points are of equal utility in designing, conducting, and reporting research.

1. What are the original data? How have they been transformed for use in the statistical analyses?
2. Is information given on uncertainty and measurement error?
3. How were the statistical analyses done, and are they accurately described in the paper?
4. Are the statistical methods used appropriate for the data?
5. Have the data or analyses been "selected," and does such selection distort the "facts"?
6. What population do the data represent? Does the design for data collection allow for the inferences and generalizations made?
7. Are there additional analyses that would be enlightening?
8. Are the conclusions sensitive to the methodologic and substantive assumptions? If so, is this acknowledged? Do reported measures of uncertainty reflect this sensitivity?

The core of the scientific method, and hence of science, is inference: learning about unobserved phenomena by studying and interpreting relevant data on observed phenomena.[14] Inference must be protected, not abused by such distorting actions as selective reporting and data-dredging. Data need to be honest and presented honestly.

ETHICS IN PUBLICATION

It is an author's responsibility to submit manuscripts that are appropriate for publication consideration and peer review. To do so means that the data need to be accurate, responsibly analyzed, and interpreted. The research design and the materials and methods used need to be clearly and fully presented. All relevant sources need full and accurate citation. As discussed in the preceding section, it is unethical and a form of deception to present data selectively, to withhold contradictory data, or to revise data for impact.

Questions often arise as to how much data should be presented in a manuscript. The goal should be to proffer the optimal publishable unit, not to disperse the data in a variety of LPUs. As tenure evaluations are turning toward quality per unit published and away from number of units published, LPUs will be a negative factor in a researcher's list of publications. When a researcher is allowed to offer five original publications for tenure consideration, the advantage will go toward a well-crafted and reasoned article rather than a single fragment of a research project.

Peer review is the prime way that science monitors itself. The scientist accepts the dual professional responsibility of submitting research for peer review and serving as an objective, ethical peer reviewer for the work of others. A reviewer assumes the responsibility of assuring the scientific integrity of published literature, and his or her confidentiality is requisite to ethical behavior toward the author. Should legitimate conflict of interests be apparent to a peer reviewer, he or she should decline to review rather than jeopardize a sound review process. It is obviously unethical to take advantage of authors by invading the confidentiality of the peer review process or by using their work before its official publication.

Error of Overgeneralizing

When interpreting and applying one's own or other researchers' data, it is tempting to over-present to the media and the public. The desire to make a point—to "feed one's bias"—to support one's preconception must not override accurate use of scientific data. As discussed, research errors resulting from sample bias, noncoverage, nonresponse, and measurement error determine, in large part, whether the data may be generalized to other populations or even to the entire study population. For example, a research study showing lower serum cholesterol levels in men who consume a low-saturated-fat diet cannot be generalized to the population at large (all other men), let alone to infants, children, adolescents, women, and the elderly. The error of overgeneralization is an error of misrepresentation to one's colleagues and to the public. To overgeneralize erodes one's credibility and erodes the credibility of science.

It is particularly disturbing when data are overgeneralized in an effort to convince others of one's prejudices or patronages. Honest differences of opinion exist; they should be stated clearly, while recognizing opposing views. However, representing one's own data or those of others inappropriately is scientifically reprehensible, as it misleads others.

ISSUES RELATED TO AUTHORSHIP

Authorship implies substantial contribution to the published article and conveys responsibility for the content. The Uniform Requirements for Manuscripts Submitted to Biomedical Journals delineates three criteria to determine whether someone has contributed sufficiently to be designated as an author. The criteria, all of which are to be satisfied, are substantial contributions to: (1) design or analysis and interpretation of the data; (2) drafting or revising the article critically for important intellectual content; and (3) final approval of the version to be published.[16] The error of misrepresentation in authorship can be avoided if the three criteria are used to determine author status.

Authorship cannot be justified for a person whose participation is limited to acquisition of funding, administration of the department or unit, or the collection of the data. General, as opposed to specific, supervision of the research group is also considered inadequate to warrant authorship. Each section critical to the main conclusions of the article must be the responsibility of one or more of the designated authors. For an article consisting of the contributions of researchers from diverse fields, only the key people responsible for the article should be specified as authors; other contributors should be recognized and thanked in an acknowledgment. Gratuitous or honorary authorship is neither appropriate nor ethically acceptable. Authorship is not a gift, but a right founded on substantial contribution to the resulting manuscript.

An author must make major contributions to the genesis and presentation of the research data. In addition, an author is not only responsible for the published data, but must be prepared to defend the data and the interpretation of the data as well. Discussion continues as to the explicit requirements that must be satisfied to qualify as an author: namely, how extensive an individual's contribution must be to qualify as an author, and how accountable to both peers and public an author must be for the paper in its entirety. One of the obvious dilemmas is the extent of accountability an author assumes when collaborating with scientists and professionals in diverse fields. At minimum, an individual author is responsible for all aspects of work that are within and proximate to his or her field(s) of expertise.

The primary or lead author has a special position that is determined from having made the major intellectual input to the article. The primary author also should have made outstanding, positive, and creative contributions; provided the major intellectual input; participated actively in the work, data tabulation, and interpretation; and provided key scientific leadership throughout the research design, conduct, analysis, and presentation.[14]

CONFLICTS OF INTEREST

Conflicts of interest occur in any situation in which financial or other personal considerations may compromise, or appear to compromise, an investigator's professional actions in designing, conducting, or reporting research. Conflicts of interest may also bias other aspects of an investigator's research activities, such as the choice of methods, length of time subjects are studied, purchase of materials, hiring of support staff, or choice of statistical analyses. Other scholarly activities are affected by conflicts of interest; for example, in the preparation of review articles, one's financial and personal interests may interfere with one's professional objectivity.

It is customary for investigators to disclose any and all possible conflicts. Professional journals expect each author's funding sources and institutional and corporate affiliations to be acknowledged on the title page of articles submitted for publication. In addition, consultancies, stock ownership, or other equity interests or patent licensing should be disclosed to the journal editor in a cover letter at the time articles are submitted.[14] The error of misrepresentation of conflict of interests is averted when such interests are disclosed to the readers of any related publication. It is important for full disclosure to be made because the *appearance* of conflict may be as professionally damaging as *known* conflict.

Fear of conflicts of interest should not deter an investigator from seeking ethical financial and corporate relations. Problems develop when financial interests are not disclosed. It is ethically irresponsible for a scientist, because of a personal conflict of interest, to repress negative data, to expose only selected findings, or in any way to distort the presentation of data because of their potentially desirable or undesirable financial impact. Financial interest should neither impinge upon professional objectivity nor drive professional activities.

RESEARCH IN AN ETHICAL CLIMATE

Discovering the unknown, expanding horizons, updating perceptions and techniques, and devising and evaluating new applications all make research exciting. The profession and society are advanced concurrently. Ethical scientific conduct of research ensures acceptance of new data and positive assessment of the data's interpretation.

Throughout the many steps of research,[17] highly ethical behavior is imperative. While selecting important questions and designing effective research protocols in which research errors are minimized, it is essential to keep in mind that the execution and presentation of the research must be accomplished in an ethical fashion. The three principles of respect for persons, beneficence, and justice are excellent guides, critical not only when considering human subjects, but when interacting with close colleagues, professional peers, clients, the public, and the media. Conflicts of interest require full disclosure to avoid misleading others. In such an ethical climate, research accomplishments will grow and survive.

The scientist values research by the size of its contribution to that huge, logically articulated structure of ideas which is already, though not yet half built, the most glorious accomplishment of mankind.

—Sir Peter Brian Medawar in The Art of the Soluble, *1967*

References

1. Code of ethics for the profession of dietetics. *J Am Diet Assoc.* 1988;88:1592–1596.
2. Dalton S. What are the sources and standards of ethical judgment in dietetics? *J Am Diet Assoc.* 1991;91:545–546.
3. Jonsen AR, Toulmin S. *The Abuse of Casuistry: A History of Moral Reasoning.* Berkeley and Los Angeles, Calif: University of California Press; 1988.
4. Issues in feeding the terminally ill adult. *J Am Diet Assoc.* 1987; 87:78–85; updated: 1989;89:1040.
5. Brody H, Noel MB. Dietitians' role in decisions to withhold nutrition and hydration. *J Am Diet Assoc.* 1991;91:580–585.
6. Silverman WA. *Human Experimentation: A Guided Step Into the Unknown.* Oxford, England: Oxford Medical Publications; 1986.
7. Garfield E, Welljams-Dorf A. The impact of fraudulent research on the scientific literature. The Stephen E. Breuning case. *JAMA.* 1990;263:1424–1426.
8. *Trials of War Criminals Before the Nuremberg Military Tribunal Under Control Council Law No. 10.* Washington, DC: US Government Printing Office; 1949;2.
9. 18th World Medical Assembly. The Helsinki Declaration of 1964. In: Reich WT, ed. *Encyclopedia of Bioethics.* New York, NY: Free Press; 1978;4:1770–1771.
10. National Commission for the Protection of Human Subjects of Biomedical and Behavioral Research. *The Belmont Report: Ethical Principles and Guidelines for the Protection of Human Subjects of Research.* Washington, DC: US Government Printing Office; 1988. DHEW publications. (05)78-0012, 78-0013, 78-0014.
11. Levine RJ. *Ethics and Regulation of Clinical Research.* 2nd ed. New Haven, Conn: Yale University Press; 1988.
12. Committee on the Conduct of Science, National Academy of Sciences. *On Being a Scientist.* Washington, DC: National Academy Press; 1989.
13. Dillman DA. The design and administration of mail surveys. *Annu Rev Soc.* 1991;17:225–249.
14. Council of Biology Editors. *Ethics and Policy in Scientific Publication.* Bethesda, Md: Council of Biology Editors, Inc; 1990.
15. Fienberg SE. Statistical reporting in scientific journals. In: *Ethics and Policy in Scientific Publications.* Bethesda, Md: Council of Biology Editors, Inc; 1990.
16. International Committee of Medical Journal Editors. Uniform requirements for manuscripts submitted to biomedical journals. *Ann Intern Med.* 1988;108:258–265.
17. Monsen ER, Vanderpool HY, Halsted CH, McNutt KW, Sandstead HH. Ethics: responsible scientific conduct. *Am J Clin Nutr.* 1991;54:1–6.

3. HOW TO WRITE PROPOSALS AND OBTAIN FUNDING

M. Rosita Schiller, PhD, RD, and Jean C. Burge, PhD, RD

Regardless of one's level of professional development, proposal writing skills can usually be enhanced. Early success at obtaining approval for research studies often triggers a lifelong pattern of grant activity characterized by increasingly larger or more prestigious awards, publication in highly reputable journals, and invitations to evaluate others' research.

This chapter offers guidelines for developing proposals that will ultimately receive both approval and funding. The information can be used in a variety of ways. Those new to the research arena can carefully follow each point to ensure optimal results. Those who have unfunded proposals can use the chapter as an evaluation checklist to identify weaknesses and pitfalls. Project leaders can offer the information as a guide to new researchers enabling them to gain valuable experience. For those who need a refresher course, this chapter may offer new insights for better preparation of proposals. Those who seek renewed motivation may find new ideas on how to prepare a high-quality proposal deserving of full funding.

THE RESEARCH PROPOSAL

Proposal development is ordinarily divided into three distinct phases: preparation, writing, and review. It takes about six months to develop a good proposal from start to finish.

Preparation

Work begins with the simple desire to conduct research, to contribute to the development of new knowledge. The preparation phase may require three to four weeks or more, depending on time spent in the library and meeting schedules.

Identify the problem area. The first challenge is generation of an idea that is clearly focused and merits investigation. Such research questions can arise from numerous sources such as those outlined by Feitelson[1]:
- untested theories
- personal observations in the work setting
- gaps in the scientific base that undergirds practice
- controversies regarding treatment
- case studies and observed trends
- questions posed by colleagues or clients

Successful researchers hone in on one area of study. All their work contributes in some way to further understanding of the specified area. Such a defined focus has several advantages. It simplifies becoming familiar with current literature and staying abreast of new developments. It helps establish one as an authority on the subject. A history of successful research projects along the same theme lends credibility to a new study and verifies importance of the work. Once an area of study is defined, one investigation easily leads to another. Findings often suggest further unanswered questions and the need to pursue new paths of inquiry.

Survey the literature. After a problem area has been identified, an initial review of literature from the past four or five years is needed to explore recent work on the topic. Reading both review articles and original reports steeps the researcher in the subject, determines whether a germinating question has been previously tested, and identifies experts in the area.[1] Such study also enables the researcher to conceptualize the theoretical framework, formulate research objectives, and delineate hypotheses.[2]

The initial survey of literature may be quite cursory. In time it will become part of an extensive literature review required for the written proposal, a topic that will be addressed later in this chapter.

Identify potential collaborators. It is possible, but difficult, to conduct research in total isolation. Dietitians can network to find others with similar research interests to share the process, stimulate new ideas, challenge poorly conceived research designs, or serve as research mentors. The best research teams are made up of people with differing backgrounds and expertise. Practitioners often benefit from collaborating with university faculty members, who generally have more extensive research experience and better access to various resources. Alternatively, faculty members gain the advantage of expanded research opportunities in practice settings. Interdisciplinary medical or health care research teams often welcome the nutrition expertise of dietitians. Membership on a multidisciplinary team generally enhances research productivity, stimulates development of research protocols, and encourages ongoing involvement in focused research studies.

Collaboration offers many other benefits.[3,4] Working together spreads the responsibilities and speeds implementation of the project. Representation from various backgrounds, such as biostatistics, epidemiology, pharmacology, nursing, or medicine, may be required to answer the research question satisfactorily. Some funding agencies give priority to interdisciplinary studies, given the complex nature of investigations involving human subjects and health care delivery systems. Collaboration with an established researcher enhances funding potential since grant awards are usually given those with a strong track record. Most funding agencies require affiliation with a university or institutional research institute, an element frequently achieved when researchers join forces.

Collaboration also has drawbacks, but these adverse effects can be minimized by addressing them up front.[5] For example, a system for frequent interaction with team members is imperative; loss of contact usually results in termination of the project. Commitment to the research is essential; collaborators who are "too busy" may disrupt momentum, delay progress, and cause missed deadlines. Divergent thinkers who are not totally sold on the research question may introduce new ideas or force compromises that are not fully acceptable to other team members. Collaborators must decide early who will serve as principal investigator and whose name will appear first on any publications. In addition, they must determine how the work will be divided and make sure everyone accepts accountability for designated assignments.

Define limits. At this point, the research collaborators are ready to formulate the research question and decide on the magnitude of the study. A key here is to think small: to pursue just one line of investigation, not to attempt to tackle simultaneously all dimensions of a multifaceted problem. The question should be as precise as possible, focusing on a single issue or group of research subjects. The examples in *Table 3.1* illustrate some clearly defined research questions and corresponding statements that are too broad or too poorly defined.

The Research Environment

Table 3.1
Sample Research Questions

Right	Wrong
Is malnutrition associated with increased length of hospitalization for patients admitted for elective hip and knee joint replacement?	Does malnutrition increase the cost of medical care?
Can blood glucose levels of tube-fed, non-stressed elderly patients with insulin-dependent diabetes be maintained within the normal range by use of a fiber-containing enteral formula?	Is there a positive relationship between blood sugar levels and dietary fiber?
Is there a unique personality profile, as assessed by the Myers Briggs Inventory, distinguishing Recognized Young Dietitians and Dietetic Technicians from other young practitioners in the field?	Are Recognized Young Dietitians characterized by a unique personality profile?
Can total meal costs be reduced by more than $1 per patient per day by converting from a three-week selective cycle menu to a one-week selective cycle menu, keeping raw food costs within the present range?	Does conversion from a three-week cycle menu to a one-week cycle menu save money?

Time limits also need to be established. For example, a five-year study probably will not be funded, so a question that can be answered in one to two years should be formulated. If sufficient subjects are unavailable or the required data cannot be collected in this time frame, the research question should be reformulated to sharpen the focus or to designate a more appropriate sample population.

Choose a potential funding agency. It is important to identify potential funding agencies before actually writing a proposal.[6] Early selection facilitates the process in several ways. Appropriate application forms and proposal guidelines can be obtained and followed right from the start. Submission deadlines are preset, enabling the group to pace its work. Eligibility can be determined and compliance with requirements confirmed in the application. The proposal can be tailored to fit funding limitations and agency priorities. Sources and techniques for obtaining research funding are considered later in this chapter.

Develop an advocate/advisory committee. It is helpful to develop a group of people who can assist in obtaining research funding. Identifying a single person as mentor is also valuable. These people can assist in providing needed skills in writing and reviewing the research proposal. They may have access to needed resources such as laboratory space or facsimile equipment. They may be able to provide introductions to individuals in federal or state agencies and foundations. Finally, they may be able to provide experience in grantsmanship, which is valuable in overcoming obstacles in achieving success.[7]

Writing the Proposal

Proposal writing is an act of persuasive communication.[8] Proposals must present a clear, accurate, and complete picture of the activity to be funded. Kennicott[8] notes that the proposal must convince reviewers that the proposed activity is:

- appropriate for support by the funding agency
- both worthwhile and highly desirable in light of funding alternatives
- both methodologically sound and likely to succeed
- in the hands of a well-qualified principal investigator who will complete the project if it is funded

To ensure achievement of these aims, the grant preparation tips outlined in *Table 3.2* should be carefully followed. Although each funding agency has its own unique guidelines, general suggestions for developing proposals and conducting research are offered in a number of resources listed in *Table 3.3*. Following is a brief overview of various sections included in a proposal.

Cover letter. As a matter of courtesy, a proposal should include a cover letter addressed to the grant coordinator, foundation president, or other appropriate individual. This letter should be brief and friendly, noting the attachment of a proposal and a designated number of copies. It also should specify whether the proposal is in response to a request for proposals (RFP), a follow up to an approved concept paper, an unsolicited initiative previously discussed with individuals at the granting agency, or a brand-new idea in pursuit of funding.

Title page. The project title should be descriptive and limited to no more than 55 typewritten spaces.[9] The project title should introduce the topic of the proposal. Key words in the title provide an introduction to the study, and they often determine where the proposal will be sent for review. Cute, magazine-type titles usually convey a flamboyant image and should be avoided.

Most grant applications provide the format for a title page, and it should be used as is, with the information typed in as requested. The form should not be retyped on a computer with spaces modified to meet individual needs. Deviations from standard formats require greater concentration from reviewers; the inconvenience may create negative feelings that might tarnish an otherwise good evaluation of the project.

Abstract or summary. This section of the proposal is written last. It offers a concise but complete overview of the entire project, including the problem statement, research objectives, research design, methodologies, timetable, and requested budget. The abstract is generally limited to one page, or the space designated in the application.

Depending on the review process, a majority of review panel members may read only the title, abstract, and significance of a proposal; they will depend on designated, in-depth reviewers for accurate assessments of the strengths and weaknesses of the study.[9] This reality accentuates the importance of drafting a descriptive title and a concise—but complete—abstract.

Table 3.2
Grant Preparation Tips

---

1. Grantwriting is not a solo activity—seek consultation and collaboration from others.
2. Have your proposal reviewed by peers before submitting it for funding.
3. Follow the directions in detail, including margins, page limits, and the use of references or appendices.
4. State ideas clearly and succinctly. Give attention to spelling and grammar.
5. Use letter-quality printing rather than dot matrix and use a good quality copier.
6. Plan ahead and develop a time frame for completing your grant. Avoid the last minute rush that will compromise the quality of your proposal.
7. Use appendices to include study instruments, procedures, or other supporting materials.
8. Include support letters from individuals who are important to the success of your study. This includes medical staff, nursing administration, consultants, and co-investigators.

From Ferrell BR, Nail LM, Mooney K, Cotanch P. Applying for Oncology Nursing Society and Oncology Nursing Foundation Grants. *Oncol Nurs Forum.* 1989;16:728–730. Used by permission.

Table 3.3
General References for Proposals and Research

Hulley SB, Cummings SR. *Designing Clinical Research.* Baltimore, Md: Williams and Wilkins; 1988.

Krathwohl DR. *How to Prepare a Research Proposal.* 2nd ed. Syracuse, NY: Syracuse University Bookstore; 1977.

Leedy PD. *Practical Research: Planning and Design.* New York, NY: Macmillan Publishing Co Inc; 1980.

Lindeman CA, Schantz D. The research question. *J Nurs Admin.* 1982;12:6–10.

Monsen ER, Cheney, CL. Research methods in nutrition and dietetics: design, data analysis and presentation. *J Am Diet Assoc.* 1988;88:1047–1065.

Oyster CK, Hanten WP, Llorens LA. *Introduction to Research: A Guide for the Health Science Professional.* Philadelphia, Pa: JB Lippincott Co; 1987.

Schantz D, Lindeman CA. The research design. *J Nurs Admin.* 1982;12:35–38.

Twomey P. Getting started in clinical nutrition research. *Nutr Clin Pract.* 1991;6:175–183.

Verhonick PJ, Seaman CC. *Research Methods for Undergraduate Students in Nursing.* New York, NY: Appleton-Century-Crofts; 1978.

Problem statement.   This part of the proposal establishes the framework for the research question. The main purpose is to justify the proposed activity and show the apparent need for conducting the study.[10] Contents may include a brief review of pertinent current literature, gaps in present knowledge of the subject, results of pilot studies, or needs assessments describing the target population. The problem statement should show how the proposed study relates to what is known and how it will advance both knowledge and practice.

Specific aims.   This section addresses the question, "What will be accomplished?" Aims should be stated as clearly and succinctly as possible. There should be an obvious coherence among aims, goals, objectives, hypotheses, and study questions, often achieved through the use of an outline format.

The writer should move from the general to the specific, clearly describing expected outcomes. Overall aims and specific objectives need to be both reasonable and attainable[11]; they should logically point toward research hypotheses, experiments, or study questions. Hypotheses should be stated for experimental studies in which relationships between variables are to be determined. A list of proposed experiments may be given under specific aims to illustrate how the desired outcomes will be achieved. Study questions, rather than hypotheses, are best used for descriptive or exploratory studies.[12]

Significance. In this section the researcher builds a foundation to support the specific aims previously stated. A thorough but concise review of pertinent literature is essential to show the researcher's familiarity with the field, the relationship of the present study to the research area, and the importance of the proposed work to extend the current knowledge base. Mackenzie[9] suggests beginning this section with the words, "The proposed research is important because. . . ." This helps the researcher to highlight immediately salient points that may otherwise get buried in the narrative.

Preliminary work. A maximum of eight pages may be devoted to this section in applications for funding from the National Institutes of Health. This specification connotes the importance given to previous research or pilot studies related to the problem area. Results of completed work can be used to report progress of previously funded projects; convey the likelihood that a project will be carried to completion; substantiate that the investigator is familiar with the techniques to be used and that he or she has the skill and qualifications to complete the proposed work; illustrate that the current study is a logical extension of earlier work; and estimate variability, experimental effect, and sample size needed for statistically significant results in the proposed study.

Various techniques can facilitate reviewer comprehension of preliminary work. For example, tables, graphs, and exhibits can present results of previous studies.[13] The section can start with an outline if several studies are to be summarized. References for published reports can be cited.

Experimental design and methodology. This is the most critical section of the proposal. Reviewers give more weight to it than any other when evaluating the proposal and calculating the total score for priority ratings. Neiderhuber[13] cautions that at least two-thirds of the time and effort of writing a proposal should be devoted to research design and methodology.

This section should parallel specific aims and contain information regarding the experimental design, subjects, measurement of variables, methodology, and statistical analysis. It should begin with a declarative statement regarding the basic research method,[1] followed by a diagram showing the flow of planned investigations.[13] Subheadings may be used to highlight major components of the research design.

Research design. If appropriate, a diagram may be used to illustrate the research model. This is especially helpful for experimental studies or proposals that contain a series of steps.

Subjects. The discussion includes the type and number of subjects to be used, as well as their availability and accessibility to the investigator. It should also describe the research setting, selection criteria, how subjects will be assigned to a random or control group, estimate of available subjects, how consent will be obtained, and the sample size (see chapter 20). The number of subjects must be sufficient to achieve desired confidence levels and statistical power, anticipated variance in the data, and potential attrition.

Measurement. The proposal should describe each variable and how it will be measured, and illustrate how each variable is linked to specific aims of the study. It is important to justify the use of measurement tools or techniques, outlining their previous use, standardization, and selection of specific tools over other available instruments or techniques. This section also should cover any measures used to assure validity and reliability of the data. A copy of data collection instruments should be included in the appendix.

Methodology or procedures. Having described what instruments or methods will be used and who will participate, the writer's next step is to explain all procedures in a step-by-step fashion, telling how data will be collected. Again, exhibits may be used to illustrate work flow, complex interventions, or sequential use of various techniques.

The following questions illustrate the wide range of information needed for this section of the proposal: Will research assistants be employed to collect data? Who will train them? What steps will be taken to enroll subjects and when will consent be obtained? When and where will data be obtained? How will the data be recorded? How will confidentiality be maintained? In what sequence will activities occur?

Statistical analysis. Use of a statistical consultant lends credibility to most studies. A consultant is essential unless the researcher has documented expertise in this area. A consultant can help an investigator think through variables, data collection techniques, organization of the data, and appropriate statistical procedures. He or she can also suggest terminology that clearly describes both statistical procedures and rationale for their use. Statistical analyses should account for all data collected, and they should answer the research questions or hypotheses. (See chapter 21.)

Timetable. Most proposal outlines require a timetable for completion of the work. If this is not required as a separate section, it should be included in a description of procedures. Reviewers want to know how long various parts of the study will take. The timetable should specify such things as preparations needed, recruitment of subjects, training of research personnel, data collection, data analysis, and preparation and presentation of reports. Provisions should appear in the timetable for items included in specific aims and anticipated outcomes of the research. Can all work be completed within the funded time frame? If not, what provisions have been made for completing unfinished work?

Budget. A researcher who has not established a track record should keep his or her request for money in a conservative range. Frequently internal funding can be obtained for a pilot study. This can serve the purpose of preparing a draft proposal, developing and testing procedures, providing preliminary data, and building a case for qualifications of the researcher.

Consultants from a research office can provide invaluable assistance in preparing the budget. An extensive discussion on estimating costs and preparing the budget is provided in the next section.

Biographical sketches. For NIH proposals, biographical sketches are limited to two pages. The reviewers will judge from the data provided whether they think the personnel can perform the proposed research. Therefore, a proposal should provide convincing information to help sway the judges. Evidence of qualifications is not limited to the curriculum vitae. Eaves[11] commented that desirable qualifications are:

> demonstrated ability to think clearly and logically, to express logical thought concisely and cogently, to discriminate between the significant and the inconsequential, to display technical prowess, to handle abstract thought, to analyze data objectively and accurately, and to interpret results confidently and conservatively.

Care should be taken to display these desirable characteristics throughout the proposal. They will place the researcher high on the list for potential funding.

Other support. Funding agencies want to know if and how much support is available from other sources and if a proposal for similar research has been submitted to another agency. What will happen if both proposals are funded? Also, if the percentage of time designated for multiple studies exceeds 100%, an explicit plan must be provided showing how requirements for each study will be met.

Resources and environment. Reviewers will not ordinarily be familiar with any specific work environment. Therefore, most proposals are strengthened by a description of the hospital, laboratory, community setting, or other factors that contribute to a supportive research environment. A proposal should give pertinent details, such as availability of specific equipment needed to carry out the proposed study, access to important information, and institutional philosophy regarding research in relation to service requirements.

Appendix. The appendix may include data that support the proposal but are too lengthy, detailed, or technical to be placed in the body of the proposal. For example, the appendix might include letters of support and endorsements, related papers published by the researcher, curriculum vitae, data collection forms, institutional ethics review committee approval, descriptive materials such as brochures and flyers, and pictures of unusual equipment or devices to be used in the study.

Appended material might not be copied for all reviewers.[9] Therefore, any material crucial to understanding the proposed research should be placed in the main body of the proposal.

Internal Proposal Review

It is a mistake to hurry through writing a proposal and to send it to a funding agency immediately. Instead, two or three seasoned colleagues should be asked to read and evaluate it. Internal reviewers can point out gaps or weaknesses in the plan, and they can give suggestions regarding organization and clarity of materials presented. Time should be provided during the development phase for peer assessment and completion of suggested revisions to make sure the proposal is "clear, concise, inclusive and understandable."[10]

Before the application is submitted it should be ascertained that a clear and documented relationship exists between the proposed research and stated priorities of the funding agency. Also, the proposal should state what will be done with the findings; for example, data may be used to generate new hypotheses for further study, develop a new treatment program, advance practice in the field, or extend development of an important database.

If the proposal is written to support a thesis or dissertation, faculty support should be documented, and the faculty advisor should be included as a co-investigator.[12]

When the research requires the use of humans or animals, approval of an institutional ethics review committee is required by most funding agencies. Sufficient lead time must be allotted for this review. The application should include evidence of institutional review committee approval and assurance of compliance with ethical guidelines of both the funding agency and the institution.

Most funding agencies require approval (in the form of signatures) of one or more institutional representatives, usually major administrators and a grant officer. These authorizations assure tacit approval for the project, release time to conduct the work, employment of designated personnel if funding is received, and fiduciary responsibility for the use of any grant support. Again, the researcher must plan ahead for unforeseen circumstances, such as vacations and business trips, to be sure the needed signatures can be obtained prior to submission deadlines.

BUDGET AND BUDGET JUSTIFICATION

The main purpose of writing a proposal is to obtain funding. Therefore, the budget is a critical segment of the proposal and should be given appropriate attention. Each agency has its own rules for what will be covered, various line item categories, and dates for the fiscal year. These specific guidelines must be followed, and if the application materials include a form, it must be used. If no forms are provided, the funding agency should be contacted for guidelines.[14] Involvement of grants officers early in the budgeting process can also save valuable time and can facilitate the budgeting process.

The budget ought to provide a detailed, precise estimate of anticipated expenses. A "padded" bottom line gives the impression of dishonesty; an inadequate budget conveys naivete or incompetence.[9] Poor budgeting can adversely affect a research study and may negatively bias future prospects for new grants. If a realistic budget exceeds the limits of a funding agency, one consideration is cost sharing of items such as donated time, equipment, or service. Multiyear projects should reflect annual increases to account for inflation.

Justification should be provided for each budget item. Sometimes this can be done on the budget form; otherwise explanations are given on a separate sheet following the budget page. Budgets ordinarily have two main sections: personnel and non-personnel. Following are descriptions of items usually included in research budgets; *Table 3.4* contains a checklist for proposal budget items.

Table 3.4
Checklist for Proposal Budget
Items

Personnel
  Academic personnel
  Research associates
  Research assistants
  Graduate students
  Interviewers
  Computer programmer
  Evaluators
  Secretaries
  Editorial assistants
  Technicians
  Hourly personnel
  Release time
  Salary increases in proposals that
    extend to a new year
Fringe benefits
  Retirement
  Insurance (hospitalization and
    major medical)
  Medicare
  Tuition/fees
Consultant services
  Consultant fee
  Travel
  Subsistence
  Supplies for consultant
Subcontracts
Computer costs
  On-line time
  Job runs
  Data storage
  Computer software
  Computer use
Equipment
  Fixed equipment
  Moveable equipment
  Office equipment
  Equipment installation
Material and supplies
  Office supplies
  Communications
  Test materials
  Questionnaire forms
  Printing materials
  Animals
  Animal food
  Laboratory supplies
  Glassware
  Chemicals
  Electronic supplies
  Report materials and supplies
  Miscellaneous
  Periodicals and books
  Instructional materials

Travel
  Administrative
  Field work
  Professional meetings
  Travel for consultation
  Auto rental/taxi/metro/train/bus
  Aircraft rental
  Foreign travel
  Per diem (hotel and meals)
  Air transportation
  Mileage
  Registration fees
Patient care
  Inpatient charges
  Outpatient charges
  Patient travel
Alterations and renovations
Other expenses
  Duplicating services (reports, etc)
  Printing
  Publication costs
  Photographic/graphic services
  Service contracts
  Space rental
  Page charges
  Equipment maintenance and
    repair
  Equipment rental
  Human subjects' payments
  Workshops
  Telephone (line charges; long
    distance and tolls)
  Postage
  Interviewers' fees
  Honoraria
Indirect costs
Cost sharing (if required)
Trainee costs
  Stipends
  Dependency allowance
  Trainee travel
  Tuition and fees
  Training supplies

From Office of Sponsored Programs Development. *Guide for Proposal Development.* Columbus, Ohio: The Ohio State University; 1988:381–382. Used by permission.

The Research Environment

Personnel. Personnel costs include wages and fringe benefits for all individuals needed to carry out the proposed work, including project directors, investigators, interviewers, research assistants, student employees, and secretaries. Each participant's expertise, precise role, and estimated time required in relation to specific aims of the project must be specified. Personnel costs often account for as much as 80% of the budget.[10]

"Release time" is often requested to free personnel from their regular duties, giving them time to conduct the proposed study. These moneys may be used to employ temporary personnel. Funding may also be sought to pay fourth-quarter salaries to faculty members who conduct the research during the "off-term" of a nine-month contract. Researchers are generally not paid supplemental wages to carry out a research project.

If graduate students are employed as research assistants, tuition and fees for designated terms may be included as expenses. Policies of the sponsoring institution should be followed in this regard.

Consultants. When weaknesses in the backgrounds or skills of the researchers are apparent , consultants can enhance success of the project. Specific roles of consultants (eg, offering statistical assistance, training research assistants, conducting interviews, managing pharmaceutical administrations, monitoring biochemical reactions) should be delineated, with approximate hours or days devoted to the project. An application is strengthened by inclusion of a letter from each proposed consultant indicating willingness to contribute the time and expertise designated.

Equipment. Durable items costing more than $500 are considered equipment. Only equipment specifically needed to conduct the proposed research should be requested. Research equipment should be budgeted in the first year of a multiyear project; this reflects need for the item and allows greatest use of it. Equipment rental and service contracts may be itemized and often receive approval. Computers, typewriters, and other office equipment should not be requested unless they are integral to a project. The sponsoring institution is expected to support these from general funds.

Costs of space rental and construction or remodeling to accommodate a specific project may be allowed by some funding agencies. It is best to clear such items prior to including them in a budget.

Materials and supplies. Accurately calculating the cost of office, laboratory, and clinical supplies is often one of the greatest challenges in budgeting. If a study involves food items, meals, or formulas, this will be a key segment of the budget, requiring careful cost projections. Funding agencies are not likely to give supplemental funding once a study has been approved; any shortfalls are the responsibility of the researcher.

Anticipated supply usage must be analyzed thoroughly. It should include such things as stamps, printing, database (Medline) searches, videotapes, telephone charges, long-distance calls, interview forms, computer time, laboratory tests, flasks and test tubes, kits for laboratory analyses, file folders, computer disks, printer paper, ribbons, letterhead, and envelopes. Researchers may wish to subcontract with a secretarial service to prepare, mail, and receive questionnaires. Specific items for the study—for example, postage and questionnaires for a survey — should be itemized. Other items can be grouped under "office supplies." Grants officers can offer advice on how best to present and justify supply costs.

Subjects.   Dietetic research will often involve the use of humans or animals. Human subjects are frequently paid a stipend to ensure compliance with the study protocol, but stipends should not be so great as to influence voluntary participation.[6] Stipends ordinarily cover the costs of travel, time involved, babysitting, and other incidentals, such as parking. On occasion, a study may require hospitalization or an overnight stay in a metabolic unit. If group sessions are planned, the funding request should cover room rental and refreshments. O her items are the costs of appropriate laboratory tests, clinical procedures, physician visits, physical examinations, and medications. Expenses for parking, mileage, bus fare, or taxi service should also be included if subjects are not paid a stipend to cover these items.

Travel.   Collaborative research may require travel for team meetings. For example, Bergstrom et al[4] describe a collaborative team comprising representatives from five states who met together annually over a five-year study period. All related costs were covered in the research grant.

Travel expenses may be extensive.   If home visits are planned those travel costs should be included in the budget. Travel expenses may also include going to a conference to present research results, attending a scientific meeting to network with others conducting similar studies, or visiting other sites to consult with experts in the field. These expenses should be described in detail, giving names of meetings or visitation sites, state airfare, and per-diem costs. Reviewers will carefully examine any unjustified expenses in this category.[9]

Other expenses.   These may include costs of computer time, telephones, reprints of journal articles, publications, graphic artwork, film, slides, photo processing, manuals, and photocopying. Sometimes these items can be moved between the "supply" and "other" sections of the budget to give balance to the overall budget.

Indirect expenses.   Some funding agencies have a policy of not paying any indirect expenses. Others designate 10% to 15% of the total budget as indirect expense.[10] Many institutions have a negotiated indirect expense rate, which may range anywhere from 25% to 67% or more of direct expenses. An institutional grants officer can assist in calculating appropriate indirect expenses.

Cost sharing.   Occasionally, a granting agency will require the institution to share the cost of conducting research. Institutions will frequently bear the costs of release time, employee benefits, office supplies, travel, equipment maintenance and repair, remodeling space, and computer time.

AGENCY REVIEW PROCESS

Although procedures differ from one agency to another, the review process generally undergoes similar steps. A grants coordinator first reviews the application for eligibility and completeness. Proposals that meet eligibility criteria are sent to a panel of 5 to 15 peer reviewers who critique the proposal for its scientific merit, following a preestablished list of evaluative criteria.

Usually the review panel meets to discuss all proposals. One or two panel members are selected to conduct an in-depth review, prepare a list of strengths and weaknesses, and present an overview of the proposed study. The panel discusses each proposal and votes for its approval or disapproval based on soundness of the research design and methodology, qualifications of the investigator(s), and overall merit of the proposal. Approved proposals are given a priority score and one panel member is given the task of writing a summary statement of the review group's comments.[15]

Applications are forwarded to a decision-making body (board of directors or trustees), which hears summary reports and votes on each proposal. Projects approved for funding may be awarded the full amount requested, or the budget may be modified to better fit priorities and resources of the funding agency.

A staff member communicates final decisions to the principal investigators and sends them summary comments of the review panel. Researchers who receive funding are sent a formal notice indicating amount of the award, starting date, and any reporting requirements.

CONTACTING FUNDING SOURCES

Researchers can use several strategies to improve their chances of getting funded. Techniques may be both informal and formal, as outlined in the following suggestions.

Networks and Personal Contacts

Some proposals receive funding on their merits alone; others are funded because the applicants are known and respected.[16] Networking both inside and outside the funding agency is one way to gain recognition.

Consultants and other successful researchers can be invaluable resources. They may share previously submitted funded proposals, which researchers can study to gain insights into strategies used in successful proposals. Influential individuals or persons from prestigious institutions may agree to serve as consultants for projects; name recognition lends significant weight to the grant proposal.

Contacts can help to both garner and document support for a proposal. Influential contacts can introduce researchers to key people who may know someone at the targeted funding agency. Mentioning the person's name at the funding agency can facilitate scheduling a meeting or getting attention by phone. Letters included in the proposal appendix from key supporters both inside and outside the institution lend credibility to a proposal. Such letters may reflect support from such individuals as the medical director of a clinical research center, a statistician or director of a research consulting center, a department whose cooperation will be needed to conduct the study, a major administrator whose unit may benefit from the project, or a publisher interested in publishing results of the study.

Before writing a proposal, a personal conversation with the designated project officer or staff person in charge of receiving proposals is in order. These names may be obtained from the RFP, agency annual reports, or foundation offices. The phone call (or meeting) can provide clues regarding staff attitudes and evaluative criteria that may be used. The discussion can cover such things as preliminary research ideas, application forms, submission dates, budget targets and guidelines, the number of proposals anticipated, how much money has been appropriated, and unwritten rules, eg, types of projects targeted to receive funding or subtle characteristics desired in winning proposals.[15,17]

Grantors may advocate a proposal. They can promote an idea within their own agency or suggest other sources of potential funding. They may also give advance information; for example, grantors often inform their contacts about impending regulations that will be published close to the deadline for proposal receipt. They can be influential in getting a deadline extended in unusual circumstances.

A researcher can establish, maintain, and expand relationships at granting agencies in a variety of ways. Such networking is a lifelong process and may include such things as meetings at the grantor's office, appointments to review panels, internships with granting agencies, attendance at meetings where grantors will be speaking, arranging for grantors to speak at the researcher's institution, and invitations to conduct site visits of the researcher's major research projects.[18]

Concept Papers

A one- to three-page concept paper, sometimes known as a prospectus or letter of inquiry, can save a lot of time in the long run. A concept paper should be prepared for all unsolicited proposals. Many agencies request concept papers as the first step in a grant cycle; the two-page papers are reviewed, and only a few researchers are selected to prepare full proposals. Agencies then spend valuable time only on the most viable ideas and proposals by the best-qualified candidates.

A concept paper offers a brief overview of the problem area, problem statement, importance, proposed research design and methods, resources and facilities, benefits of the research results, qualifications of the researchers, a timetable, and budget figure.[16] This short paper should be compelling and persuasive. It forces the researcher to be cogent and concise and may prevent preparation of a proposal that has no possibility of being funded.

MATCHING PROJECTS WITH FUNDING AGENCIES

A successfully funded proposal can start a lifelong career in nutrition research. Locating appropriate funding sources for a project enhances the potential for successful funding. Even the best written and best thought out proposal will not be funded if it arrives at the wrong agency. Funding priorities are a fact of life for every agency. It is part of the researcher's job to ascertain that each proposal meets the goals of the selected funding agency. Therefore it is important to know as much as possible about the "giving history" of a particular agency. This information, as well as agency goals and priorities is widely available, but it must be sought. This section provides steps to follow when searching for an appropriate agency to fund a research proposal.

Define the Project

A research proposal should clearly identify the gap between what knowledge or technology exists today and what should exist. A project should be defined carefully, looked at in as many ways as possible, and related to other subject areas. This activity will help to identify agencies that may benefit from funding the project and will simplify the next step.

A project that proposes to study the effect of early nutrition intervention on the birthweight of infants born to adolescent mothers might seem to be very straightforward. However, looking at it in a different light might generate the following questions:

- Does the project involve nutrition education to the client or training physicians or other health professionals who might be asked to intervene? If the latter is true, the proposal might be submitted to an agency that funds professional education in nutrition.
- Does the project involve the use of special supplements or provision of additional milk to the mother? If so, a dairy association or a pharmaceutical company might be a funding possibility.
- Will the project involve the school system in any way? A department of education may support the study.
- Will the project involve public assistance programs? A department of health might be a source of possible funding.
- Is this a model project? A local foundation may be receptive to funding the project.

Identify Constituency Groups

During the investigation of a project, it is important to identify who will benefit from its results. Funding agencies also have constituencies and will usually set funding priorities accordingly. The project on nutrition intervention described earlier would have several possible constituencies. Infants born of adolescent mothers is the most obvious. The adolescent will also benefit. Agencies that serve these clients may be a less obvious constituency group. Efforts to improve birth outcomes should decrease costs of neonatal care and may decrease hospital care costs. If the outcome is positive, fewer federal dollars may be spent in postnatal care of these infants. Physicians and nurses who observe and/or participate in the project may benefit from improved nutrition knowledge and therefore may become another constituency group.

Search for Key Words

Once the idea is defined and subject areas are explored, it is important to begin searching for key words. A project titled "The effect of early nutrition intervention on the birthweight of infants born to adolescent mothers" might generate the following key words: *nutrition, pregnancy, adolescent pregnancy, infants, birthweight,* and *prenatal nutrition.*

The process of identifying key words allows a researcher to begin access to a funding source database. IRIS (Illinois Research Information Services)* and SPIN (Sponsored Program Information Network),† the two major databases available, list agencies, both federal and private, that fund projects. Access to these agencies is based on a search for key words listed in the agency descriptions of funding priorities and limitations. IRIS has a key word list of approximately 2500 words.

Limitations of the database systems are that, although both attempt to update frequently, their information may not be current. Both databases are

---

*IRIS, Campus Wide Research Services Offices, University of Illinois at Urbana–Champaign, 901 S Mathews Ave, Urbana, IL 61801.
†SPIN, The Research Foundation of SUNY, PO Box 9, Albany, NY 12201.

"term sensitive" and may list numerous funding agencies that, in fact, do not match given research criteria. Nevertheless, from the generated list, several agencies can be identified for potential research funding.

Access to these databases usually requires a university affiliation. Subscriptions are expensive, and few private institutions have the resources and the need to justify purchasing access. Many universities are willing to make database information available to researchers in the local community.[19]

Target Appropriate Funding Agencies

Funding agencies can be separated into five distinct types, as shown in *Table 3.5* and described below. Addresses for various agencies are provided in *Table 3.6*.

Table 3.5
Funding Agencies

Type	Examples
Federal	National Institutes of Health, Department of Health and Human Services, Agency for International Development
State and local	Department of education, department of human services, arts council, local school districts
Foundations	Ford Foundation, Spenser Foundation, Rockefeller Foundation
Nonprofit organizations	American Diabetes Association, The American Dietetic Association
Industry	IBM, Eli Lilly, Ross Laboratories, Mead Johnson

Table 3.6
Sources of Information on
Funding Agencies

Foundations
IRIS, Campus Wide Research Services Offices, University of Illinois at Urbana–Champaign, 901 S Mathews Ave, Urbana, IL 61801
Sponsored Programs Information Network (SPIN), The Research Foundation of SUNY, PO Box 9, Albany, NY 12201
The Foundation Center, 79 Fifth Ave, New York, NY 10003 (800/424-9836)

COMSEARCH
The Foundation Directory
The Foundation Grants Index
The National Directory for Corporate Giving
The National Guide to Funding in Aging

Government
Catalogue of Federal Domestic Assistance, Superintendent of Documents, Government Printing Office, Washington, DC 20402
Federal Register, Superintendent of Documents, Government Printing Office, Washington, DC 20402
Commerce Business Daily, Superintendent of Documents, Government Printing Office, Washington, DC 20402
NIH Guide for Grants and Contracts, Office of Grants Inquiries, Room 499, Westwood Building, NIH, Bethesda, MD 20894 (301/496-7441)
National Institute for Occupational Safety and Health, Center for Disease Control, 255 E. Paces Ferry Rd NE, Room 321, Atlanta, GA 30305 (404/262-6575)

Federal agencies. Federal agencies still provide the greatest proportion of research funding. Most nutrition research money comes from the NIH through its various individual institutes. Additional sources of federal funding would be the Department of Agriculture, the Department of Health and Human Services, and the Department of Education.

Federal funding may be in the form of an investigator-initiated research grant submitted to an agency for consideration of funding or a response to an RFP. Requests for proposals are developed by research agencies for completion of specific research projects. For federal agencies, RFP guidelines are published in the *Federal Register*. These guidelines may be very specific, including a brief review of the literature and prescribed methodology. Other RFPs may be less specific in methodology, allowing the investigator more latitude in the implementation of the project. Those who carefully follow the *Federal Register* can obtain advance notice of pending RFPs. Frequently, the preliminary guidelines will be published several months ahead so that public comment can be generated prior to finalizing the RFP guidelines. Attention to the preliminary guidelines and the discussions generated at public hearings can give valuable lead time to a research team wishing to respond. The submission date for an RFP is usually less than two months after the final guidelines are printed. However, first publication of the proposed RFP may be six months or longer.

State and local agencies. State and local agencies are another source of potential funding for research projects. Giving clear documentation on how a research project will uniquely benefit a particular local population greatly improves the likelihood of funding. Many state agencies also generate RFPs for projects important to a given area. Personal contact should be established with personnel at state and local agencies that may potentially fund research. Such contacts often give access to information regarding pending agency interests. They also provide the agency with potential researchers who may be contacted when projects are under consideration.

Foundations. *Table 3.7* identifies the different types of foundations and characterizes their usual funding priorities.[16] Foundations are an increasingly important source of research funding as federal research dollars are decreasing. Identifying the appropriate foundation for a proposal takes homework.

Table 3.7
Foundations

Type	Approx. No.	Examples	Funding Priorities
Community	300	San Francisco Foundation	Generally fund projects in local area only
National (multi-purpose)	100	Ford Foundation	Fund large model projects that have national impact
Special purpose	100	National Kidney Foundation	Fund projects specific to discipline
Family	> 10 000	Small Family Foundation	Fund diverse projects; each operates independently with own set of criteria, which may change frequently
Corporate	> 10 000	Burroughs Wellcome Foundation Marriott Foundation	Fund projects that have potential benefit to corporation profits and/or community image

Several reference sources provide information about private foundations. *The Foundation Directory* and *The Foundation Grants Index* are two that are available in most university libraries. Foundations are required to submit annual reports that include their net worth and the amount of funding provided in the past year. A foundation's mission statement, also found in these documents, offers a clue to funding priorities. If a report does not list grantees and titles of funded projects, such information usually can be requested from the foundation.

Foundations usually require less detailed proposals than those demanded by federal agencies. But foundations generally expect concept papers or letters of intent to be submitted before the completed proposals. Contacts with and personal visits to a foundation may enhance funding. A researcher should begin with a telephone call to the foundation to obtain information about funding priorities and limitations. When planning a visit to a foundation, the researcher should organize an agenda beforehand to obtain information regarding funding priorities, size of grants funded, and evaluation criteria. Offering to provide service to the agency in the form of grants review will give both valuable insight into criteria for successful funding and demonstrate a researcher's willingness to support foundation goals.

Nonprofit organizations. Nonprofit organizations, such as The American Dietetic Association, the American Institute of Nutrition, and the American Diabetes Association may also fund research. The dollar amount of funding is usually small, and the research must specifically benefit the association's constituency. Information regarding grant possibilities can be obtained by contacting the individual associations.

Industry. Industry also funds research by independent investigators.[20] Working with industry may involve a research proposal, but more often than not involves a contract, a binding agreement to provide research in a specific area for a specific amount of money. Although it may be similar to a research proposal, it may have strings attached. Contracts may provide for delay of publication of research results to give the corporation time to patent the findings. Difficulties and delays in publication may develop in situations in which the findings do not support the corporation's products. It is important to define clearly the research to be done and publication rights and procedures prior to acceptance of the contract. University grant offices usually have experienced personnel who are familiar with preparing contracts and have the researcher's interest in mind.[10]

Most industry grants are for smaller dollar amounts and cover a shorter period than do federal and foundation grants. However, industry can provide products and services that may comprise an important dimension of research in nutrition and dietetics.

COPING WITH REJECTION

Every successful investigator has had to deal with a rejected proposal, usually several. In fact, a researcher who has never had a proposal rejected probably has never submitted one. The ability to deal with rejection may be the difference between a successful investigator and one who is not.

A researcher who receives a rejection letter should take several positive steps before deciding to abandon the proposal.

Avoid discouragement. Rejection of a proposal to which numerous hours and untold personal energy have been committed can be devastating. After all, how could an agency not recognize the effort and the uniqueness of the research proposal? There are numerous reasons for rejections and few, if any, pertain to a researcher personally. It is important for the successful investigator to realize that rejection of a proposal by an agency does not mean that the research is without merit. The first step after the rejection of a proposal is to take a break and then regroup.[21]

Ask for a pink slip.   Federal agencies provide a critique of each proposal they review for funding. This critique is printed on pink paper, which is why it is called a pink slip. This document is a valuable resource; it summarizes the strengths and—more importantly—the weaknesses of the proposal. If the funding agency has not provided a pink slip, a researcher should ask for it. Careful review can provide suggestions to improve the proposal for a second submission. Subsequent submissions of improved proposals have a much greater chance of funding.[22]

Table 3.8 lists the most frequent problems with unfunded proposals. Reviewing rejected proposals and pink slips can often pinpoint the problem area. These clues are extremely helpful when preparing subsequent proposals.[21]

Obtain a list of funded research.   A list of successful grants funded by the agency in the current funding cycle is always available; however, a researcher may need to request it. Agency priorities can usually be identified from this list. Perhaps the research question needs to be refocused or funding needs to be sought from a different source.

Successful grantees are usually willing to share their proposals. These may provide insight into problem areas and possible revisions that could increase funding potential.

Ask for a list of reviewers.   Granting agencies will also provide a list of proposal reviewers. By identifying the individuals who read his or her proposal, the researcher may be able to determine if the proposal was written in the appropriate language. It is possible that a proposal was too technical for the reviewers to understand. Reviewers with very little nutrition background may not appreciate the significance of the research. Knowing the reviewers greatly improves the possibility of effective and persuasive communication.

New researchers may find it helpful to resubmit a proposal to a reviewer for comment prior to submission of the completed proposal to an agency. Such prior review significantly improves the chances of having the proposal funded.[23]

SUMMARY

Both new and experienced dietetic researchers can improve both their grantsmanship and ability to receive research funding. Diligent adherence to techniques for preparation, writing, and internal review can improve chances for positive external reviews for proposed investigations. An accurate, precise, complete, and reasonable budget adds to the merit of a persuasive proposal. The likelihood of being funded can be advanced by effective use of strategies for establishing and maintaining strong ties with funding agencies, matching projects with funding priorities, and targeting sources most likely to fund specific projects. If at first a proposal is not funded, it is appropriate find out why, take steps to address problem areas, and resubmit the proposal. Good research requires tenacity; sustained funding for research demands both persistence and ingenuity.

Table 3.8
Shortcomings of Disapproved
Research Grant Applications*

Type of Problem	Percentage
Class I: Problem (58%)	
1. The problem is of insufficient importance or is unlikely to produce any new or useful information.	33.1
2. The proposed research is based on a hypothesis that rests on insufficient evidence, is doubtful, or is unsound.	8.9
3. The problem is more complex than the investigator appears to realize.	8.1
4. The problem has only local significance, or is one of production or control, or otherwise fails to fall sufficiently clearly within the general field of health-related research.	4.8
5. The problem is scientifically premature and warrants, at most, only a pilot study.	3.1
6. The research as proposed is overly involved, with too many elements under simultaneous investigation.	3.0
7. The description of the nature of the research and of its significance leaves the proposal nebulous and diffuse and without clear research aim.	2.6
Class II: Approach (73%)	
8. The proposal tests, methods, or scientific procedures are unsuited to the stated objectives.	34.7
9. The description of the approach is too nebulous, diffuse, and lacking in clarity to permit adequate evaluation.	28.8
10. The overall design of the study has not been carefully considered.	14.7
11. The statistical aspects of the approach have not been given sufficient consideration.	8.1
12. The approach lacks scientific imagination.	7.4
13. Controls are either inadequately conceived or inadequately described.	6.8
14. The material the investigator proposes to use is unsuited to the objectives of the study or is difficult to obtain.	3.8
15. The number of observations is unsuitable.	2.5
16. The equipment contemplated is outmoded or otherwise unsuitable.	1.0
Class III: Personnel (55%)	
17. The investigator does not have adequate experience, training, or both, for this research.	32.6
18. The investigator appears to be unfamiliar with pertinent literature, methods, or both.	13.7
19. The investigator's previously published work in this field does not inspire confidence.	12.6
20. The investigator proposes to rely too heavily on insufficiently experienced associates.	5.0
21. The investigator is being spread too thin and would be more productive by concentrating on fewer projects.	3.8
22. The investigator needs more liaison with colleagues in this field or in collateral fields.	1.7
Class IV: Other (16%)	
23. The requirements for equipment, personnel, or both are unrealistic.	10.1
24. It appears that other responsibilities would prevent devotion of sufficient time and attention to the research.	3.0
25. The institutional setting is unfavorable.	2.3
26. Research grants to the investigator, now in force, are adequate in scope and amount to cover the proposed research.	1.5

*Found in study section review of 605 disapproved applications to the National Institutes of Health.

From Office of Sponsored Programs Development. *Guide for Proposal Development.* Columbus, Ohio: Ohio State University; 1989;9-5–9-7. Used by permission.

References

1. Feitelson M. Integrating research into clinical dietetic practice. *Dietitians in Nutrition Support Newsletter.* June 1987;9:4,10–11.
2. Meyer KA, Zaporozhetz LE. Writing the review of literature for the research proposal: problems and solutions. *Grants Magazine.* 1987;10:153–157.
3. Evers SE. Competitive grant applications: some guidelines. *J Can Diet Assoc.* 1987;48:74–76.
4. Bergstrom N, Hanson BC, Grant M et al. Collaborative nursing research: anatomy of a successful consortium. *Nursing Res.* 1984;33:20–25.
5. Boykoff, SL. Coauthorship: collaboration without conflict. *Am J Nurs.* 1989;89:1164.
6. Hodgson, C. Tips on writing successful proposals. *Nurse Pract.* 1989;14:44–54.
7. Dimino ER. Acquiring foundation funds for health related projects. *Pediatr Nurs.* 1987;13:363–364.
8. Kennicott PC. Developing a grant proposal: some basic principles. *Grants Magazine.* 1983;6:36–41.
9. Mackenzie RS. Grant writing and review for dental faculty. *J Dent Educ.* 1986;50:180–186.
10. Pagonis JF. Successful proposal writing. *Am J Occup Ther.* 1987;41:147–151.
11. Eaves GN. Preparation of the research-grant application: opportunities and pitfalls. *Grants Magazine.* 1984;7:151–157.
12. Ferrell BR, Nail LM, Mooney K, Cotanch P. Applying for Oncology Nursing Society and Oncology Nursing Foundation grants. *Oncol Nurs Forum.* 1989;16:728–730.
13. Niederhuber JE. Writing a successful grant application. *J Surg Res.* 1985;39:277–284.
14. Bagley CS. The process of preparing a grant: part I. *Oncol Nurs Forum.* 1987;14:113–114.
15. Carty RM, Silva MC. Writing effective federal grant proposals. *Nurs Econ.* 1986;4:74–79.
16. Wood JB. Grantsmanship: winning foundation funding. *Nurs Econ.* 1986;4:80–82.
17. Shapek RA. Do's and don'ts in proposal writing: how to increase your probability of obtaining federal funding. *Grants Magazine.* 1984;7:51–58.
18. Sladek FE, Stein EL. Funding agency contacts: letting them help. *Grants Magazine.* 1983;6:19–31.
19. Bagley CS. The process of preparing a grant: part II. *Oncol Nurs Forum.* 1987;14:110–112.
20. Larson E. Guidelines for collaborative research with industry. *Nurs Econ.* 1986;4:131–133.
21. Clinton J. Rejected proposal: what next? *Image J Nurs Scholarship.* 1988;20:54.
22. Cuca JM, McLoughlin WJ. Why clinical research grant applications fare poorly in review and how to recover. *Cancer Invest.* 1987;5:55–58.
23. Levy M, Aschenbrener TD, Morse JA. Tips from the other side: a firm knowledge of the grant application review process will improve your chances for a successful funding request. *Biomed Commun.* 1981;9:18–19, 26–28.

PART 3
DESCRIPTIVE
RESEARCH

Descriptive research is an effective way to obtain information germane to devising hypotheses and proposing associations. As stated in chapter 1, descriptive research cannot test or verify; analytical research is required to evaluate hypotheses or ascertain cause and effect. Major examples of descriptive investigations are qualitative research studies and descriptive epidemiologic research.

Qualitative research generates narrative data, ie, data described in words instead of numbers (chapter 4). A variety of techniques are suitable for securing qualitative data. Observation, in-depth interviews, focus group interviews, the Delphi technique, free elicitation, and cognitive response task are among approaches specified in chapter 5. Such data may produce graphic and dramatic responses to research questions. Impressive applications of descriptive research may be seen in program planning, identification of population needs, and development of educational materials. New methods, some computer-based, for analyzing and comparing qualitative data are being developed. Future research will explore strategies for appraising "confirmability" of qualitative data (akin to evaluating reliability of quantitative data).

Epidemiologic research is descriptive when data detailing person, place, and time are collected (chapter 6). Descriptive epidemiologic research encompasses correlational studies, case reports, case series, and surveys.

In research, we often consider two distinctly different parameters: *incidence* (referred to as *incidence density* or *cumulative incidence*), ie, the number of new cases over a given period; and *prevalence*, ie, the total number of cases at a specified time point or period. These data are useful in describing populations and in monitoring programs.

Two other sets of terms need differentiation: *reliability* and *validity*, and *sensitivity* and *specificity*. Reliability indicates whether the results are repeatable or reproducible, and validity indicates whether the test measures what it is designed to measure, and whether the measured value agrees with the "true" value. Sensitivity indicates the proportion of subjects with a given condition who test positive for that condition (greater sensitivity means that there is less likelihood that a negative result will misclassify an individual).

Specificity indicates the proportion of subjects without the condition who test negative (there is less likelihood of misclassifying an individual with a positive test if the test has greater specificity).

Questionnaires are ubiquitous research instruments. They are used extensively in qualitative research and epidemiologic research. When a new client is asked to fill out a form, it is usually a type of questionnaire. The design and construction of a questionnaire are critical to its successful use. Chapter 2 discusses research errors that have a high degree of association with questionnaire formation and use. Chapter 7 presents critical issues to consider in developing and validating questionnaires. Pilot tests are invaluable because they encourage refinements in language and response options that can increase the reliability and validity of the instrument and its applicability to the specific research setting. Future research will likely emphasize enhanced reliability and validity, computer questionnaire administration, incorporation of video technology, and expansion of questionnaire utilization to a broader range of settings.

ERM, Editor

4. THE COMPONENTS AND USE OF QUALITATIVE RESEARCH

Cheryl L. Achterberg, PhD, and Sandra K. Shepherd, PhD, RD

Qualitative research has always been an integral part of cross-cultural comparisons and descriptions of food habits in the nutrition and anthropology literature,[1,2] but it has also become routine in food product development and sensory evaluation,[3] food and nutrition marketing, and nutrition education materials development[4,5] and evaluation.[6,7] The unique assumptions underlying qualitative research, the various approaches that may be used, and types of information that they can produce are of importance to dietitians. The purpose of this chapter is to define qualitative research, to describe when and why it should be conducted, and to correct some common misconceptions often associated with it. A subsequent chapter reviews particular qualitative methodologies.

WHAT IS QUALITATIVE RESEARCH?

Precise definitions for qualitative research are rarely found in the literature. Most of the ones that are offered are complex and based on philosophical perspectives that contrast qualitative and quantitative research.[8,9] The distinction, however, is artificial,[10] and a purely dichotomous approach (ie, quantitative versus qualitative) tends to obscure the differences that exist among the qualitative methods themselves.[9,11] Moreover, one need only scratch the surface of the literature to find that the terms *qualitative* and *quantitative* are themselves misleading.[12]

The authors, as qualitative researchers, depart from the traditional or purist approach because we are more pragmatic than most, and our purpose is more application-oriented. We simply define qualitative research as any data-gathering technique that generates narrative data (ie, words) rather than numerical data (ie, numbers).[13,14] For example, a qualitative approach to consumers' understanding of the word *cholesterol* would generate a large number of definitions in their own words, which may vary greatly from a quantitative approach that uses a set of definitions generated by dietitians in a multiple-choice survey questionnaire. The primary caveat in qualitative research is that the words must reflect the study participant's—or "native's"—point of view, *not* the researcher's.[15,16] In other words, qualitative research is based on the assumption that human interaction, thinking, and behavior are understood and more scientifically valid when seen from the *inside out* than when seen from the *outside in*. This definition allows us to broaden the scope of qualitative techniques and to offer a greater selection of methodologies to our readers.

THE RANGE OF QUALITATIVE RESEARCH

Qualitative research is not a homogeneous enterprise: A multitude of qualitative approaches exist.[9,12] Lincoln and Guba[8] allude to this in their discussion of a continuum between qualitative and quantitative research approaches, with pure analytic induction at one extreme and standardized measures and statistical protocols at the other. However, according to our pragmatic definition of qualitative research, standardized measures of words or word production and statistical protocols (as applied to the analysis of words or narrative) *can* be used in certain qualitative inquiries. Thus, as Firestone and

Dawson[17] note, the question of when a study may properly be considered qualitative is becoming increasingly difficult, especially when combined techniques are used. We prefer to depict qualitative and quantitative research approaches on separate, but parallel continua (*Figure 4.1*). From this perspective, the two approaches have obvious similarities, as well as differences.

The most important similarity is that qualitative and quantitative research approaches share the view that the world can be known through empirical observation. This view values systematic, scientific inquiry and is in dramatic contrast to other world views, which may hold, for example, that knowledge (or truth) is either God-given or produced only within the self. Because the latter views do not promote scientific inquiry, debating a qualitative or a quantitative research approach is irrelevant for some people, because they see neither as a legitimate enterprise. The authors believe that if the operation of one research approach is viewed as legitimate, then the operation of the other must be viewed as legitimate also, and for the same fundamental reasons. Both studies can provide and produce knowledge that will add conceptually to the theoretical base of the field, add functionally to the methodological base, contribute meaningful information to policy makers, and/or provide useful information to practitioners. However, the appropriateness, fit, scope, and quality of the data produced by qualitative or quantitative studies will vary according to the particular issue of interest. For example, qualitative approaches are seldom appropriate in astrophysics, but almost always appropriate to social situations.

As indicated in Figure 4.1, both qualitative and quantitative approaches may be descriptive, evaluative, theory-building, hypothesis-testing, and context-sensitive, at least at certain points along the continua. Only at the extreme ends are the differences between the research approaches greater than the similarities. It is also important to point out that, whereas qualitative researchers start out with words, they often end up using numbers to describe their results. By the same token, quantitative researchers may start out with numbers, but they end up using words to describe their results. Thus, researchers from both traditions use words and numbers, and both use interpretive analyses in one form or another. One of the advantages of qualitative research, however, is that qualitative data can be analyzed as such and they can be subsequently converted to quantitative data for further analysis, eg, by simply ranking or counting the number of statements within each category. Quantitative data rarely, if ever, exhibit such versatility.

Glaser and Strauss[18] maintain the extreme position that qualitative research generates theory, whereas quantitative research does not. However, concept and observation are interdependent in both approaches.[10] In other words, "Theories are not developed deductively or inductively, but *both* deductively and inductively."[10] No qualitative researcher is able to observe from a blank slate, and no quantitative researcher should be blind to any unanticipated data a given experiment produces. Thus, the theory-generation value of both qualitative and quantitative studies depends on the particular data in hand and the researcher's insight and creativity.

However, research can be performed "atheoretically" in both qualitative and quantitative inquiries. In the atheoretical approach, the underlying theory

Figure 4.1
Qualitative and quantitative research approaches represented as parallel continua and illustrated by hypothetical studies about increasing fiber intake in a nursing home.

QUALITATIVE APPROACH

(less quantitative)

Description

Purpose: description, theory-building
Hypotheses: none
Concepts: fluid, emergent
Setting: natural, unobtrusive, uncontrolled
Research-subject relationship: intentionally interactive
Context: emphasized
Validity: very good
Reliability: questionable
Primary data: words
Analysis: constant comparative method, emergent coding/ categorization, analytic induction, no statistical analysis

Purpose: evaluative, theory-building, and hypothesis-testing
Hypotheses: some are explicit
Concepts: emergent as well as informed by theory
Setting: natural with some modifications
Research-subject relationship: researcher is cognizant of and tries to minimize interaction
Context: emphasized
Validity: good
Reliability: can be good
Primary data: words, sometimes numbers, eg, based on enumeration of comments within each category
Analysis: coding based on predetermined categorical schemes, descriptive statistics, nonparametric and group comparisons

(more quantitative)

QUALITATIVE APPROACH

Examples

Ethnography, participant observation: eg, researcher lives in nursing home taking meals in cafeteria with other residents, observing consumption of high-fiber sources and listening to any related discussion

Researcher *observes* nursing home resident in cafeteria at mealtime selecting/rejecting fiber sources

Focus groups with nursing home residents discussing fiber and related programming materials

Researcher *interviews* nursing home residents about fiber before and after programming that is designed to increase consumption of fiber sources using *open-ended questions*

Researcher *interviews* nursing home residents about fiber before and after programming designed to increase consumption of fiber sources using *closed-ended questions*

Cognitive responses with nursing home residents reviewing program materials and/or menus with fiber sources

Mail or telephone *survey* or nursing home residents using closed-ended questions to determine knowledge, attitudes, and behavior re fiber

Researcher *measures* fiber consumption before/after programming by controlling serving size and measuring plate waste

---

QUANTITATIVE APPROACH

(more naturalistic)

Description

Purpose: hypothesis-testing, evaluative, descriptive
Hypotheses: usually explicit
Concepts: may or may not be informed by theory
Setting: artificial, sometimes obtrusive
Research-subject relationship: not of critical importance
Context: may or may not be of concern
Validity: can be questioned
Reliability: usually good
Primary data: numbers, sometimes words
Analysis: descriptive, group comparisons, sometimes multivariate

Purpose: hypothesis-testing
Hypotheses: precise
Concepts: operationally defined in precise terms
Setting: artificial, controlled environment
Research-subject relationship: intentionally noninteractive; researcher is not cognizant of reactivity
Context: artificial
Validity: should be questioned
Reliability: very good
Primary data: numbers
Analysis: always statistical

(less naturalistic)

QUANTITATIVE APPROACH

---

is not made explicit before or after the study and, thus, is not open to verification, analysis, discussion, or development. This limits the study in terms of explaining the events or behavior of interest and prohibits conceptual development within the field of study.[19] Theoretical research relies on theory to guide study design, interpretation of results, or both. The theory provides a conceptual framework for approaching the research problem, understanding the results, and relating them to the real world. Atheoretical research lacks that conceptual framework. Therefore, each study is designed and interpreted independently with no common ground on which to base generalization. For example, when no comprehensive theory exists as to why diet, smoking, stress, gender, age, and even beard growth are related to cholesterol levels and heart disease, it is not surprising that the results are variable from study to study.[20] If, however, a theory-based, ecological approach were used to relate these variables together, then we may come to a better understanding as to why some variables are related to a given outcome in some circumstances, but not in others. Both qualitative and quantitative approaches may provide valuable data in this respect.

It may be easiest to combine qualitative and quantitative approaches within a study in the area where the two continua overlap (see Figure 4.1), and more difficult philosophically and logistically in the areas where there is no overlap.

WHY DO QUALITATIVE RESEARCH?

The most common answer to this question is that qualitative research "enables researchers to ask new questions, answer different kinds of questions and readdress old questions."[12] But this answer is so vague as to be almost useless to the novice. One of the main reasons an interest in qualitative research has grown in community settings is that the more traditional, quantitative methods[21] may be impractical, eg, it is difficult to keep treatment cells balanced due to unequal assignment and/or attrition, and the very complex nature of real-world events often introduces confounding variables that cannot be controlled. Qualitative methods often present a more pragmatic approach to conducting research in a natural setting.

Researchers may also turn to qualitative methods if they feel they are constantly trying to force "round data into square holes,"[10] analyzing variables that are measurable but irrelevant,[23] ignoring categories of data that are important to the respondent but unanticipated by the researcher, producing results that are not useful because they were generated under artificial or invalid conditions, or using theories that explain the measurable outcomes of interest.[15] In some instances, researchers may suspect that they have fallen victim to type III error, the most common validity error made in research, by asking the wrong research questions.[16] In these situations, qualitative methods can be used to "discover" pertinent questions and variables, concepts and problems, and to generate hypotheses and, perhaps, theories that are more pertinent to the practitioner-researcher.[18,24]

Other reasons for choosing a qualitative approach include:
- When a research problem is so new that it is "pretheoretical" (ie, not enough is known about a situation to formulate testable hypotheses and/or to select a suitable theory to address it).[25]
- The researcher is as interested in process variables as he or she is in outcome variables (ie, evaluators wish to know how and why a given outcome happens).
- When the evaluation needs to be extremely audience-specific and/or very detailed in nature (eg, needs assessment for a group of women in whom both diabetes and bulimia are diagnosed).

Descriptive Research

- The researcher needs data on social context, structure, and interactions within which a particular behavior pattern can be understood. This last may be particularly important for the understanding of aberrant dietary behavior expressed by either individuals or groups, eg, pica, anorexia, nonorganic failure-to-thrive, and binge eating.

In some cases, quantitative survey data may be difficult to collect from certain groups of people, such as young children and those who are functionally illiterate or unfamiliar with testing procedures. Others may refuse to answer survey questionnaires because they distrust questionnaires, the source of the questionnaire (eg, private industry or government), or researchers in general. Yet all of these groups may readily participate in the more intimate and interactive data collection procedures offered by qualitative methodologies.

A small, in-depth qualitative study may also provide more useful information than a large-scale quantitative study during formative evaluations (ie, design and development testing of new products or programs) when the details provide insight as to how a future intervention program or product might be improved before further investments of time, personnel, and money are made. This can result in an economy of effort in the long run, whether the product is a new gastric tube, hospital menu, pamphlet, or weight-loss program. Similarly, qualitative methods are most productive when the research must be tailored to the specific needs, abilities, and realities of the target population.

Ideally, investigators should not use qualitative research methods unless they have training and experience with the methods, or a consultant can train and supervise staff appropriately. An in-depth study of the literature and some pilot work may also provide suitable background.

MYTHS AND MISCONCEPTIONS

There are many widespread myths and misconceptions about qualitative research. Some of these are discussed below.

Qualitative Research Uses No Theory

The major premise on which our use of qualitative research rests is that qualitative data analysis can be theory-driven,[19] theory-generating,[18] or both. Analysis is considered theory-driven when theory is used to guide the collection, analysis, and interpretation of data. An example is when pre-existing categories, based on theoretical concepts and their relationships, are used to organize the data for analysis and interpretation. Analysis is considered theory-generating when the researcher constructs theory from data that have already been collected and analyzed. An example is when the investigator has no preconceived notion of categories for organizing the data and subsequent interpretation but, instead, allows categories and their relationships to emerge naturally from the data set itself. As noted by Walker,[25] "Many would argue that in practice, each approach involves elements of theory creation and testing." An example of a hybrid approach is when the investigator starts out with theoretical categories, then proceeds to shape, mold, and possibly reconceptualize those categories based on the discovery of naturally occurring categories, patterns, or regularities that seem to emerge from the data set. Again, our premise is that qualitative analysis can proceed in either or both ways.

Qualitative Research Is Not Fundable

Numerical output is more easily funded at this point in time, although national funding agencies are becoming increasingly receptive to qualitative inquiry.[23] For example, the USDA's Human Nutrition Information Service has funded several major qualitative investigations over the past five years.[4,26-28] Many foundations and smaller agencies are more receptive to qualitative, grassroots evaluations and inquiries than they are to quantitative, impersonal approaches. Our recommendation is to choose agencies and requests for proposals (RFPs) carefully. We also urge investigators to combine qualitative and quantitative methods whenever it makes sense. When agencies become acquainted with the usefulness of the qualitative data, they often become more receptive to its methods in future inquiries. They may never become acquainted, however, unless researchers take a pragmatic approach and provide quantitative data along with the qualitative data.

Qualitative Research Is Not Publishable

Research journals in education, nutrition, human development, home economics, and social science are publishing more qualitative studies. Several journals, such as *Qualitative Health Research,* have dedicated themselves entirely to qualitative research. In short, there are many opportunities to fund and publish qualitative research. If at first you don't succeed, try somewhere else.

Qualitative Research Is Not Objective

Several authors, even within the qualitative research literature, have emphasized the need to standardize—ie, objectify—qualitative research data. Sandelowski[11] suggests that investigators find ways in which "qualitative research can be made as rigorous as it is relevant." Fetterman[12] concurs: "Efforts to establish standards commensurate with the mainstream of scientific inquiry serve to further institutionalize qualitative approaches, anchoring them in the fertile soil of educational evaluation." Miles[29] sums it up nicely, saying that "the nuisances [of qualitative research] can be reduced by thoughtful methodological inquiry—most centrally into the problem of analysis and how it can be carried out in ways that deserve the name of science. Without more such inquiry, qualitative research. . .cannot be expected to transcend story-telling and we will be stuck with the limitations of numbers."

At the same time, "it is not possible to extract human judgment from any research process."[22] Objectivity has been associated traditionally with numerical data because numerical data are not considered subject to different interpretations. But subjective decisions are always made in the interpretation of numerical data.[30] For example, significance levels are typically set at a 0.05, rather than 0.06 or 0.10, α level, primarily on a subjective basis.

Thus, the important issue is not whether qualitative research is objective, but how its subjectivity is managed. If subjectivity is hidden or unrecognized, it can interfere with good science. If, however, it is made explicit and systematically identified, its impact on the research should not be burdensome.[31]

Some measures that can be taken to diminish any bias from subjectivity include using a research partner who plays devil's advocate to question the researcher's analyses critically, searching constantly for negative cases, checking and rechecking the data for possible testing of rival hypotheses, devising tests to check analyses, and making the data retrievable so that other researchers can challenge and reanalyze the data.[15]

Qualitative Research Is "Soft" and Less Desirable Than Quantitative Research, Which Is "Hard"

This statement is similar to the previous one regarding objectivity. Numerical information is considered highly reliable because it is replicable, and therefore more trustworthy or "hard." The fact that such data may not be valid is often overlooked. Qualitative data, on the other hand, are rarely replicable, and are therefore considered untrustworthy or "soft."[10,16] Once again, the authors take a pragmatic stand. Because this bias exists, it is useful to provide some numerical information so that readers do not automatically dismiss the results produced in narrative form. We have, for example, calculated inter-rater reliabilities on the number of positive, negative, and neutral statements made in our interviews,[26] focus groups,[28] and cognitive response tasks.[27] We have found that once these results are produced, most of the ensuing discussion turns on the substance of the qualitative results, rather than the appropriateness of our research methods. Kirk and Miller[16] may summarize it best, stating that qualitative work will "reasonably go ignored" if attention is not given to the issue of reliability.

Research Design Is Not an Issue in Qualitative Research

Design choices for both qualitative and quantitative studies are made on certain untestable assumptions[32] that dictate how a researcher frames questions, chooses data collection sites, and handles data collection, analysis, and write-up. All those who undertake qualitative studies must make design choices at least to this extent, and these choices should never be arbitrary. When qualitative studies involve hypothesis-testing (see Figure 4.1), design issues may become more complex and similar to those associated with quantitative studies. Thus, as with other types of research, the value of any qualitative results depends largely on the quality of the research design.

Qualitative and quantitative research approaches have one major difference in terms of design. In qualitative research, the investigator retains the right to modify, alter, and change the study design in the field, depending on the need to reassess issues that become apparent only when in the field.[15] In quantitative research, the design is seldom if ever altered, regardless of circumstances.

Qualitative Research Can Only Be Performed in a Natural Setting

Natural context is central to the philosophy of qualitative research because the qualitative approach tries to maximize validity by collecting data as close to real life as possible. However, context can be defined on a micro- or macro-level, and it should vary according to the phenomena of interest.[33] If, for example, a researcher is interested in how a person reacts mentally to an educational brochure, the important data are the thoughts and feelings (in words) that the person has upon exposure, whether they are observed in a simulated physician's office or their own physician's office. In this case, the natural setting is inside the respondent's mind. If, however, the researcher is interested in family interaction around the dinner table, the natural context and setting is probably the home or, perhaps, a fast-food restaurant. Thus, natural settings are important to qualitative research, but depending on the research question, they can include laboratory studies as well as field studies.

Qualitative and Quantitative Methods Are Incompatible

The incompatibility thesis holds that the distinctions (eg, about truth, reality, and the relationship between the investigator and the subject) between qualitative and quantitative methods are so important that the methods will always be separate.[8] We, as does Howe,[32] hold that in the most important sense, the approaches are inseparable. Ultimately, most qualitative research involves some kind of quantitative claims and quantitative studies always involve qualitative judgments. Thus, we again take the pragmatic approach and urge the combination of methods *when it makes sense to do so*, but to keep them separate otherwise.[7]

Qualitative research has its own limitations. Perhaps the most obvious is that generalizations cannot be made from any one data set to larger populations, and it is often difficult to compare qualitative studies because they are so context-bound. In addition, qualitative data do not lend themselves to meta-analysis. Data collection is very dependent on personnel (as opposed to equipment), and data quality subsequently depends entirely on the quality and training of personnel. Data analysis tends to be time-consuming and tedious. When qualitative and quantitative methods are used together, it is sometimes difficult to complete the qualitative analysis in time to be useful to the quantitative process. Finally, qualitative studies often require longer write-ups that stretch the page limits of many research journals.

CONCLUSIONS

The purpose of this paper is to introduce readers to the premises, products, strengths, and limitations of qualitative research, particularly in relation to the more commonplace quantitative approach. Neither approach is inherently superior, and each can make important scientific contributions to nutrition and nutrition education research. There are many similarities as well as differences between them.

Human events are far too complex to be viewed or analyzed from any single perspective.[32,33] We urge dietitians, therefore, to explore the variety of methodologies offered by the qualitative approach to research, especially to resolve applied problems in clinical or community environments. The results will undoubtedly be useful.

References

1. Grivetti LE, Pangborn RM. Food habit research: a review of approaches and methods. *J Nutr Educ.* 1973;5:203.
2. Wilson CS. Food custom and nurture. *J Nutr Educ.* 1979;11(suppl 1): 211.
3. Marlow P. Qualitative research as a tool for product development. *Food Technology.* Nov 1987:74,76.
4. Shepherd SK, Sims LS, Cronin FJ, et al. Use of focus groups to explore consumers' preferences re: content and graphic design of nutrition publications. *J Am Diet Assoc.* 1989;89:1612.
5. Crockett SJ, Heller KE, Merkel JM, et al. Assessing beliefs of older rural Americans about nutrition education: Use of the focus group approach. *J Am Diet Assoc.* 1990;90:563.

Descriptive Research

6. Edwards PK, Mullis RM, Clarke B. A comprehensive model for evaluating innovative nutrition education programs. *J Nutr Educ.* 1986;18:10.
7. Achterberg C. Qualitative methods in nutrition education evaluation research. *J Nutr Educ.* 1988;20:244.
8. Lincoln YS, Guba EG. *Naturalistic Inquiry.* Beverly Hills, Calif: Sage Publications; 1985.
9. Jacob E. Qualitative research traditions: a review. *Rev Educ Res.* 1987;57:1.
10. Bulmer M. Concepts in the analysis of qualitative data. *Soc Rev.* 1979;27:651.
11. Sandelowski M. The problem of rigor in qualitative research. *Adv Nurs Sci.* April 1986:27–37.
12. Fetterman DM. Qualitative approaches to evaluating education. *Educ Res.* Nov 1988:17–23.
13. Knafl KA, Howard MJ. Interpreting and reporting qualitative research. *Res Nurs Health.* 1984;7:17.
14. Miles MB, Huberman AM. Drawing valid meaning from qualitative data: toward a shared craft. In: Fetterman DM, ed. *Qualitative Approaches to Evaluation in Education: The Silent Scientific Revolution.* New York, NY: Praeger; 1988:222.
15. Marshall C, Rossman GB. *Designing Qualitative Research.* Newbury Park, Calif: Sage Publications;1989.
16. Kirk J, Miller ML. *Reliability and Validity in Qualitative Research.* Beverly Hills, Calif: Sage Publications; 1986:1.
17. Firestone WA, Dawson JA. Approaches to qualitative data analysis: intuitive, procedural and intersubjective. In: Fetterman DM, ed. *Qualitative Approaches to Evaluation in Education: The Silent Scientific Revolution.* New York, NY: Praeger; 1988:209.
18. Glaser BG, Strauss AL. *The Discovery of Grounded Theory: Strategies for Qualitative Research.* New York, NY: Aldine Publishing Co; 1967: 1–271.
19. Achterberg CL, Novak JD, Gillespie AH. Theory-driven research as a means to improve nutrition education. *J Nutr Educ.* 1985;17:179.
20. Dean K. Nutrition education research in health promotion. *J Can Diet Assoc.* 1990;51:481.
21. Campbell DT, Stanley JC. *Experimental and Quasi-Experimental Designs for Research.* Skokie, Ill: Rand McNally;1963.
22. Hamilton JA. Epistemology and meaning: a case for multi-methodologies for social research in home economics. *Home Econ Forum.* 1989;4:12.
23. Patton MQ. *Qualitative Evaluation Methods.* Beverly Hills, Calif: Sage Publications; 1980:9–379.
24. Reeder LG. Social epidemiology: an appraisal. In: Jaco EG, ed. *Patients, Physicians and Illness.* New York, NY: Free Press; 1972: 97–101.
25. Walker R. Evaluating applied qualitative research. In: Walker R, ed. *Applied Qualitative Research.* Brookfield, Vt: Gower Publishing Co; 1985:177–198b.
26. Achterberg CL, Bradley E. Bulletin features found most and least appealing to an extension audience. *J Nutr Educ.* 1991;23:244.
27. Shepherd S, Sims LS. Employing cognitive response analysis to examine message acceptance in nutrition education. *J Nutr Educ.* 1990;22:215.
28. Trenkner LL, Achterberg C. Use of focus groups in evaluating nutrition education material. *J Am Diet Assoc.* 1991;91:1577–1581.
29. Miles MB. Qualitative data as an attractive nuisance: the problem of analysis. *Admin Sci Quart.* 1979;24:590.
30. Pelto PJ, Pelto GH. *Anthropological Research: The Structure of Inquiry.* 2nd ed. Cambridge, England: Cambridge University Press; 1978.
31. Peshkin A. In search of subjectivity—one's own. *Educ Res.* October 1988:17.
32. Howe KR. Against the quantitative-qualitative incompatibility thesis. *Educ Res.* Nov 1988:10.
33. Achterberg C. Contexts in context. *J Nutr Educ.* 1988; 20:180.

5. QUALITATIVE RESEARCH METHODOLOGY: DATA COLLECTION, ANALYSIS, INTERPRETATION, AND VERIFICATION

Sandra K. Shepherd, PhD, RD, and Cheryl L. Achterberg, PhD

This chapter provides a basic overview of qualitative techniques so that researchers and practitioners in dietetics may be better equipped to apply and evaluate qualitative research. It will include classic approaches, such as participant observation, in-depth interviews, and content analysis, as well as the relatively newer methods, including focus group interviews, free elicitation, cognitive response tasks, and the Delphi technique. While observation and one-on-one interviewing remain the core techniques used in qualitative research,[1] the newer methods described in this chapter serve as additional tools for the researcher interested in using qualitative methods.

QUALITATIVE METHODS OF DATA COLLECTION

Qualitative data collection may take a variety of forms, some more structured than others. The following is a brief description of the most common techniques.

Participant observation. This special form of observation demands first-hand involvement in the study setting and entails systematic description of events, behaviors, and artifacts in that setting.[1] Involvement may include interaction between the researcher and subjects in the study setting, but not necessarily.[2] For example, to determine how the homeless might best be served through nutrition policies and programs, a researcher might live on the street for a period, experiencing homelessness, observing other homeless people, talking with them, and learning to view the world through their eyes.

In-depth interview. The interview technique involves a face-to-face meeting at which one person systematically obtains information from another via questioning and observation.[3] This has long been recognized as the most penetrating method available for assessing a person's knowledge and/or attitudes.[4] For example, this technique might be used to determine how bulimics feel about their condition, how they deal with it emotionally, what problems they encounter, and what types of nutrition interventions might be most helpful to them.

Content analysis. Content analysis is any technique that provides an objective and systematic description of the presence, intensity, or frequency of a characteristic (eg, word, concept, phrase) in samples of text.[5] Its purpose is to make valid inferences from multiple examples of text to characterize the authors (individuals, institutions, groups, or societies) along certain parameters.[6] For example, one might apply content analysis to weight-control articles from representative samples of women's magazines dating from 1950 to 1990 to determine whether any trends exist with respect to women's views on weight control over that period.

Focus group interview. This is a group technique involving 7 to 12 participants who are representative of a specified target audience and discuss among themselves topics introduced by a trained moderator.[7-9] The goal is to elicit the respondents' personal perceptions of a defined area of interest through carefully planned, semistructured discussion.[10] For example, a researcher interested in defining optimal topics and formats for nutrition classes for the elderly might conduct focus group interviews with members of the target audience to determine their perceived needs and preferences regarding nutrition classes.

Free elicitation. With this technique, participants are instructed to state as rapidly as possible all thoughts that come to mind when they are presented with a stimulus cue. The stimulus cue is typically one or two words (eg, the name of a consumer product) carefully selected to activate or trigger that part of the respondent's cognitive structure (memory) in which cue-related information resides.[11]

The resulting responses are thought to represent the content of a respondent's most salient cue-related knowledge. Furthermore, the sequence and timing of responses may be used to infer organization of that knowledge in the respondent's memory.[12] For example, an investigator interested in adolescents' conceptualization of cholesterol might conduct free elicitation sessions with boys and girls 14 to 16 years old. The technique would be used to determine what concepts tend to be closely associated with cholesterol in the minds of respondents, and how those closely associated concepts relate to other, more distal concepts to form a network of salient knowledge about cholesterol.

Cognitive response task. A variation of free elicitation, the cognitive response task involves a stimulus cue that typically takes the form of a persuasive message (eg, a message encouraging moderation of dietary fat), rather than a single word or concept. The thoughts elicited by exposure to a stimulus message are labeled *cognitive responses* and are presumed to mediate persuasive impact of the message.[13-16] The primary difference between free elicitation and the cognitive response task is that the former focuses on cognitive structure (content and organization of memory),[17] while the latter focuses on cognitive processes (eg, the process whereby incoming information is critically analyzed in light of existing knowledge, beliefs, values, and so forth that are already stored in memory).[18] For example, a researcher investigating consumers' use of information on food labels might use the cognitive response task to "observe" consumers' thoughts as they compare labels from two different breakfast cereals.

Delphi technique. The Delphi technique is a method of soliciting and consolidating expert opinion regarding phenomena for which few data are available and history seems irrelevant.[19,20] An investigator using the Delphi technique typically selects a variety of experts with diverse but relevant backgrounds and requests that each provide written comments on the point in question.[21] Each expert operates on an individual basis and provides feedback through the mail. They are not informed of the identities of the other participating experts so their judgments are free from social pressure and other negative aspects of small group dynamics.[22] Responses from all participants are summarized and then resubmitted to the individual experts for the purpose of reevaluation and further comment in light of the group response.[23] This process is reiterated until some degree of agreement is reached.[24] An example of a case in which the Delphi technique might be useful is in investigating the potential role of registered dietitians in the year 2050.

PRELIMINARY CONSIDERATIONS RELATED TO DATA COLLECTION

Preliminary considerations related to the collection of qualitative data often include sampling; interview scripts, forms, and protocols; selection and training of interviewers/observers; use of electronic recording equipment; and transcription of verbalizations.

Sampling

Qualitative research is rarely based on probability samples; purposive sampling is typically used instead. Purposive sampling seeks participants with specified characteristics, experiences, or behaviors who represent one or more perspectives deemed relevant to the research goals.[25] The sample is often small because the nature of qualitative research demands intensive and prolonged contact with participants, yielding an enormous amount of data per person.[26] Furthermore, the sample need not always be specified in advance. Sampling for qualitative research is often done incrementally as initial findings suggest the need for additional input from the same or different perspectives.[25,26] This is referred to as a *phased approach* to sampling.[27] It may also be referred to as *theoretical sampling* if the sampling decisions are dictated by a developing theory.[28] With the phased or theoretical approach, sampling continues until additional interviews fail to provide fresh insight into the phenomenon under investigation, or until the benefit of additional insights is outweighed by the cost of obtaining them.[25]

In sampling for group interviews, additional considerations related to group dynamics may apply. For example, it is often advisable to assemble relatively homogeneous groups (eg, with respect to age, educational background, ethnic group, or income) so that group members are comfortable expressing their views. If a variety of perspectives is required, additional groups may be formed, each representing a different perspective. By the same token, it may be best for group members to be strangers to one another so that the social liability of candid discussion is minimized.[27]

The important points are that sampling decisions be made explicit in describing qualitative research, that the decisions be adequately justified, and that generalizations be made only to the extent allowable on the basis of the sample involved.[28,29]

Interview Scripts, Observation Forms, and Protocols

Qualitative research is, by definition, open-ended. During data collection, it is acknowledged and accepted that the researcher and respondents will interact with and affect each other. While this precludes the possibility that any two observations will be identical, it is acceptable as long as investigators can later identify certain regularities across the data set.[4]

A semi-structured interview script (*Table 5.1*) provides a general guide that is uniform enough to generate comparable responses, but flexible enough to accommodate the variety of people encountered in an interview setting. In other words, it provides the interviewer with a basic framework for covering all topics of interest, while allowing him or her the latitude needed to approach interviewees as individuals and to follow up on unanticipated questions and issues raised during the encounter. An excellent example of this concept is provided by Kirk and Miller.[30]

Table 5.1
Excerpt From a Semistructured Interview Script

This script is used to elicit reactions of focus group participants to a proposed set of nutrition print materials on fat, cholesterol, sodium and fiber. This part of the discussion focuses on content, and it should last for 20 minutes.

One of the booklets you received earlier looks like this. Do you need a few minutes to look it over before you discuss it as a group? [*Allow five minutes for review*].

What did you think of it? [*If they try to respond to you directly, remind them again that they are here to discuss it* among themselves; *that you are only here to suggest topics and distribute related materials.*]

Should more or less scientific evidence be presented (to support the recommendations about diet)?

What did you like the best about this one?

What did you like the least?

Was there anything that should be eliminated?

[*If these topics did not emerge naturally, ask:*]

How did you feel about the "Did You Knows," the quick facts highlighted in yellow and sprinkled throughout the booklet? [*Turn to one in the material and display it.*]

Did you do the "Food Choice Check Up" on page 6? [*If nobody responds right away, move on to the next topic.*]

Do you think you'll use the recipe? [*If the participants hesitate, ask if they ever use recipes from nutrition materials. If not, skip the remaining questions on recipes and move on to the next subject area.*]

How do you use a recipe like this? [*If examples are needed, use the following:* Do you use it as is, or do you just get ideas from it, use it to make changes in your own recipe, or what?]

How would you handle a recipe printed in a brochure like this? [*If examples are needed, use the following:* Would you cut it out, copy it onto one of your own recipe cards, just remember it, just remember where it is, or what?]

What would be the *best* way to present recipes in a brochure like this?

Any other comments on this piece before we move on?

A semistructured observation form (*Table 5.2*) is similar in nature to an interview script and serves the same purpose when the objective is observation. Such forms can help multiple observers know what to look for, based on the research objectives, and describe what they observe in common terms so that subsequent comparisons are possible.[31] At the same time, it allows observers the flexibility needed to include observations that do not fit into preconceived categories.

Pilot-testing of interview scripts, observation forms, and protocols is extremely important. Pilot-testing of an interview script and its corresponding protocol can help ensure that: the questions are mutually understood by respondents and interviewers, the terms used in formulating questions are not offensive to respondents, the time allocated for each interview is adequate, the

Table 5.2
Semistructured Observation
Form

To describe shoppers' physical reactions to an educational exhibit on comparing food labels, observers are required to record observations for every tenth shopper who passes within 3 ft of the front of the exhibit. The 3-ft limit is marked on the floor with masking tape.

Return shoppers (those who have passed by or have already stopped at the exhibit during the observation period) are not counted a second time.

Times 1, 2, 3, and 4 on the record form below refer to repeat reactions within one stop at the exhibit. For example, if a shopper looking at the exhibit picks up cereal 1 and reads the label, puts it down, then comes back to it before leaving the exhibit, the amount of time spent the first time he or she examines cereal label 1 is recorded in the column labeled Time 1. The amount of time spent the second time she or he examines cereal label 1 is recorded in the column labeled Time 2.

Observer #_____ Shopper #_____

Physical Reaction	Amount of Time Spent (in seconds)			
	Time 1	Time 2	Time 3	Time 4
Passed by without stopping (check here _____)	N/A	N/A	N/A	N/A
Examined textual panels				
Examined cereal label 1				
Examined cereal label 2				
Compared cereal labels				
Examined salad dressing label 1				
Examined salad dressing label 2				
Compared salad dressing labels				
Examined tipsheet				
Did the shopper take a tipsheet? _____ yes _____ no				

protocol facilitates rapport, and the interview produces the expected quantity and quality of information desired. Pilot-testing of an observation form and protocol can help ensure that the form is sufficiently detailed and comprehensive to capture the essence of the phenomenon observed without overburdening observers, the observations are as unobtrusive as possible, and the research objectives underlying observations can be met.

Finally, it is important that the investigator describe the protocol and provide (or have available) samples of the interview script or observation form when reporting the research.[27] This information is crucial to the reader in both understanding the responses or observations and evaluating the plausibility of conclusions drawn by the author.

Selection and Training of Interviewers/Observers

Two factors that should be considered during the selection of interviewers are gender and safety issues. First, an interviewer's gender can affect respondents' replies. In some cases, cross-sex interviewing has been shown to help reduce bias,[32] but other researchers have shown that bias effects due to gender depend on the topic and context of the interview.[33] In our work it was apparent that men opened up more readily to other men and women to other women. This may be due to the fact that neither likes to display any perceived ignorance or other sensitivities to the opposite gender.[34] Safety issues also must be considered if meetings are to take place outside the university or worksite environment. Men may have an easier time in some neighborhoods, although two women together might collect better information from other women in those same neighborhoods.

Regardless of gender, the interviewer must be thoroughly familiar with the material to be covered.[4] This means more than memorizing the interview script (which is not necessary at all). It implies that interviewers have enough training and expertise in the subject matter to enable them to probe respondents intelligently and competently. In our field, this usually means that they should be dietitians or nutritionists.

Selection of interviewers and observers is followed by thorough training. Formal training can help ensure that scripts and observation forms are used as intended and that the protocol is consistently followed. Training can also provide interviewers and observers the opportunity to practice communication and observation skills necessary for successful completion of the task.

Trained interviewers and observers should produce consistent, comparable data across a target audience. The amount of time required to achieve this quality may vary considerably with the circumstances, but even when experienced personnel are employed, training and pilot testing are critical.

Training should include four components: reading, discussions with experienced interviewers, one-on-one supervised experiential instruction, and practice. Reading should include literature reviews, "how-to" articles, and a wide variety of actual transcripts. It is helpful to analyze and discuss those transcripts in detail with the original interviewer (if possible) or another interviewer with experience using similar protocols among a similar target group. Discussions are important, even if they are only anecdotal. They provide a wealth of background information for problem-solving during interviews when interviewers have to work without the aid of any resources other than their own knowledge and intuition. We have found that instruction proceeds most efficiently when the trainee is videotaped while conducting an interview. The trainee and trainer together can review the tape immediately after the interview, stopping whenever it is appropriate to comment. The process can be repeated as many times as necessary, but dramatic improvements between interviews are commonplace.

No amount of training, however, can replace practice. The authors have found that eight to ten one-on-one interviews or three to four group interviews using the same interview guide with participants from a single target group are required for a consistent, relaxed performance. Even after training, however, occasional quality control checks are advised. For example, the trainer may review every tenth interview. In cases in which an interview is not up to standard, the problem can be addressed before further interviews are completed. Billiet and Loosveldt[35] provide further suggestions.

Use of Electronic Recording Equipment

Electronic recording equipment is often used by qualitative researchers to document interview encounters and observations. This relatively new technology offers many advantages.[36] One of the primary advantages for qualitative researchers is the opportunity to increase both reliability and validity of the data.

Audiotaping and videotaping can eliminate the shortcomings of manual note-taking, which can yield incomplete and sometimes inaccurate data. These shortcomings include limited memory capacity and attention spans, perceptual bias, and unsystematic recording formats.[37] Audiotaping and videotaping also allow the investigator to employ multiple observers and/or coders, thereby enhancing the potential for reliable and valid data analysis.

Although the use of electronic recording equipment is beneficial in many ways, it also has one distinct liability: It introduces an extraneous element that may cause a certain degree of social reactivity or confounding to occur. How serious is this?

The effects of audiotaping and videotaping on subjects in experimental situations have received some limited attention in the literature. Published studies, including an attempted assessment of the effects of observation procedures (not including videotaping) on subject behavior, were reviewed by Weick.[38] He concludes that observation interference is "not extensive" and that, when it occurs, its effects are usually limited to a brief period at the beginning of the experimental session.

The potential reactivity of videotaping per se on conversational behavior of subjects in a typical laboratory setting has been empirically investigated by Wiemann.[39] Wiemann's findings are that the conversation behaviors examined were not significantly affected by knowledge of being videotaped; behaviors associated with the communication of relaxation or anxiety and responsiveness were not significantly affected by various levels of obtrusiveness of the videotaping procedure; and anxiety peaked during the first minute of the session, then dropped significantly and stabilized by the end of the third minute. Consequently, Wiemann concluded that videotaping procedures, in and of themselves, are not reactive.

Niebuhr and associates[37] draw the same conclusions from a review of the literature on the use of videotape technology in behavioral research. These authors note, however, that one-way glass and adaptation periods can reduce reactivity. Other methods for potentially reducing reactivity to audio or video recording equipment might include use of cordless, remote microphones, so that recording equipment need not be positioned within eyeshot of the subject, and use of equipment sensitive enough to pick up very low voice levels so that the respondents need not be asked to speak up. An audio consultant can be especially helpful in identifying specific equipment that meets these needs.

Naturally, respondents are always informed when they are being audiotaped and/or videorecorded. A release form is typically used to relay that message, to assure respondents that the source of any information provided will be kept confidential, and to give the investigator the legal and ethical basis to use that information in relation to the study.

Finally, with respect to electronic recordings, good-quality equipment and tapes always should be used. Ninety-minute audiocassettes (45 minutes per side) are recommended. Longer tapes tend to be thinner to the point that quality can suffer and breakage is more likely. Shorter tapes require more frequent handling, which can result in irritating interruptions and increase the obtrusiveness of the recording.[27] Of course, new technologies emerge onto the market regularly, so a review of all available options is advised.

Some additional tips that facilitate transcribing and coding of the information later are:
- To speak clearly toward the microphone and encourage respondents to do so as well.
- To avoid rustling papers, which can easily drown out voices.
- To watch for breakage or tangling of tapes, and to keep replacements handy.
- To conclude each recorded interview with a taped message that identifies participants by code, indicates that the interview is complete, and notes any informal observations or insights that might be helpful in evaluating and interpreting the data at a later date, eg, observations regarding contextual issues that might have influenced the session.

Transcription of Verbalizations

In most cases in which researcher-subject encounters are electronically recorded, a typewritten transcript is subsequently produced. Transcripts are usually verbatim accounts designed to preserve, as much as possible, everything that was said during the encounter. Transcripts do not, however, preserve non-linguistic data such as emphasis, mood, tone of voice, and other descriptive information that can be so crucial in elaborating meaning.[40,27] Because of this, Jones[40] warns against the temptation to let reading transcripts become a substitute for listening to tapes.

Transcribing tapes is very time-consuming and, therefore, costly. Miles[41] estimates that a 60- to 90-minute tape takes approximately six to eight hours to transcribe. Morton-Williams[27] offers a rule of thumb of four to six hours per transcript for individual in-depth interviews or group interviews. Our experience places transcription time somewhere within these same ranges.

If someone else is employed to transcribe the tapes, he or she should be trained so that the product meets the researcher's expectations and needs. A written set of instructions can be used to establish the format of the transcript. The best way to determine what should be included in instructions to transcribers is for the researcher to thoroughly pilot-test the process. The experience is invaluable in establishing guidelines and in estimating the amount of time (and cost) that should be allotted per transcript.

We have also found it critical that the original interviewer edit each typed transcript carefully to check for accuracy, to fill in the gaps using notes taken during and after the interview, and to annotate the transcript appropriately. For example, annotations may be needed to clarify ambiguous situations, eg, "the numerous, intermittent comments regarding this issue were provided by a single respondent who kept repeating her position, rather than several different respondents in consensus."

Finally, from our own experience, professional dictation equipment is especially helpful in making the transcription process less onerous. High-quality headphones can make the difference between capturing or losing hard-to-hear text, and a foot pedal frees both hands for uninterrupted work on the keyboard. Use of a computer, instead of a typewriter, is also a major advantage.

QUALITATIVE DATA ANALYSIS

Qualitative data analysis is characterized by Jones[40] as the "breaking down and building up of analytic structure in the data," and by Walker[25] as "fracturing data into lumps of meaning and a subsequent restructuring, firstly by categorization and then by development of relationships between categories." Qualitative analysis can proceed both inductively (moving from particular cases to generalizations) and deductively (moving from general cases to the particular). This is eloquently described by Lachenmeyer[42]: "There is constant interplay between the observation of realities and the formation of concepts, between research and theorizing, between perception and explanation. The genesis of any theory is best described as a reciprocal development of observational sophistication and theoretical precision."

Our discussion of qualitative analysis rests on three basic premises outlined in the previous chapter. These may be summarized as follows:
1. Qualitative data analysis may be theory-driven, theory-generating, or both.
2. To mature as a science, qualitative data analysis must be standardized to some extent.
3. Analysis follows a continuum that ranges from purely qualitative (involving no numbers) to quantitative.

These premises should serve as a foundation for understanding the nuts and bolts of qualitative analysis as described below.

Unitizing

Unitizing is the process by which a recorded stream of verbalization (usually in the form of a transcript) is segmented into units amenable to categorization.[43,44] Units may be defined in terms of time (eg, 20-second units), speaker (eg, all statements made by one speaker while holding the floor), or content (eg, each complete phrase, statement, or group of statements that express a single, coherent thought). Pilot testing should help determine which type of unit is most appropriate for a given project and how the units will be recorded. In most cases, predefined symbols are penciled directly onto the transcript to signal the beginning and end of each unit, rather than using a separate unitizing form.

Unitizing occurs as a formal process primarily in cases in which qualitative data is destined for quantitative analysis.[43] For example, if the investigator plans to count the number of units in each category, it is important that they be standardized according to some predefined concept of what constitutes a unit. Furthermore, as with any data handled quantitatively, it is a basic requirement that the investigator assess the degree of reliability, or in this case, interrater agreement. For example, Shepherd and Sims[16] used two independent judges to unitize transcripts into individual cognitive responses. Interrater agreement was determined by dividing the number of agreements by the total number of judgments (agreements plus disagreements). Other methods for assessing interrater agreement among multiple unitizers have been offered in the literature.[44,45]

Coding

Coding is a data reduction strategy in which a voluminous amount of qualitative data, usually in the form of unitized verbalizations, is subsumed into a more manageable number of representative categories.[46] It is the process of identifying "conceptual frameworks within which the analysis can be organized."[27] Coding (or categorizing) helps the investigator extract meaning from qualitative data in a systematic way, uncovering patterns or themes that might otherwise be obscured by the sheer mass of information. Coding facilitates storage, retrieval, and analysis of data, and may even suggest the need for further data collection.[41] As noted by Patton,[29] "A classification system is critical; without classification there is chaos."

Order and structure may be imposed on qualitative data in a number of ways, depending on the researcher's philosophy and objectives.[25,27] Coding schemes may be driven by existing theory, or they may be developed inductively. If the phenomenon under investigation has already been described by theory, the existing theory may be used as a conceptual framework for developing categories prior to data collection. In such cases, the terminology of the theoretical model is used to label those categories.[43] If no existing theory describing the phenomenon is available or existing theory is considered inadequate, the inductive approach may be more applicable. With an inductive approach, the researcher allows categories to emerge from the data naturally. This is accomplished by pulling together quotations and observations that reflect similar underlying concepts and placing them in categories based on those concepts.[29]

Finally, a combination of deductive and inductive approaches may be used, as suggested by Bulmer[47]: "The way to approach the paradox of categorization is to focus on the interdependence of theory and observation." With this approach, the researcher attempts to shuttle back and forth between theory and data to evolve a comprehensive set of categories that accurately reflects both. An excellent example of this hybrid approach is provided by Jones.[40]

Other potential frameworks for organizing or coding qualitative data may include research questions developed during the design of the investigation[27,29] and those that emerge during analysis; policy questions posed by funding agents in commissioning the research[40]; and results from task analyses (for coding cognitive processes involved in problem-solving tasks).[43] An example of a case in which this last framework might be applied would be a task that asks participants to think aloud as they use food label information to calculate the percentage of calories provided by fat.

The actual mechanics of organizing or coding data is a creative process that varies from researcher to researcher and from project to project. There is no formula.[29] Furthermore, pilot work is needed to refine the system and make sure that it works.[43] An investigator may start with a very elaborate coding scheme, only to find it too cumbersome to be practical.[41] In contrast, an investigator may begin with a very simple scheme but find that it fails to cover or describe certain types of data adequately.[43] In either case, refinement of the coding system is necessary.

The important point is that the researcher should have a rationale for coding data in a certain way and that the rationale for coding be made explicit.[48] In specifying the rationale and criteria by which data are coded, the investigator fosters consistency and reliability in the coding process[43] and exposes the process to personal and peer scrutiny.[48]

Once a coding system has been established, it may be judged according to two criteria outlined by Guba[49]: internal homogeneity and external heterogeneity. The former refers to the extent to which all data within a category reflect the concept represented by that category. In other words, do the data within each category go together in a meaningful way? The latter refers to the extent to which the categories are mutually exclusive. In other words, are the differences between categories obvious?

There is some disagreement in the literature with respect to the external heterogeneity criterion proposed by Guba.[49] For example, Bogdan and Taylor[48] contend that the categories used to organize qualitative data need not be mutually exclusive. They even suggest that using mutually exclusive categories may, in fact, decrease the researcher's ability to develop an integrated picture showing relationships between hypotheses (when hypotheses are used to structure the categorization). Multiple coding of verbalizations thus may be appropriate in some cases just as multiple responses are accepted in surveys.

For example, in coding a transcript for misconceptions about nutrition, the following comment was categorized as a misconception about the food grouping system *and* as a misconception about carbohydrates:
So I guess we do need to eat from all of those [food] groups, but as far as the breads and cereals, we could probably eat less. We don't need to eat six slices of bread a day. Probably one would be substantial.

To classify the quote as one or the other (a misconception about the food grouping system *or* a misconception about carbohydrates) would have resulted in a considerable loss of information. On the other hand, a redefinition of categories would have been unwarranted, especially given that each category had already been used extensively and this was the only verbalization that satisfied both. Again, the important point is that the researcher be explicit about the criteria for multiple coding and consistent in applying that criteria.

Use of context in coding.   One question that often arises in coding unitized verbalizations is whether the context surrounding a unit should be brought to bear on the coding or categorization of that unit. Oral prose is often choppy, ungrammatical, and fraught with partial phrases or even single words.[43] A fragment of normal speech may express a complete thought—and thus constitute a unit—but only if the surrounding text is used to derive its meaning. Consider the following example:
Speaker 1: I like the one with the pictures of food on the cover.

Speaker 2: Yeah, me too.

Speaker 2 has expressed a complete thought, but without the preceding text it would be uninterpretable and, thus, defy categorization.

Context can help make coding less ambiguous, thereby promoting objectivity—a primary concern in using verbal reports as data.[43] Furthermore, context is what makes qualitative data so rich and meaningful. To remove it from that context would "deprive it of its essential holistic nature,"[27] transforming it to something more akin to quantitative data. As Patton[29] asserts, "Keeping things in context is a cardinal principle of qualitative analysis." Miles and Huberman[46] concur: "We do not rule out converting the data into numbers or ranks, provided that the numbers, and the words used to derive the numbers, remain together in the ensuing analysis. That way one never strips the data at hand from the contexts in which they occur."

Both the protocol and the level of abstraction represented by the coding system help determine the amount of context that must be considered in assigning verbalizations to categories.[43] The key is to address this issue formally as instructions for coders are developed.

Second-tier coding. In some cases, a second round of coding may be advisable to describe the data further or to help determine the relative confidence the investigator has in the various units of data. Shepherd[50] used a second-tier coding scheme to describe the magnitude of certainty expressed by subjects in their cognitive responses. This was accomplished by identifying specific words and phrases representing "weak" versus "strong" expressions. According to this scheme, a strong response might be, "I really love the one with pictures of food on the cover." A weak response might be, "I kind of like the one with pictures of food on the cover."

Patton[29] recommends crossing initial categories to create a second-tier coding matrix. For example, if focus group participants are asked to react to six versions of a proposed nutrition education poster, the responses to each version might be categorized in terms of the desired qualities of a poster, eg, perceived intelligibility, memorability, visual appeal, capacity to elicit behavior change, and usefulness. On the second round of coding, two categories, intelligibility and visual appeal, might be crossed to yield a dimension that encompasses both. The investigator would then search the data for responses reflecting this hybrid category, eg, "The way this one is designed to look like a target with the lowest-fat foods in the middle makes it flashier *and* easier to understand than the other ones."

Once categories are crossed, data can be reassigned to appropriate cells of the matrix, possibly generating new insights and exposing themes not readily apparent in the original analysis. As Patton[29] points out, each cell of the matrix may not be filled, but the process itself should promote the "ongoing search for understanding through description."

Bogdan and Taylor[48] suggest a second-tier coding process that may help the investigator determine the relative confidence placed in various units of data once they are categorized. This coding scheme may differentiate verbal reports according to whether they are:
• solicited or unsolicited (volunteered)
• made in a group or in a one-on-one situation with the observer
• made by the subjects in question or by their significant others
• made in a "comfortable" interview versus one in which the subjects appear to be very "guarded"
• made at the beginning or the end of the interview

Data may also be differentiated according to whether they are direct statements or indirect inferences derived by coders from fragmentary verbalizations. Although indirect inferences can provide valuable insight, analysts may invest greater confidence in direct statements.

Again, the goal is description. Careful scrutiny of verbalizations in context and a constant search for insight should result in distinctions that will capture the essence of verbal reports and enhance the analysis and interpretation.

Interrater reliability of coding. The coding of qualitative data can be a very subjective process requiring considerable judgment on the part of coders unless specific steps are taken to avoid it. For this reason, we recommend extensive piloting of the process to generate a well-defined set of instructions that will reduce subjectivity and enhance objectivity. As pointed out by Ericsson and Simon,[43] "Without appropriate safeguards, the encoder, exposed to a series of ambiguous verbal statements, may encode them with a bias toward his own preferred interpretation."

While most researchers would agree that objectivity is the hallmark of "good" science, some disagreement exists as to the extent to which this criterion should be applied in the analysis of qualitative data. An unpublished memorandum quoted by Miles,[41] states that "there is an inherent conflict between validity and reliability—the former is what [qualitative research] is specially qualified to gain, and increased emphasis on reliability will only undermine that unique function" (Sieber SD. Memorandum; 1976). In the same vein, Guba,[51] as quoted by Miles,[41] stresses that qualitative data be evaluated in terms of being more or less "auditable," "confirmable," and "credible," rather than reliable or valid in the sense typically applied to quantitative data.

We propose a compromise between the view expressed by Ericsson and Simon and that represented by Sieber and Guba. The compromise rests on whether or not the data is destined for quantitative analysis. In those cases in which the units of analysis are to be counted, ranked, subjected to statistical analyses, or all three, reliability of the coding process should be established. In general, this is done by using multiple, independent coders and monitoring the extent to which their codes agree or disagree. Ericsson and Simon[43] report that interrater reliabilities of 0.8 or 0.9 have been achieved by coders who understood the task and used context to code segments of verbalized data. An excellent summary of various strategies used to determine interrater reliability or agreement of subjective judgments is offered by Tinsley and Weiss.[52]

Displaying the Data Visually

Data display is defined as "an organized assembly of information that permits conclusion-drawing and action-taking."[46] Raw qualitative data typically occurs as narrative text—bulky, sequential, highly dispersed and difficult to manage in terms of analysis and interpretation.[53] Consequently, it is often useful to develop matrices, flow charts, concept maps, and other nomographic networks to organize and simultaneously display the data in a visual form. Firestone and Dawson[54] and Jones[40] describe some of the benefits of developing visual displays of qualitative data:
- It promotes completeness in that it may help the investigator recall data that might otherwise be overlooked.
- It facilitates cross-comparisons between cases and events that may be isolated under a simple categorization process.
- It may suggest new interpretations of the data as the display reveals relationships that may not have been obvious before.
- It requires "intense immersion" in the data, thereby fostering the development of categories, relationships, and conclusions firmly grounded in observations.
- It helps the investigator retain a holistic view of the data—a view that may be easily obscured when the same data are parceled into categories.
- It can promote understanding on the part of those who review the research.

While "spatially compressed" displays have been proposed as "a major avenue to improving qualitative data analysis,"[46] they are subject to drawbacks. Besides being "laborious and tedious,"[40] visual displays necessarily limit the amount of information that may be included.[46] In developing displays, it is often necessary to summarize raw data or restrict the display to especially illustrative examples. This requires a great deal of subjective judgment on the part of the researcher, who must take care that his or her displays represent the bulk of the data accurately and adequately. As with coding, investigators are advised to record and report decision rules used to selectively display data so that the process remains open to scrutiny.

Computer Analysis of Qualitative Data

The use of computers to manage and analyze qualitative data is a relatively new advance and one that appears promising for qualitative research.[25] Conrad and Reinharz[55] outline the advantages (and in some cases, the implications) of an automated approach to qualitative analysis. These include: speedy data entry and coding via keyboard, easy sharing of data among researchers via modem, conservation of space in data storage, and fast, efficient data retrieval. Automated analysis might also increase the potential for standardization of analytic procedures and for integrating qualitative analysis with quantitative analysis through automated systems common to both.

Walker[25] addresses the advantages of computerized qualitative analysis in more global terms: "The advent of sophisticated text management systems...expands the boundaries of qualitative research, both with respect to the complexity of relations that can be explored within the data and perhaps also to the scale of qualitative studies that can be envisaged."

Some of the drawbacks of automated qualitative analysis include the possibility that available analytic programs will dictate research goals and design and the potential risk of violating confidentiality of data stored in systems accessible to others.[55] One additional drawback is that the aesthetics of presentation (especially in creating visual displays) may become more important than interpretation of results.

An excellent compilation of articles related to the use of computers in qualitative research is provided in a special double issue of *Qualitative Sociology* (volume 7, 1984). The authors comment on issues and dilemmas that arise in considering automated qualitative analysis, criteria for assessing systems, and potential uses of computer programs for content analysis. An annotated bibliography of current literature is also included. Ericsson and Simon[43] and Hiemstra and colleagues[56] add to this body of literature by specifically describing some of the programs now in use.

INTERPRETATION AND VERIFICATION

Interpretation of Data

According to Patton,[29] interpretation involves "attaching meaning and significance to the analysis, explaining descriptive patterns, and looking for relationships and linkages among descriptive dimensions." In structuring this chapter, we have separated analysis from interpretation for the sake of discussion. In reality, however, the two often proceed simultaneously to some extent. For example, the investigator involved in organizing and categorizing data will almost always find himself or herself discovering insights, coming up with hunches, and developing preliminary hypotheses for interpreting the data. Indeed, preliminary interpretation may provide direction for further data collection and analysis.

The key word here, though, is *preliminary*. The final interpretation must rest on a comprehensive evaluation of all the data. This may require a reconceptualization of hunches formed during analysis and possibly the revision or discarding of pet theories developed early in the process.[30] It is often difficult to abandon preliminary interpretations that fail to be supported when all the data are in. At the same time, doing so can lead to important, unanticipated discoveries.

Whereas informal interpretation may occur during data collection and analysis, formal interpretation begins when the analysis is complete. Again, interpretation involves identifying regularities and themes in the data, searching for links between concepts, and posing hypotheses for explaining them.[41] The goal is understanding what the data mean in terms of the researcher's objectives.

Verification of Interpretation

Once an interpretation is made, the researcher is ready to proceed with verification of the interpretation. The primary criterion for evaluating interpretation of qualitative data is that it accurately reflect the reality represented by those data.[57] Verification involves a systematic evaluation of conclusions drawn through interpretation to see whether they meet this primary criterion.

Verification of an interpretation is considerably strengthened if a variety of data collection strategies and analytic techniques have been used and yield comparable conclusions. This concept is known as *triangulation* (assuming the use of at least three different techniques), and is probably the best defense against criticism of investigator bias or subjectivity in qualitative research.[58] Triangulation may involve multiple qualitative and/or quantitative methods. The more diverse the methods used and the greater the number involved, the better.

Several steps have been suggested for verifying interpretation of qualitative data. These steps constitute a process sometimes referred to as *provisional hypothesis testing* in which one seeks to disqualify the hypothesis.[41] Since qualitative research is not designed to test causal propositions, interpretation typically amounts to data-based speculation and generation of hypotheses.[29] The interpretation is then subjected to verification *not* by seeking confirmation, but by actively seeking disconfirmation through intense and systematic scrutiny. Miles[41] and Miles and Huberman[46] provide some tactics for applying this scrutiny.

Look for concomitant variation and assess conditions making for greater or lesser concomitant variation. Does the pattern of variation observed in one part of the data hold true across all the data and/or across data reported by other researchers? If not, what are the circumstances (eg, settings, sources, occasions) under which the pattern of variation seems to hold most consistently? What are the circumstances under which the pattern of variation is weaker or not observed?

Look for negative cases. Are there data that seem to contradict a conclusion? If so, what is the extent and relative trustworthiness of these data?

Rule out spurious or confounding factors. What are possible alternative explanations for the data? Are the alternative explanations supported by the data in part or in whole?

Descriptive Research

Look for intervening variables. Are there potential intervening variables without which patterns of concomitant variation would evaporate?

Make predictions and search for violations. What else would be true if this prediction were correct? Is it true according to the data? What would not be true if this prediction were correct? Is it "not true" according to the data?

Get feedback from informants. Does the interpretation ring true to those who provided the data?

Miles and Huberman[46] noted that, while getting feedback from informants can be fraught with difficulties, it has "particular confirmatory power" in terms of validation.

As is the case with all the processes described in this chapter, the methods used to verify interpretation of qualitative data should be reported. Firestone and Dawson[54] emphasize this point with the following comment, "Even if suggestions such as these are followed, the results [of provisional hypothesis testing] remain suspect when the process is not made public. Ways need to be found to make this process of generation and rejection of explanations more public."

CONCLUSION

The objective of this chapter was to offer researchers and practitioners in dietetics a basic overview of qualitative techniques so that they are in a better position to apply and evaluate qualitative research. We provided practical guidance on how to conduct qualitative research systematically and rigorously without compromising the qualitative nature of the endeavor, for this is what makes qualitative research unique in its contribution to understanding the world around us.

In conclusion, we offer the following ten criteria suggested by Marshall and Rossman[1] for developing and evaluating qualitative research proposals and reports:
1. Data collection methods are explicit.
2. Data are used to document constructs.
3. Negative instances of findings are displayed and accounted for.
4. Biases are discussed, including biases of interest (personal, professional, policy-related) and theoretical biases and assumptions.
5. Strategies for data collection and analysis are made public.
6. Field decisions altering strategies or stubstantive focus are documented.
7. Competing hypotheses are presented and discussed.
8. Data are preserved.
9. Participants' truthfulness is assessed.
10. Theoretical significance and generalizability are made explicit.

This list of criteria summarizes much of what has been said in the foregoing pages and reinforces many of the key points that we have tried to make. We hope that our comments will stimulate more investigators to consider qualitative research as an option and that our suggestions will promote a more rigorous approach to the conduct and reporting of qualitative investigations.

References
1. Marshall C, Rossman GB. *Designing Qualitative Research.* Beverly Hills, Calif: Sage Publications; 1989.

2. Walker R. An introduction to applied qualitative research. In: Walker R, ed. *Applied Qualitative Research.* Brookfield, Vt: Gower Publishing Co; 1985:3.

3. Lipchik E. *Interviewing.* Rockville, Md: Aspen; 1988.

4. Novak JD, Gowin DB. *Learning How to Learn.* Cambridge, England: Cambridge University Press; 1984.

5. Carney TF. *Content Analysis. A Technique for Systematic Inference From Communications.* Winnepeg, Manitoba, Canada: University of Manitoba; 1972.

6. Weber RP. *Basic Content Analysis.* Beverly Hills, Calif: Sage Publications; 1985.

7. Calder BJ. Focus groups and the nature of qualitative marketing research. *J Marketing Res.* 1977;14:353.

8. Bellenger DN, Bernhardt KL, Goldstucker JL. Qualitative research techniques: focus group interviews. In: Higginbotham JB, Cox KK, eds. *Focus Group Interviews: A Reader.* Chicago, Ill: American Marketing Association; 1979.

9. Shepherd SK, Sims LS, Cronin FJ, Shaw A, Davis CA. Use of focus groups to explore consumers' preferences for content and graphic design of nutrition publications. *J Am Diet Assoc.* 1989;89:1612.

10. Krueger RA. *Focus Groups: A Practical Guide for Applied Research.* Newbury Park, Calif: Sage Publications; 1988.

11. Olson JC, Muderrisoglu A. The stability of responses obtained by free elicitation: implications for measuring attribute salience and memory structure. In: Wilkie WL, ed. *Advances in Consumer Research.* 1979;6:269.

12. Kanwar R, Olson J, Sims L. Toward conceptualizing and measuring cognitive structures. In: Monroe KB, ed. *Advances in Consumer Research.* 1981;8:122.

13. Petty RE. The importance of cognitive responses in persuasion. In: Perreault WD, ed. *Advances in Consumer Research.* 1977;4:358.

14. Wright P. Message-evoked thoughts: persuasion research using thought verbalizations. *J Consumer Res.* 1980;7:151.

15. Lutz RJ, MacKenzie SB. Construction of a diagnostic cognitive response model for use in commercial pretesting. In: Chasin J, ed. *Straight Talk About Attitude Research.* Chicago, Ill: American Marketing Association; 1982:145.

16. Shepherd SK, Sims LS. Employing cognitive response analysis to examine message acceptance in nutrition education. *J Nutr Educ.* 1990;22:215.

17. Olson JC, Reynolds TJ. Understanding consumers' cognitive structures: implications for advertising strategy. In: Percy L, Woodside AG, eds. *Advertising and Consumer Psychology.* Lexington, Mass: Lexington Books; 1983:77.

18. Wright PL. The cognitive processes mediating acceptance of advertising. *J Marketing Res.* 1973;10:53.

19. Chambers JC, Mullick SK, Smith DD. How to choose the right forecasting technique. In *Harvard Business Review: On Management.* New York, NY: Harper and Row; 1975:501.

20. Wallace KM. The use and value of qualitative research studies. *Industrial Marketing Management.* 1984;13:181.

21. Adams EE Jr, Ebert RJ. *Production and Operations Management: Concepts, Models, and Behavior.* Englewood Cliffs, NJ: Prentice Hall Inc; 1978.

22. Wheelwright SC, Makridakis S. *Forecasting Methods for Management.* 3rd ed. New York, NY: John Wiley and Sons; 1980.

23. Linstone HA, Turoff M. *The Delphi Method: Techniques and Applications.* Reading, Mass: Addison-Wesley Publishing Co; 1975.

24. Spears MC, Vaden AG. *Foodservice Organizations: A Managerial and Systems Approach.* New York, NY: John Wiley and Sons; 1985.

25. Walker R. Evaluating applied qualitative research. In: Walker R, ed. *Applied Qualitative Research.* Brookfield, Vt: Gower Publishing Co; 1985;177.

26. Sandelowski M. The problem of rigor in qualitative research. *Adv Nurs Sci.* 1986;1:27.

27. Morton-Williams J. Making qualitative research work: aspects of administration. In: Walker R, ed. *Applied Qualitative Research.* Brookfield, Vt: Gower Publishing Co; 1985:27.

28. Knafl KA, Howard MJ. Interpreting and reporting qualitative research. *Res Nurs Health.* 1984;7:17.

29. Patton MQ. *How to Use Qualitative Methods in Evaluation.* Beverly Hills, Calif: Sage Publications; 1987.

30. Kirk J, Miller ML. *Reliability and Validity in Qualitative Research.* Beverly Hills, Calif: Sage Publications; 1986.

Descriptive Research

31. Churchill GA Jr. *Marketing Research: Methodological Foundations.* 3rd ed. New York, NY: Dryden Press; 1983.
32. Bailey KD. *Methods of Social Research,* 2nd ed. New York, NY: Collier Macmillan; 1982.
33. Riessman CK. When gender is not enough: women interviewing women. *Gender and Society.* 1987;1:172.
34. LaBorde GZ. *Influencing with Integrity.* Palo Alto, Calif: Syntony; 1983.
35. Billiet J, Loosveldt G. Improvement of the quality of responses to factual survey questions by interviewer training. *Public Opinion Quart.* 1988;52:190.
36. Smith RL, McPhail C, Pickens RG. Reactivity to systematic observation with film: a field experiment. *Sociometry.* 1975;38:536.
37. Niebuhr RE, Manz CC, Davis KR Jr. Using videotape technology: innovations in behavioral research. *J Management.* 1981;7:43.
38. Weick KE. Systematic observational methods. In: Lindzey G, Aronson E, eds. *The Handbook of Social Psychology.* 2nd ed. Reading, Mass: Addison-Wesley; 1968;2.
39. Wiemann JM. Effects of laboratory videotaping procedures on selected conversation behaviors. *Human Communication Res.* 1981;7:302.
40. Jones S. The analysis of depth interviews. In: Walker R, ed. *Applied Qualitative Research.* Brookfield, Vt: Gower Publishing Co; 1985: 56.
41. Miles MB. Qualitative data as an attractive nuisance: the problem of analysis. *Admin Sci Quart.* 1979;4:590.
42. Lachenmeyer C. *The Language of Sociology.* New York, NY: Columbia University Press; 1971.
43. Ericsson KA, Simon HA. *Protocol Analysis: Verbal Reports as Data.* Cambridge, Mass: MIT Press; 1984.
44. Folger JP, Hewes DE, Poole MS. Coding social interaction. In: Dervin B, Voight M, eds. *Progress in Communication Sciences.* Norwood, NJ: Ablex Publishers; 1984;4.
45. Guetzkow H. Unitizing and categorizing problems in coding qualitative data. *J Clin Psychol.* 1950;6:47.
46. Miles MB, Huberman AM. Drawing valid meaning from qualitative data: toward a shared craft. In: Fetterman DM, ed. *Qualitative Approaches to Evaluation in Education: The Silent Scientific Revolution.* New York, NY: Praeger; 1988:222.
47. Bulmer M. Concepts in the analysis of qualitative data. *Sociological Rev.* 1979;27:651.
48. Bogdan R, Taylor SJ. *Introduction to Qualitative Research Methods.* New York, NY: John Wiley and Sons; 1975.
49. Guba EG. *Toward a Methodology of Naturalistic Inquiry in Educational Evaluation.* Los Angeles, Calif: UCLA Center for the Study of Evaluation; 1978.
50. Shepherd SK. *An Information Processing Approach to the Evaluation of Nutrition Education Materials.* University Park, Pa: Pennsylvania State University; 1987. Doctoral dissertation.
51. Guba EG. Investigative journalism as a metaphor for educational evaluation. Portland, Ore: Northwest Regional Educational Laboratory; 1979. Paper.
52. Tinsley HEA, Weiss DJ. Interrater reliability and agreement of subjective judgments. *J Counseling Psychol.* 1975;22:358.
53. Miles MB, Huberman AM. *Qualitative Data Analysis: A Sourcebook of New Methods.* Beverly Hills, Calif: Sage Publications; 1984.
54. Firestone WA, Dawson JA. Approaches to qualitative data analysis: intuitive, procedural, and intersubjective. In: Fetterman DM, ed. *Qualitative Approaches to Evaluation in Education: The Silent Scientific Revolution.* New York, NY: Praeger; 1988:209.
55. Conrad P, Reinharz S. Computers and qualitative data: editors' introductory essay. *Qualitative Sociol.* 1984;7:3.
56. Hiemstra R, Essman E, Henry N, Palumbo D. Computer-assisted analysis of qualitative gerontological research. *Educational Gerontol.* 1987;13:417.
57. Hirschman EC. Humanistic inquiry in marketing research: philosophy, method, and criteria. *J Marketing Res.* 1986;23:237.
58. Achterberg CL. Qualitative methods in nutrition education evaluation research. *J Nutr Educ.* 1988;20:244.

6. DESCRIPTIVE EPIDEMIOLOGIC RESEARCH

Bettylou Sherry, PhD, RD

Epidemiology is defined as the study of the distribution and determinants of disease. The epidemiologic methods for study design, data collection, and analysis provide the conceptual framework for describing the distribution of disease and for testing etiologic hypotheses for a disease or health consequence.

Descriptive epidemiologic studies focus on the enumeration and description of person, place, and time. These studies can be used to quantify the extent and location of nutrition problems within a population and suggest associations between diet and disease that can be evaluated in analytic research.

Person-associated characteristics can provide valuable insights into disease etiology. By examining who gets a disease, one can determine whether a particular age, gender, racial, or cultural group is more likely to be at risk. Other person-associated attributes such as socioeconomic status, family size, marital status, birth order, and personality traits may be important to consider as well. For example, family income and education both show a strong inverse association with the prevalence of iron-deficiency anemia in women of child-bearing age.[1]

Place may provide valuable insights about potential risk factors when describing nutrition-associated problems. For example, major geographic differences exist in cardiovascular disease mortality: Japan and France have very low rates in comparison with Northern European countries, New Zealand, and the United States.[2] This kind of data leads researchers to investigate reasons for the differences. Another example of the importance of place is that urban or rural living may affect availability and price of food items. Even with our modern food distribution system, the availability and price of highly nutritious, perishable foods such as fruits, vegetables, and fish vary dramatically by geographic region. This variability may have a significant impact on the poor. In poverty-stricken, inner-city areas, neighborhood groceries charge higher prices than do suburban supermarkets, making it more difficult for poor people to include adequate amounts of these foods in their diets.

Time factors can also impact disease. Seasonal and interannual fluctuations in cumulative incidence, as well as secular trends, may indicate patterns that help elucidate causation. Timing and length of exposure to a risk factor or the duration of latency period also may be important to consider.

This chapter focuses on descriptive epidemiologic research measurements and study designs applicable to nutrition and dietetics. The advantages and limitations of measurements and designs are presented.

Supported in part by grant MCJ 009043 from the Department of Health and Human Services.

DISEASE FREQUENCY

Disease frequency measures the amount of disease or morbidity in a population and is expressed as incidence or prevalence. In practice, the amount of disease translates into risk of disease and becomes the foundation for all descriptive and comparative work. For example, knowledge of the amount of a given disease in different populations can be used to compare the relative importance of this disease in these populations, or it may be used as a basis for comparing populations with different exposures to possible etiologic factors.

In addition to disease frequency, measures of vital statistics are used to provide more information about a disease or health consequence. The most commonly used indicators are infant mortality, birth rate, and death rate.

Measurements of Incidence

Cumulative incidence. *Cumulative incidence* (CI), or *incidence rate,* as it was formerly called, is the term used to describe disease frequency in a population. Cumulative incidence is the number of new cases of a disease occurring in a population at risk within a specified time interval. Frequently, the observed period is one year. It is defined as

$$\text{Cumulative incidence} = \frac{\text{No. of new cases}}{\text{Population at risk}} \times \text{Time period}$$

Cumulative incidence is normally expressed as the number of cases per 100 000 per year, however, it can also be described as the risk of disease (*Figure 6.1*). The population at the midpoint in the period of study is used as the population at risk. Technically, the denominator should include only those still at risk of disease, so the cases that have occurred in the population at risk should be subtracted. However, in large studies of relatively rare diseases, this is not usually done.

Figure 6.1
Calculation of cumulative incidence (CI).

$$CI = \frac{\text{No. of persons in whom the disease develops}}{\text{Population at risk}} \times \text{Time period}$$

$$= \frac{\text{No. of new cases of colon cancer in county A}}{\text{Midyear population of county A}} \times 1 \text{ yr}$$

$$= \frac{20 \text{ new colon cancer cases in county A in 1991}}{995\ 000 \text{ population } 7/1/91} \times 1 \text{ yr}$$

$$= \frac{20}{995\ 000}$$

$$= \frac{2.01}{100\ 000}$$

or the risk of colon cancer in 1991 in county A is 0.002%

When CI is calculated, the denominator is based on a population defined by geographic area, and it can have an even more specific focus such as a particular gender, age, or ethnic group. For example, the population at risk could be the state of Washington or the number of 14- to 17-year-old black girls in Boston, Mass. The use of a large population base such as these makes the results of a study generalizable to other populations that have similar characteristics to the study population. This means that the results of the study would have a more widespread use than if the study were conducted on a small, distinct group within a population, such as that of a small town.

Cumulative incidence is useful for documenting the relative importance of a disease in a population and to track changes in the occurrence of a disease over time. For example, changes in rates of premenopausal breast cancer are tracked by monitoring CI over time. Cumulative incidence can also provide etiologic clues. By comparing CI for populations that have different sex distributions, age groupings, ethnicities, or geographic locations, population groups with low or high rates of disease can be identified. This allows one to target high-risk groups for etiologic studies of a disease.

A specific application of CI for nutritionists and dietitians is to quantify the attack rate of an outbreak of food poisoning. *Attack rate* is the term substituted for CI when the period of observation is of short duration. In this situation, the population would be at risk for a short time, and the study period would encompass the entire epidemic. A good example would be an outbreak of salmonella infection in a public school. An outbreak investigation would seek to identify the food contaminated with *Salmonella* organisms by documenting what food was more likely to be eaten by those who became ill in contrast to those who remained well.

Incidence density. Sometimes the study population in a research project is dynamic. Subjects may be lost due to death or migration, or they may have acquired the disease and therefore are no longer at risk. To account for this loss of subjects, one can calculate *incidence density*, a term similar to CI, but calculated in a slightly different manner. As in the calculation of CI, the numerator includes the number of new cases of a disease. The denominator, however, is different. It includes the total amount of time each person in the study is at risk for disease (*Figure 6.2*). Incidence density is calculated as

$$\text{Incidence density} = \frac{\text{No. of new cases}}{\text{Person-time observed}} \times \text{Time period}$$

Figure 6.2
Calculation of person-time and incidence density.

Subject	1984	1985	1986	1987	1988	1989	1990	Total No. of Years at Risk
A		•————	——————	—X				2.0
B			•————	——————	——————	——————	——————	5.0
C					•————	——————	——————	3.0
D			•————	—X				1.0
						Total time at risk		11.0

• = Enrollment in study
— = Follow-up
X = Onset of disease

$$\text{Incidence density} = \frac{2 \text{ cases}}{11 \text{ person-years}}$$

$$= \frac{18 \text{ cases}}{100 \text{ person-years}}$$

Good resources for more in-depth discussions on the calculation of incidence density include Rothman[3] and Hennekens and Buring.[4]

Incidence density calculations would be useful in studies of osteoporosis in postmenopausal women in which the subjects might die or move from the study area. The advantage of using incidence density is that it permits inclusion of all of the time that each person participates in the study. If CI were used, only the subjects enrolled in the study for the entire project period would be included in the calculation of the rate. Thus, incidence density calculations tend to use participant time in a study more efficiently.

Measurements of Prevalence

Prevalence is the proportion of the population that is affected by a certain disease or condition at a given time, and it includes both new and existing cases. Technically, prevalence is not an incidence rate because it does not quantify the number of new cases of disease occurring within a specified period of time.

Prevalence can be expressed either as point or period prevalence. Point prevalence depicts one point in time, as in a cross-sectional survey, and unless otherwise specified, it is how the term generally is defined. Point prevalence is calculated as

$$\text{Point prevalence} = \frac{\text{No. of new and existing cases}}{\text{Total population at risk}} \times \text{Time}$$

Where time = one point in time.

In contrast,

$$\text{Period prevalence} = \frac{\text{No. of new, existing, and recurring cases}}{\text{Total population at risk}} \times \text{Time}$$

Where time = a period of time.

Sometimes incidence data are not available for a disease, so prevalence data are calculated. This is an acceptable alternative as long as the person interpreting the numbers clearly understands that incidence is the number of new cases within a certain period and prevalence is the number of old and new cases within a period. This lack of understanding of the difference between incidence and prevalence is one of the most common mistakes in scientific writing.

Prevalence data are advantageous for assessing the frequency of diseases or conditions that do not have an acute onset. Anemia and obesity are good examples of conditions that can best be described in this manner. Breastfeeding is generally expressed in terms of prevalence.

Prevalence is useful for targeting and planning health services because prevalence describes the burden of a disease or condition to a population. For example, National Health and Nutrition Examination Survey (NHANES) II data show that between the ages of 25 and 44 years, 13.8% of white women and 43.7% of black women have hemoglobin concentrations less than 120 g/L,[5] the lower limit of the accepted reference interval for this indicator.[6,7] Thus, these prevalence data indicate that many more black women than white women of child-bearing age have low or deficient concentrations of hemoglobin, suggesting that this group should be targeted for special services.

Prevalence is applicable for monitoring control programs for chronic illnesses such as anemia. A series of cross-sectional studies that document point prevalence can be used to track changes in the burden of a disease to a population.

The difference between incidence and prevalence can introduce important sources of bias when evaluating the effect of a screening program. In a screening program, both the issues of identification of cases and the effectiveness of intervention need to be examined. An initial survey of the prevalence of anemia before the implementation of a screening program may be compared with a follow-up survey that includes prevalent plus incident cases. The prevalence of the anemia may be the same at the two points in time. However, the important consideration is whether the same people were included in the "before" and "after" surveys or if old cases were being cured and new ones identified. Thus, because prevalence includes subjects who have survived, as well as new incident cases, more information is needed to make an evaluation meaningful. This example shows that prevalence can produce a biased view of disease, favoring chronic disease and underestimating short-term infectious diseases.

Measurements of Vital Statistics

In addition to disease frequency, vital records data can improve the understanding of disease or health consequences. Vital records data are obtained from birth certificates, death certificates, and census data. By law, birth and death certificates must be filed by the birth attendant or attending physician at the local town or city clerk's office. These data are forwarded to county and state offices for compilation and reporting. Census data are collected by the federal government at the beginning of each decade.

Birth and death certificate data are readily available from the vital records offices of a county or state. State vital statistic reports are published annually and can be obtained from the state office. They are also available in the public documents area in public, college, or university libraries.

In many states it is now possible to use computer data tapes that link birth and death records. This allows a researcher to obtain a more complete report of a newborn, in addition to information about the parents.

These data are especially useful for documenting the relative importance of a disease or health problem. For example, cause-specific maternal mortality rates can be used to identify the primary causes of maternal deaths. This would permit targeting the major problem areas such as maternal hypertension. This would in turn lead to the development of intervention strategies to reduce the risk of death from this problem.

The calculation of commonly used indices are summarized in *Table 6.1.*

SCREENING TESTS

Screening tests are designed to identify people who either have a disease that can be effectively treated in the early stages or who are at high risk for a disease and therefore can benefit from intervention measures to reduce their risk. Dietitians and nutritionists utilize screening tests at the community level, for example, to target children with anemia for iron supplementation. In a clinical setting, the screening of newborns for phenylketonuria is a routine practice. A

Descriptive Research

screening program may be established in a clinical setting to identify patients who are at high risk for a poor nutritional outcome to target them for special care to avoid or minimize their risk of nutritional depletion.

Reliability and Validity

Tests that are used for screening must be both reliable and valid. A reliable test is one that gives the same results when the test is repeated on the same person several times. In other words, a reliable test gives reproducible results. A valid test is one that measures what it is designed to measure. For example, a glucose tolerance test is used to diagnose diabetes mellitus; an increase in serum glucose concentration is indicative of diabetes. Validity is also used in epidemiologic studies to assess various methods of interest to dietitians, such as dietary assessment and anthropometric measures.

Table 6.1
Commonly Used Indices of Vital Statistics

Crude birth rate (per 1000 population)	=	$\dfrac{\text{No. of live births during year}}{\text{Average (midyear) population}}$
Infant mortality rate (per 1000 live births)	=	$\dfrac{\text{No. of deaths of children} < 1 \text{ year of age during year}}{\text{No. of live births in same year}}$
Neonatal mortality rate (per 1000 live births)	=	$\dfrac{\text{No. of deaths of children} < 28 \text{ days of age during year}}{\text{No. of live births in same year}}$
Fetal death ratio (per 1000 live births)	=	$\dfrac{\text{No. of fetal deaths}^{*} \text{ during year}}{\text{No. of live births in same year}}$
Fetal death rate (per 1000 live births and fetal deaths)	=	$\dfrac{\text{No. of fetal deaths during year}}{\text{No. of live births and fetal deaths in same year}}$
Maternal (puerperal) mortality rate (per 100 000 or 10 000 live births)	=	$\dfrac{\text{No. of deaths from puerperal causes during year}}{\text{No. of live births in same year}}$
Crude death rate (per 1000 population)	=	$\dfrac{\text{No. of deaths during year}}{\text{Average (midyear) population}}$
Age-specific death rate (per 1000 population)	=	$\dfrac{\text{No. of deaths among persons of a given age group during year}}{\text{Average (midyear) population in specified age group}}$
Cause-specific death rate (per 100 000 population)	=	$\dfrac{\text{No. of deaths from a stated cause during year}}{\text{Average (midyear) population}}$

* > 20 weeks' gestation

Sensitivity and Specificity

Two parameters used to assess the validity of a test are sensitivity and specificity. Sensitivity is the proportion of persons with the disease or condition who test positive. The greater the sensitivity of a test, the less likely it is that a negative result will misclassify a person. Specificity is the proportion of people without the disease or condition who test negative. The greater the specificity, the less likely it is that a positive test will misclassify a person. These tests are schematically described in *Figure 6.3.*

These parameters are used to establish cutoffs or reference interval limits for a test. The goal is to maximize both sensitivity and specificity to minimize false positive and false negative test results, but in reality there usually must be a compromise. A natural biological variability results in a spectrum of test values in any population. A few people with abnormally high or low values for a diagnostic test nevertheless will not have a disease. The converse will also occur: some people with a normal test result will have the disease. Where the normal reference range cutoff points are set will affect the number of false negatives and false positives. This in turn will affect the sensitivity and the specificity. Detsky et al[8] discuss how reference intervals are established to maximize sensitivity and specificity in their comparison of nutrition assessment techniques.

Figure 6.3
Schematic description of screening test indices and the calculation of these indices.

	Test Result	
	Positive	**Negative**
Disease or Condition Yes	a	b
No	c	d

Sensitivity = Proportion of those with a disease who have a positive test

$$= \frac{a}{a+b}$$

Specificity = Proportion of those without a disease who have a negative test

$$= \frac{d}{c+d}$$

Predictive Value

The predictive value of a test is its ability to accurately measure the proportion of the population with or without the disease or condition. Thus, the positive predictive value is the probability of disease, given a positive test; negative predictive value is the probability of no disease, given a negative test (*Figure 6.4*).

Predictive values are strongly affected by the number of people with and without disease. For example, if sensitivity and specificity are constant, the differences in predictive values positive for a test for anemia in populations of different sizes with prevalences of 25%, 3.3%, and 0.3% are notable (*Figure 6.5*). This example using a highly sensitive and specific test shows that in a population where anemia is rare, this screening test has a very low positive predictive value. In this situation, the screening test may not be of value for public health purposes.

For screening to be effective, it must have a major role in improving the outcome of illness. Thus, in addition to a screening test with a high positive predictive value, there must be an effective treatment or intervention for the disease or condition of interest. A protocol for following up with treatment for people identified as being at risk for disease by the test is an important part of the effectiveness of any screening program.

Descriptive Research

Figure 6.4
Schematic diagram of the
calculation of the predictive
value of a screening test.

		Test Result	
		Positive	**Negative**
Disease or Condition	**Yes**	a	b
	No	c	d

Predictive value positive = Proportion of those with a positive test who have a disease

$$= \frac{a}{a + c}$$

Predictive value negative = Proportion of those with a negative test who do not have a disease

$$= \frac{d}{b + d}$$

Figure 6.5
Comparison of predictive
values positive in populations of
different sizes and different
prevalences of anemia.

		Population = 400 Prevalence = 25%		Population = 3100 Prevalence = 3.3%		Population = 30 100 Prevalence = 0.3%	
		Test Result		Test Result		Test Result	
		+	−	+	−	+	−
Anemia	+	97	3	97	3	97	3
	−	10	290	100	2900	1000	29 000

Sensitivity	$= \frac{97}{100} = 97\%$	$\frac{97}{100} = 97\%$	$\frac{97}{100} = 97\%$
Specificity	$= \frac{290}{300} = 97\%$	$\frac{2900}{3000} = 97\%$	$\frac{29\,000}{30\,000} = 97\%$
Predictive value positive	$= \frac{97}{107} = 90.6\%$	$\frac{97}{197} = 49.2\%$	$\frac{97}{1097} = 8.8\%$

Diseases or conditions appropriate for screening are those that have serious consequences, a detectable preclinical phase, an effective treatment, and a high prevalence of preclinical disease in the population.

Phenylketonuria meets all but one of these criteria: It has a low prevalence of preclinical disease in the population, occurring in approximately 1 of 15 000 live births.[9] However, in affected infants, the elimination of all but the essential requirement of phenylalanine in the diet of an infant will prevent mental retardation. The social and economic costs of caring for a mentally retarded child are high. In contrast, the cost of screening all newborns is low, and the test is highly sensitive. In this example, a highly effective available treatment makes the cost of screening for a rare disease in a population justifiable.

It is also worthwhile to consider the practical qualities of a screening test. A suitable screening test is inexpensive, easy to administer, provides minimal discomfort to the patient, and has reliable, valid results.

Three biases must be considered in evaluating the limitations of screening programs. The first bias is that of volunteers or self-selection. On average, volunteers have a better health status than that of the general population. This means that in a screening program that includes only volunteers, the proportion with preclinical disease may be less than that of the general population. The second bias is that of lead time. Lead time refers to the amount of time the diagnosis is advanced by a screening program. Early diagnosis might make the treatment more effective. This would shorten the amount of time an affected person would have to suffer the consequences of a disease. This is an important consideration when evaluating the change in morbidity and mortality as a result of screening. Third, length bias must be considered. This refers to the length of the preclinical phase of disease. In a cross-sectional screening survey, cases that have a long preclinical phase of disease will be overrepresented.

DESCRIPTIVE RESEARCH DESIGN

Descriptive studies are the simplest of all research designs. They are simply a reporting of the characteristics of person, place, and time of a disease or a condition of interest. They may report on country-wide populations, small geographic areas, small groups of people, or individual subjects.

These studies are valuable for identifying potential associations between risk factors and a disease, as well as for elucidating patterns among particular population groups, places, or time periods and a disease. Frequently descriptive studies are cheaper and take less time than analytic studies because they use precollected data such as the National Food Consumption Survey, NHANES I, II, and III, vital statistics, or clinical records. Results from this type of research can form the basis of hypotheses for analytic research.

Correlational Studies

Correlational studies are beneficial for examining patterns relating a possible risk or causative factor in a disease. Often data from several countries are examined to identify these relationships. A good example of the application of this type of study to nutrition and dietetics is the international documentation of the relationship between diet and mortality from coronary heart disease (CHD) by Keys.[10] Using data from seven countries, Keys found a significant correlation between the proportion of calories from saturated fat and death from CHD. Keys' results suggested a causative relationship between saturated fat and CHD, but his findings could not document the biological process or evaluate the effect of other potential confounding factors such as physical exercise, obesity, and genetics. Analytic studies must be used for confirming these process-oriented relationships.

Case Reports and Case Series

Unique experiences of a patient or a group of patients with a similar diagnosis are reported in the literature as case reports or series. Accounts of this nature can provide the basis for an analytic approach to examining the factors of interest. These brief documentations also alert health care professionals as to possible, but not proved, beneficial or life-threatening aspects of a disease or its treatment. Historically, case reports or case series were used to document the beginning of an epidemic. A case series is of greater value than a single case report because it gives more documentation of evidence for the suggested hypothesis.

Surveys

Surveys provide a cross-sectional assessment of exposure to possible risk factors and prevalence of disease or health problems in a population at one point or period of time. These data provide an indication of the health of the population surveyed. In turn, this information can be used for the identification of health problems and for public health care planning.

Many national surveys have been done and are repeated periodically. Examples include the National Food Consumption Survey, NHANES I, II, and III, the Pediatric Nutrition Surveillance Survey, and the Health Interview Survey. All have sophisticated sampling frames to provide representative information from all segments of the population or special, high-risk population groups.

The advantage of cross-sectional surveys is that they can offer a representative overview of the health of a population. Their limitation is that the data cannot provide answers to questions of disease etiology. When a population is surveyed at one point in time, there is no way to determine whether exposure to a risk factor came before a disease. The only exception would be a one-time exposure, such as the nuclear accident at Chernobyl, or a genetic risk factor, such as eye color, or an enzyme defect.

For further discussion of surveys and using these large databases, see chapter 12.

SUMMARY

The two primary measures of disease frequency are incidence and prevalence. Cumulative incidence measures the rate of either the morbidity or mortality of a disease in a population over a specified period. Incidence density is similar to CI, but it uses person-time as the denominator. In contrast, prevalence describes the burden of a disease to a population: It reflects the number of cases, both existing and new, at a specified point or period in time.

Screening tests are used to document the amount of disease that can be affected positively by early intervention. These tests must be reliable and valid. Specificity and sensitivity are used to measure validity. The predictive value of the tests assesses its ability to accurately predict the proportion of the population with and without a disease. Predictive values are strongly influenced by disease prevalence.

The major descriptive study designs include correlational studies, case reports or series, and cross-sectional surveys. The primary uses for descriptive studies are to provide information to develop priorities for health care planning and to generate hypotheses to be tested in analytic research.

References

1. Life Sciences Research Office, Federation of American Societies for Experimental Biology. *Nutrition Monitoring in the United States—An Update Report on Nutrition Monitoring. Prepared for the US Department of Agriculture and the US Department of Health and Human Services.* Washington, DC: US Public Health Service, US Government Printing Office; 1989:144. DHHS publication PHS 89-1255.
2. Inter-Society Commission for Heart Disease Resources. Optimal resources for primary prevention of atherosclerotic diseases. *Circulation.* 1984;70:153A–205A.
3. Rothman KJ. *Modern Epidemiology.* Boston, Mass: Little Brown and Co; 1986:26–29.
4. Hennekens CH, Buring JE; Mayrent SL, ed. *Epidemiology in Medicine.* Boston, Mass: Little Brown and Co; 1987:58–60.
5. National Center for Health Statistics, *Hematological and nutritional biochemistry reference data for persons 6 months–74 years of age: United States, 1976–80.* Washington, DC: US Dept of Health and Human Services; 1982:41. DHHS publication PHS 83-2682. Series ll, no. 232.
6. O'Neal RM, Johnson OC, Schaefer AE. Guidelines for classification and interpretation of group blood and urine data collected as part of the National Nutrition Survey. *Pediatr Res.* 1970;4:103.
7. *Ten-State Nutrition Survey Reports, I–V.* Atlanta, Ga: Centers for Disease Control; 1972.
8. Detsky AS, Baker JP, Mendelson RA, Wolman SL, Wesson DE, Jeejeebhoy KN. Evaluating the accuracy of nutritional assessment techniques applied to hospitalized patients: methodology and comparisons. *JPEN J Parenter Enteral Nutr.* 1984;8:153–159.
9. Poskanzer DC. Neurological disorders. In: Clark DW, MacMahon B, eds. *Preventive and Community Medicine.* Boston, Mass: Little Brown and Co; 1981:265–291.
10. Keys A. *Seven Countries: A Multivariate Analysis of Death and Coronary Heart Disease.* Cambridge, Mass: Harvard University Press; 1980.

Further Reading

Hennekens CH, Buring JE, Mayrent SL, ed. *Epidemiology in Medicine.* Boston, Mass: Little Brown and Co; 1987.
Mausner JS, Kramer S. *Mausner and Bahn: Epidemiology—an Introductory Text.* 2nd ed. Philadelphia, Pa: WB Saunders Co; 1985.
Rothman KJ. *Modern Epidemiology.* Boston, Mass: Little Brown and Co; 1986.
Weiss NS. *Clinical Epidemiology: The Study of the Outcome of Illness.* New York, NY: Oxford University Press; 1986; 11. Monographs in Epidemiology and Biostatistics.

7. DESIGN AND USE OF QUESTIONNAIRES IN RESEARCH

Judy Perkin, DrPH, RD

The questionnaire is an important tool in dietetics descriptive research, just as it is in other descriptive research areas such as marketing and political science. Some of the areas in dietetics recently surveyed by questionnaires are: attitudes and symptoms of eating disorders, enteral nutrition formulary practices, vitamin and mineral supplementation practices, productivity in clinical dietetics, and third-party reimbursement.

Defined by Berdie et al,[1] as a "series of predetermined questions," a questionnaire can provide important information about behaviors, attitudes, beliefs, and characteristics of populations. It may be completed with the aid of an interviewer (in person or by telephone) or by the respondent alone (in person or by mail).[2] There are general considerations and suggestions that may be applicable to all questionnaires, but there are no hard and fast rules that apply in every situation. Each questionnaire is a product of survey design and is unique, depending on survey factors such as population sample, objectives, methods, timetable, and budget. As Sheatsley[2] notes, questionnaire design, construction, and use involve both intellectual work and trial and error. The purpose of this chapter is to help provide guidance to the dietitian who wishes to use the questionnaire as a tool in research, practice, or both.

STEPS IN THE QUESTIONNAIRE PROCESS

As described in this chapter, the questionnaire process consists of six steps: conceptualization, design and construction, pre-testing, administration, analysis and reporting of results, and utilization of results to affect knowledge and/or action.

Step 1: Conceptualization

A common problem related to the questionnaire process is lack of attention paid to conceptualization. Conceptualization should encompass both survey goals and the questionnaire instrument needed to achieve these goals. Thinking through the questionnaire process to visualize the end knowledge or action product is very important, and although it may seem at first time-consuming, conceptualization actually can conserve time and resources in the overall study process. Surveys that use the questionnaire as an instrument should have defined, meaningful goals. Issues addressed by the questionnaire should relate to the survey goals.

How the questionnaire results will be utilized should be part of the conceptualization process. For example, what are the conclusion options that will be chosen based on questionnaire answers? The focus should be in terms of "need to know" answers rather than "nice to know" answers. "Nice to know" answers usually are only tangential to survey goals and often are never analyzed. They have the further disadvantage of lengthening the questionnaire. Study or survey goals should be relevant, and questions in the questionnaire instrument in turn need to be relevant to these goals.[3] Important to defining relevance are knowledge of the conceptualized questionnaire subject matter (eg, in dietetics, nutrients, food habits, and food beliefs and behaviors); and knowledge of the population to be surveyed. In other words, is the questionnaire asking questions that really need to be answered to increase knowledge or decide about action? Are the right people being asked these questions?

Specifying "the right people" to answer questions in the conceptualization stage usually involves defining respondents on the basis of one or more characteristics such as age, sex, race, location, health status, occupation, socioeconomic status, and/or educational level. The knowledge *and* the ability of potential respondents to answer questions should be determined.[2] Assessment of ability to answer questions should take into consideration education level, literacy status, ability to recall information, language or languages spoken, and the physical ability to hear, see, speak, and write. Environmental factors related to ability are also important. Does the proposed respondent population receive mail or have telephones? Can they be accessed for an interview in their home or at another site?

McClendon and O'Brien[3] suggest two principles related to ability that should be considered: recency and cognitive accessibility. Their recency principle states that, in terms of more accurate respondent recall, recent use or thought about a piece of information is more important than when it was acquired. In other words, recency of thought about a topic is more important than the time when it was first learned in terms of recall ability. The principle of cognitive accessibility states that respondents will respond with the most easily accessed information they have on a topic. Applying these principles in assessment of ability has definite implications for questionnaire design.

Mode of questionnaire administration (interviewer versus respondent self-administration) and questionnaire administration location (in person, by phone, or by mail) are just two examples of design that are influenced by knowledge of respondent abilities. These and other respondent population considerations relevant to ability will be discussed under step 2.

These general thoughts about the scope and content of relevant survey questions, the appropriate population to be asked these questions, and the best means of asking the questions according to respondent ability need to be placed in the context of the survey's budget and timetable as the actual design and construction of the questionnaire begins.

Step 2: Design and Construction

Mode of administration. An important, initial design consideration is whether the questionnaire is to be administered by an interviewer, completed by the respondent, or administered by computer in an interactive mode with the respondent.

Interviews offer the following advantages: (1) flexibility (ability to repeat, probe, and make on-site distinctions about question appropriateness); (2) higher response rate; (3) ability to standardize and control the environment (including ability to record the time of the answer); (4) ability to control question order; (5) ability to observe nonverbal behavior; (6) ability to record spontaneous answers; (7) assurance that only the designated respondent answers the questions; and (8) enhanced ability to ensure that all questions are answered.[4] Bailey suggests that a more complex questionnaire (ie, one with detailed

Descriptive Research

instructions, multiple areas to be skipped, and many charts) may be better handled by interview.[4] Interviews also may be the only option for administration if a respondent population is illiterate, semiliterate, or physically disabled to the extent that questionnaire self-administration is difficult or impossible.

The option of completion of the questionnaire by the respondent also has its own advantages, among them: (1) cost (the interview format entails more labor costs); (2) speed (enhanced ability to administer questionnaires simultaneously to large numbers of subjects); (3) greater convenience for the respondent; (4) ability for respondents to remain anonymous; (5) ability to standardize wording completely; (6) ability to allow for the respondent to consult, review records, or conduct research as part of the answer process; and (7) greater accessibility to respondents with regard to both numbers and location.[4] Advantages 6 and 7 seem particularly relevant to the mailed self-administered questionnaire. A further advantage of the self-administered questionnaire is that it excludes the possibility of interviewer bias or error.[4]

Administration suggestions for use of both interviews and self-administered questionnaires are discussed further under step 4.

Computer administration of questionnaires is also a possibility.[5,6] O'Brien and Dugdale[5] found that the computer may elicit more candid answers than a personal interview. Computer questionnaire administration may also be more cost-effective and be less restrictive in terms of hours available for subject response.[5,6]

Language and readability. Once the mode of administration has been chosen, the researcher or practitioner can make design decisions about the language or languages to be used. These considerations should include not only the use of foreign languages along with or instead of English, but also the need to use braille, sign language, or other language forms appropriate to the defined respondent population. Another important decision consideration for dietitians involves appropriate reading levels for all questionnaire words, particularly for health-related terms. For example, given the defined respondent population, which would be the most appropriate term, *bed sores* or *decubitus ulcers*? Can such words as *delineate* or *verify* be used with the assurance that respondents will understand their meaning?

Achieving appropriate reading level, or using understandable terms, should be a goal in questionnaire design. Readability (or comprehension level) can be estimated through a variety of formulas. Examples include the SMOG formula,[7,8] the FOG index,[9] the Lorge and Flesch readability formula,[10] the Cloze procedure,[11] and the Flesch-Kincaid formula.[12] Several computer programs that assess readability are also available.[12]

Design visualization. Questionnaire length, layout, visual design (including paper color), print type, and issues related to respondents' anonymity or identification can be anticipated in the early phases of the design process. These factors will be discussed more extensively in the latter part of this section. The results of question construction will influence many of the same factors as the mode of administration decision discussed earlier. Question order or placement is a design factor that needs to be addressed once individual questions have been constructed. Question order is crucial to producing a document that flows logically and in a way that encourages response. Specific suggestions for question placement are discussed later in this chapter.

Question construction. Relevance of questions is a key point to remember at all times when proceeding to question construction. Three strategies can be employed to ensure that questions are worded or presented in ways that are relevant to the respondent:

1. If appropriate and necessary, multiple questionnaires tailored to specific characteristics of the respondent population (eg, male/female, patient/caregiver, vegetarian/omnivore) can be used.
2. Multiple wording can be used to enable the respondent to choose the appropriate term.
3. Contingency or skip questions can be used (eg, "If you answer No, proceed to question 4").[4]

Caution should be exercised if the multiple wording option is used in a self-administered questionnaire to ensure that the answer is clear and the problem of double-barreled questions is avoided. A double-barreled question is a question worded so that it includes two questions, for example, "Do you like milk and ice cream?" The researcher or practitioner might conclude that neither food is liked when, in fact, the respondent is answering that he or she does not like the combination or that he or she likes one food but not the other. Double-barreled questions are common mistakes[3] and provide problems for both the respondent and questionnaire analyst.

Another consideration in the construction of questions is the attempt to minimize ambiguity.[4] One way this can be accomplished is by providing definitions of terms in the questionnaire instrument. Terms such as *rural*, *urban*, and *poor* are subjective and need to be defined. Sentences also may be ambiguous. A poorly written, ambiguous question composed by this author for a diet-related questionnaire was "Do you read food labels?" To dietitians, this usually means reading the portions of the food label listing ingredients and nutrition information. Most respondents, however, interpreted this question to mean "Do you read the front of the label?" or "If you wish to purchase corn, do you read the front of the label and check that it says *corn*?" The question is ambiguous.

Question length is an important variable.[2] One researcher has advised keeping questions to 25 words or less[13] while some would say that a magic limit on word number is not critical, but that brevity is important.

Wording questions to avoid "loading" or "leading" in general is a good practice.[2,4] Loaded questions are ones that encourage or suggest an answer to a question and put the onus on the respondent if he or she wishes to deviate from the subtly prompted response. An example of a loaded question that inappropriately suggests an answer is "Do you binge?" The respondent may hesitate to admit to this behavior, so the hidden suggested response is "No." Nevertheless, if worded appropriately, sometimes loading can be effective in dealing with sensitive areas in which the respondent may not feel comfortable admitting an activity. For example, a loaded question that may be helpful is "How often do you binge?" The respondent could say, "never," but potentially would feel comfortable responding with a number.

Double negatives should be avoided in questions because they are confusing.[2] An example of a question using a double negative is "Do you favor or oppose passage of a USDA regulation not allowing food stamps to be used to purchase peanut butter?"

Another rule of questionnaire construction is that in general, factual questions are better than abstract questions.[2] For example, "How would you rate your overall diet—good, fair, poor?" is a difficult question for a respondent to answer. The answer is also difficult for the investigator to interpret. The concept of "overall diet" is unclear: Is this diet throughout the life span or for one year? The rating scale is also both abstract and subjective. One person's "fair" may be another person's "good."

Response formats.   Once a question that would seem to elicit a needed response to accomplish survey goals has been constructed, the issue of response format should be addressed. The two major response formats categorize questions as either open-ended or closed-ended. The response format to an open-ended question is not specified, whereas the response format to a closed-ended question is specified. Some questionnaires include both types of response formats, while some use only one. Study or survey goals, budget, and timetable all influence choice of response format.

Both major response format types have advantages and disadvantages. Open-ended questions, for example, may be useful in preliminary survey work when the researcher does not know all possible answers or believes that all answers cannot be anticipated.[2] Responses from an initial open-ended question may later give the researcher more confidence in constructing a closed-ended question on the topic. Another potential advantage to the use of the open-ended question is that it can be helpful when the number of potential responses is large. For example, asking "What vegetables do you eat more than three times per week?" and leaving a blank space for response would be simpler than listing all potential vegetables that could be cited. In this case, use of an open-ended question also shortens questionnaire response time for the respondent. Another advantage of the open-ended question is that it can allow for creativity, complexity, and clarity in response.[4] Some respondents may feel more assured that they have answered a question more accurately and may appreciate the chance to express themselves in a way that is not structured by the researcher.

One potential disadvantage of an open-ended question is that it may not be truly reflective of a response, since persons with better writing skills are at some advantage when faced with this type of question.[4] Geer[14] states, however, that subject interest is a more important factor than writing ability in generating a good open-ended response. Other cited drawbacks of open-ended questions relate to potentially increased costs with use, coding difficulties,[14] and collection of irrelevant information.[4] Open-ended questions also may be perceived as too time-consuming or laborious by some potential respondents.[4] Those choosing to use open-ended questions in dietetic research may wish to consult with a sociologist or statistician trained in techniques for coding open-ended questions. Use of specified procedures may increase the reliability of coding open-ended questions.[15]

Closed-ended questions have their own set of advantages and may be desirable to use in mailed or self-administered questionnaires.[4] Advantages of closed-ended questions are that responses are in standard categories and are easier to code and analyze, and that responses are usually relevant to the question as defined by the intent of the person or persons constructing the questionnaire. Respondents also may be able to ascertain question intent more easily if they see response categories. Another important advantage is that some respondents may perceive this question type as simpler to answer.[4]

Disadvantages of closed-ended questions are possible guessing or random responses, inability or unwillingness of a respondent to answer within categories provided, and the possibility of forcing choices and therefore not describing or seeing the potential true level of response variation in the respondent population.[4]

Open-ended questions usually are followed by a blank space for a response.[4] The response formats for closed-ended questions fall into one of several types, depending on elicited response content: interval, ratio, nominal, and ordinal.[4] An interval response is one that is ordered and for which there is equality among all ranks. A ratio response format is an interval measure for which there is a set zero point. A nominal response is defined as one that is discrete (non-overlapping) and nonnumerical; it is not a graded scale. (Nonnumerical overlapping responses will be discussed later, with suggestions for clarification.) An ordinal response format uses rank-ordered categories (such as excellent, good, fair, and poor) and therefore has a directional meaning. Examples of the four response format types for closed-ended questions are shown in *Table 7.1*. A general rule of construction for all closed-ended formatted responses is that all potential answers should be included in an uncluttered fashion, and that all potential answers should have clear meaning.[4]

For interval and ratio responses, all potential responses can be listed, but for reasons of both space and utility, interval and ratio responses are more commonly grouped, as in income response categories. Two errors should be avoided when grouping responses.[4] One is overlapping responses (eg, asking the individual's income and providing the ranges of $10 000–$15 000, $15 000–$20 000, and $20 000 or above). People who earn $15 000 or $20 000 would be placed in a quandary as to which response to give. Another error to be avoided is failing to include all potential responses (eg, asking about money spent each week for food and providing as response categories $0–$10, $11–$20, $21–$30, and so forth). The person who spends $20.50 has no category to check unless he or she has been instructed to round to the nearest dollar. It should also be kept in mind that while grouping of continuous variables may be useful in some instances, it does pose limitations for subsequent statistical analyses.

Nominal responses are generally formatted with a blank or box to be checked or crossed. Assigning a number to a nominal response and requesting that the number be circled is another option. Nominal response categories are most frequently listed one above another, but side-by-side placement can be used with appropriate spacing, dots, or parentheses.[4] Berdie and associates[1] recommend vertical over horizontal placement, since respondents sometimes mark blanks incorrectly because they are not sure if they are to mark before or after their desired response. *Figure 7.1* illustrates the formatting of nominal responses both vertically and horizontally.

When a respondent is asked to check all nominal responses that apply, the term *inventory* is used to describe the format. Inventory placement is usually also in vertical categories.[4]

Categories that are nonnumerical and potentially not mutually exclusive were mentioned earlier. Use of "other" or "none of the above" as responses, or having the respondent check all that apply (ie, inventory format) may be helpful in these instances.[1] Questions about race or ethnicity have response options that are not mutually exclusive and are nonnumerical. Biracial respondents, for example, have particular difficulty with questions about race or ethnicity if they are forced by question format to mark only one choice.

Ordinal response categories may be formatted similar to nominal categories (boxes or blanks to be checked, numbers to be circled), but they also may be shown as continua with scored labels at the continuum endpoints. Care must be taken in designing the scoring system for such continua. Too few categories may not distinguish these differences among respondents but too many categories can be confusing.[4] Berdie and associates[1] recommend that an equal number of options be placed on each side of the midpoint.

Ordinal variables may also be presented vertically and respondents asked to rank-order them. If possible, such vertical listings should be randomly assigned, as order of vertical listing may affect response.[4]

One issue pertinent to all categories of response is whether to include such options as "don't know," "no opinion," and "can't decide."[1,2] Berdie et al[1] recommend inclusion of the "don't know" option rather than risk the chance of obtaining incorrect information by forced choice. Sheatsley[2] cautions that there is no universal rule about inclusion or exclusion of these options, and that some respondents may view them as quick and easy choices and fail to answer more thoughtfully and potentially more accurately. Poe and colleagues[16] recommend that "don't know" not be included as a potential response to factual questions. In analyzing pretest results from a mortality survey conducted under the auspices of the National Center for Health Statistics, these researchers found that the exclusion of the "don't know" option resulted in a greater number of useable responses without altering the substance of responses. They also note that exclusion of the "don't know" option made their questionnaire less cluttered and slightly shorter.

Another issue to be considered when asking questions about frequency and magnitude of dietary intake is whether the options as constructed could lead to underreporting. Research on questionnaire use with alcoholics, for example, indicates that providing response options indicative of greater intake and frequency are most effective[17] in avoiding the problem of underreporting.

Question placement. Once questions and response categories have been formulated and formatted, the process of question placement or question ordering can begin. Some suggestions for question placement:
- Nonthreatening, simple-to-respond-to questions should come first.[1,2] Berdie and associates[1] suggest that it also helps if these questions have interest value and are not perceived of as dull.
- Sensitive or difficult questions should be placed close to the end of the questionnaire.[2] Some researchers recommend that demographic questions also be placed at the end of a questionnaire.
- A logical content order to question sequence should be established.[1,2]
- Within content categories, broad questions should start, and more specific questions should follow.[2]
- Transitional phases or visual distinctions should be provided between content sections.[1]
- Important items should not be placed last on the questionnaire, as they may be overlooked or left unanswered.[1]
- The question numbering system must be clear, not confusing.[1]

Questionnaire length. At this point, the investigator should assess the appropriateness of questionnaire length. Questions should be reviewed again for relevance to study goals. In general, the longer the questionnaire, the more costly it will be in terms of supplies, resources, and time.[2] It is thus important to ensure that all information requested is needed and will be used. Although the effect of questionnaire length on response rate is debatable,[18] it seems reasonable that there is a length limit beyond which persons will fail to respond.[1] Berdie et al,[1] however, make the point that interest value of a questionnaire may be more important than length in determining response.

The role of computers. Computers can play a vital role in the questionnaire design and construction phase as well as their more familiar use in data analysis.[19] A word processor can eliminate cutting and pasting of typed material throughout the various draft stages. In addition, once all questions and response categories have been constructed and placed in order, information needed for later computer processing can potentially be placed directly on the form. Karweit and Meyers[19] highly recommend consultation with computer staff during the design phase. Berdie and associates[1] introduce a note of caution and warn that accommodating requirements to computerize should not overshadow the need to make the questionnaire "respondent friendly."

Design considerations. Some further design considerations relate to self-administered questionnaires, particularly ones that are mailed. Dillman[20] outlines one process called the Total Design Method (TDM), the general principles of which involve booklet format, size, question placement, and visual cues. He reports that 28 studies that followed his method in its entirety earned a mean response rate of 77%.[20] This rate is excellent, given that a 50% return rate for mailed questionnaires is considered adequate.[4]

Berdie and associates[1] make the following suggestions regarding visual appearance and enhancement of design for self-administered questionnaires:
- Instructions should be concise and clear. Better yet, if a change in question wording can eliminate the need for instructions, the question should be changed.
- The areas where answers are to be marked should be as close to the questions as possible.
- The term *questionnaire* should not appear on the form itself. The term may have a bad connotation if a respondent has previously received poorly designed questionnaires.
- The word *over* should be included at the bottom of the front side of a two-sided form.
- Too many questions should not be placed on one page, creating a crowded appearance.
- If the questionnaire is to be mailed, a name and return address should be printed directly on the questionnaire, even when a self-addressed return envelope is included, since the envelope may be misplaced or lost.

Another design consideration for the self-administered questionnaire is paper color. Berdie,[1] Fox,[21] and their respective colleagues believe that colored paper can add interest and increase response rate.

Berdie et al[1] also recommend that printing and paper for questionnaires be of the best quality possible within the limits of the study budget. Investigators need to convince respondents of the quality of their studies and respondents are influenced by these visual cues.

A final design consideration for the self-administered questionnaire is determining whether respondents are to be anonymous or identified. Bailey[4] believes that unless knowledge of identity is important to ensure response clarity, allowing respondents to be anonymous is the best decision. Anonymity, as defined by Bailey,[4] is when "the researcher is unable to link the respondent with the questionnaire he or she answered." If follow-up while assuring anonymity is desired, Bailey[4] states that a note may be sent to all potential respondents worded as follows:

> If you have already mailed your questionnaire, please disregard this notice. We have no means of identifying respondents, as all replies are anonymous. Thus, we are sending this reminder to all, since we have no way of knowing whether or not you have responded already.

One potentially less costly alternative is to assure the respondent that only the researcher will have identity information and that answers will be kept confidential. Questionnaires can be assigned numbers to which only the researcher has coded names. Another relatively inexpensive alternative is to instruct respondents to return a separate postcard listing their names and addresses after completing and returning the questionnaire.[4] Both Bailey[4] and Berdie et al,[1] advise against techniques such as writing identification numbers in invisible ink.

Not all researchers in the area of questionnaire design have found that anonymity increases response rate or influences response. Fuller,[22] for example, found little difference between respondent answers in anonymous versus identity-known situations. Researchers should keep in mind that confidentiality can be maintained even if respondents are not anonymous to the researcher. A system of code numbers linked to names on only one document kept by the researcher is one method of accomplishing this. Use of aggregate information for publication or report purposes also aids in maintaining confidentiality for individual respondents.

There are also design considerations unique to questionnaire forms that are to be used in an interview setting. Berdie and colleagues[1] suggest the following:

- Different type styles or some distinctive device should be used to separate parts of the questionnaire to be read to the respondent from parts not to be read to the respondent.
- Questions should be printed only on the front of pages.
- Sufficient instructions should be provided to the interviewer to allow him or her to proceed in the desired question sequence. This is particularly important if a questionnaire includes skip or contingency questions.
- Enough space should be allowed on the form so that the interviewer may record pertinent additional information.
- Response options should be limited to a number that the respondent can easily remember.
- The interview should end with a closed-ended, rather than an open-ended, question. This will aid the interviewer in closure.

Step 3: Pretesting

The third step in the questionnaire process is the pretest phase. Pretesting ideally should be conducted with persons typical of the respondent population. Sheatsley[2] recommends pretesting with 12 to 25 people, and using several interviewers for the pretest if more than one will be administering the questionnaire. For mailed or interview questionnaires, it may be have respondents or the interviewer record the amount of time take questionnaire. Bailey[4] urges that respondents also be encol questions. Questionnaires should be pretested using the m tion specified for the final questionnaire product.[4]

120

Clues to problems in questionnaire design and construction that may become apparent in the pretesting phase may include: a large number of non-responses not attributable to contingency or skip questions; a pattern of small variation in response; many responses given with qualifications; and responses perceived as meaningless.[4] These clues need to be examined critically to determine if they are indicative of problem areas. Hunt and associates[23] report that pretests are particularly useful in detecting missing alternate responses.

Once the questionnaire has been pretested, the designer needs to review the results and make appropriate changes in question wording, response categories, question order, instructions (including definitions), and questionnaire length. If major changes are made at this point, the revised questionnaire also should be pretested to ensure that the appropriate changes were made.[2]

Step 4: Administration

Achieving a good (or high) response rate is a major goal of the administration phase. Response rate should be defined prior to questionnaire administration and when reporting results. Kviz[24] suggests that response rate be defined as C/E where C is the number of completed questionnaires and E is the number of persons sampled by the questionnaire. Even this definition is problematic because all questions on a questionnaire might not be answered, and how one defines the population sampled is not always clear. For instance, do questionnaires returned for incorrect address count as mailed questionnaires?[4] The best course is for the researcher to both define and report response rate in research reports.

The definition of an adequate response rate to a questionnaire is not absolute. Obviously, the higher the response rate, the better because a greater representation of the population is achieved. Some researchers define a 50% response rate as adequate,[4] while others seek a 90%+ response rate.[1] Mailed surveys are more likely to have response rates in the 30% to 50% range, while interviews typically yield response rates of more than 70%.[25] Techniques to increase response rates will be discussed later, but it should be kept in mind that nonresponse may produce bias in results.

Another consideration prior to questionnaire administration is obtaining approval from the appropriate institutional review board dealing with human subjects. Some boards may require that participants sign a consent form before the questionnaire is administered or, in some instances, boards may decide that completion of the questionnaire after the purpose is explained denotes implied consent. Use of a questionnaire is a form of human research and does need appropriate review. Researchers also should be aware that questionnaires mailed to another institution for distribution will most likely need to be reviewed again by the appropriate secondary institutional review board.

Informed consent may affect response rate if sensitive issues are being surveyed. Singer[26] reports that in one instance, 8% of a national probability sample indicated they were willing to be interviewed, but refused to sign a consent form.

Mailed questionnaires. Mailed questionnaires should be accompanied by a one-page cover letter stating the purpose of the research, how results will be used and sponsorship of the project. The researcher also should indicate that individual responses will be maintained in confidence. Any plans for publication of questionnaire data should be stated. If questionnaire responses will be anonymous, it should be so stated in the cover letter. If not, reasons for needing to know the respondents' identities should be given.[4] Berdie and associates[1] recommend inclusion of a phrase such as "Please complete as soon as you can" to prompt respondents to avoid procrastination, rather than a deadline. A deadline date can be used, however, and if used, it should be given in the cover letter. The cover letter also should give information related to questionnaire return. If a stamped return envelope is included, the cover letter should make note of it. Most importantly, the cover letter should indicate the value of appreciation for the respondents' cooperation in completing and returning the questionnaire.

Fox et al[21] identify several factors that appear to increase response rate to mailed questionnaires: colored paper (as opposed to white), inclusion of a stamped return envelope, first-class postage, a prenotification letter, sending a follow-up postcard, and mentioning a university as questionnaire sponsor. Not all researchers agree that first-class postage is necessary. McCrohan and Lowe,[27] for example, found no difference in return rates between return envelopes bearing third-class and first-class postage.

Follow-up letters, postcards, or calls can increase response rates to mailed questionnaires. A follow-up letter to a nonrespondent can include another copy of the questionnaire.[1] The technique for follow-up in an anonymous survey has been discussed previously.

Interviews. Completion of an interview questionnaire involves contacting the respondent and conducting the interview. The respondent population must be understood to facilitate the process of contact. Contact by telephone may necessitate six to seven callbacks.[1] The purpose of the interview and other information that would be conveyed in a cover letter accompanying a mailed survey needs to be reviewed verbally upon respondent contact.

Using an interview questionnaire also may mean training the interviewers. Fowler and Mangione[28] discuss interview training in detail, and they outline four general rules:
1. Read questions exactly as worded.
2. Probe inadequate answers nondirectly.
3. Record answers without interviewer discretion.
4. Maintain an interpersonally neutral, nonjudgmental relationship with the respondent.

Frank and associates[29] recommend interviewer training when using the 24-hour recall for research purposes. Their report emphasizes the importance of interviewers' being familiar with and consistent in the use of criteria for naming foods, recording food quantities consumed, and coding foods. These researchers recommend conducting duplicate recalls to a quality assurance technique.

Telephone interviewing is a relatively new technique being explored for dietary questionnaire administration.[30,31] Krantzler et al[31] report that the telephone interview can obtain dietary information similar in quality to the information obtained in a personal interview. Computerized interviewing discussed earlier[5,6] is another option for interview administration.

Other. Dietitians may administer questionnaires in a way not typically discussed in social science methodology texts. For example, questionnaires may be distributed in a clinic or educational setting to be completed by the respondents and returned on site. In these cases, the cover letter may be attached to the front of the questionnaire or read aloud to the respondent or respondents. This form of administration combines many of the advantages of the interview and the self-administered questionnaire. Knowledge of population literacy and vocabulary still remain important design issues. Having writing instruments on site will facilitate response.

Stage 5: Analysis and Reporting of Results

This stage of the questionnaire process falls under the rubric of statistical analysis and research reports discussed elsewhere in this volume; however, it is appropriate to discuss in this chapter the concepts of validity and reliability as they relate specifically to questions and questionnaires.

Question validity is usually approached using the constructs of face validity, criterion validity, or both.[4] Face validity is defined by researcher judgment and is an assessment of whether the question truly measures a behavior, attitude, or opinion. Criterion validity involves measuring the question against "the truth" derived by another measure. An example would be trying to assess the truth about food consumed by assessing whether two measures of food consumption (such as the 24-hour recall and the three-day diet record) agree.

Reliability is a measure of consistency. Berdie et al[1] define a reliable question as one "that consistently conveys the same meaning to all people in the population being surveyed." Cronbach[32] describes retesting and parallel testing methods used to assess reliability. Use of statistical formulas for testing reliability such as Kuder-Richardson formulas and the Guttman lower bounds formulas are also reviewed in this reference, to which readers are referred for details.

The analysis phase involves assessment of the reliability and validity of questions. Have the questions elicited consistent as well as accurate and relevant data? If the answer is yes, questionnaire results can be utilized to affect knowledge and action.

Stage 6: Utilization of Results to Affect Knowledge and Action

Questionnaire results can provide important information for policy- and decision-makers as well as for researchers. Questionnaire results may provide knowledge that has impact on management of foodservice operations, clinical practice, or community programming and service delivery. Questionnaire (or survey) research can set the stage for development of laboratory or clinical experiments, and questionnaires can be useful in determining knowledge and attitudes as both preface to and evaluation of educational efforts. When appropriately constructed, administered, and analyzed, questionnaires can advance knowledge and provide the framework for constructive action plans.

EXAMPLES OF COMMONLY USED DIETARY QUESTIONNAIRES

It is useful to look at the 24-hour recall and the food frequency questionnaire as examples of questionnaires commonly used in dietetic research. This section will focus on reliability and validity of instruments as used in previous research.

The 24-hour recall is generally administered in an interview setting. Its construction in practice settings may be loose (ie, no form and simply asking and recording the foods and beverages that were consumed the preceding day). For research purposes or in practice settings that demand precision, the 24-hour recall should be formatted carefully and consistently using question construction techniques previously discussed. The 24-hour period must be defined and used consistently. Questioning about quantification also needs consistency, and food models or photos may be used as aids. Readers are again referred to Frank et al[29] for a discussion of interview technique in the 24-hour recall. Although clinicians may express judgment while conducting a 24-hour recall for client counseling purposes, the dietetic researcher should not. Judgmental statements may bias the respondent.

The food frequency questionnaire is used both in interview and self-administered situations. Major design considerations relate to choice of foods, categorization of consumption frequency, and whether and how to quantify consumption.

In one publication specifically focusing on dietary instruments, reliability has been defined as "representativeness," ie, in terms of both interrespondent and intrarespondent data.[33] Reliability of dietary questionnaires is also a function of measurement accuracy. This dimension of reliability defined as "the ability of a procedure to give the same results when used repeatedly in the same situation"[34,35] is compromised by measurement error (in both the data collection and analysis phases).

The 24-hour recall is considered to be fairly reliable in terms of obtaining information related to mean nutrient intakes for populations, but to obtain reliability because of individual, day-to-day diet variation, it is recommended that data from several 24-hour recalls be used (ie, serial use). As summarized by Block,[36] there is research indicating that, to reflect a person's daily mean caloric intake within ± 20% for a one-year period, a survey would need "to obtain four 24-hour recalls for the least variable half of the population and nine 24-hour recalls for 90% of the population." Beaton et al[37,38] note that study patterns of variance can be helpful in data interpretation. These researchers particularly note the problem of intraindividual variation in the 24-hour recall, which may result in the improper classification of subjects with regard to their usual diet intakes. Rush and Kristal[34] point out that the smaller the intraindividual variance and the larger the interindividual variation, the greater the reliability of a dietary measure such as the 24-hour recall. Reliability of dietary measurement of the 24-hour recall has been tested in various populations—pregnant women[34] and the elderly[39] are just two examples.

Reliability of the food frequency questionnaire has also been studied. Willett and colleagues[40] published in 1983 an evaluation of the reliability (or reproducibility) of a semiquantitative food frequency questionnaire. These researchers administered the questionnaire two times in a one-year period to 173 respondents (female nurses). Intraclass correlation coefficients ranged from 0.49 for vitamin A to 0.71 for sucrose and were comparable to intraclass correlation coefficients computed from repeated one-week diet records completed by these same respondents. Pietinen et al[41] tested the reproducibility of a food frequency questionnaire that included a booklet containing photographs of portion sizes. In this study, the questionnaire was completed three times at intervals of three months. The range of intraclass correlation was 0.56 (vitamin A) to 0.88 (alcohol). In 1988, Pietinen and associates[42] published the results of a reliability test of a qualitative food frequency questionnaire containing 44 food items. One hundred seven respondents completed the questionnaire three times at intervals of three months. The intraclass correlation range was from 0.52 for vitamin A to 0.85 for polyunsaturated fat. Reproducibility was best for both foods consumed infrequently and foods consumed daily. Smith-Barbaro et al[43] examined the influence of varying the format of a food frequency questionnaire on reliability. These researchers concluded that a food frequency questionnaire that contained broad food categories ordered by meal and that was administered at one-month intervals was associated with greatest reliability.

Validity of the 24-hour recall and the food frequency questionnaire has been studied extensively. Validity, or the ability of the instrument to measure what it in fact purports to measure, has been assessed in several ways for dietary intake study instruments. One approach to measuring validity of reported intake is to observe actual intake.[36] Another approach compares intake as reported by the respondent with respondent intake information obtained from another person (eg, spouse or parent). A third approach, one that is commonly used, is to compare one measure of dietary intake with another.[36] Rush and Kristal[34] caution against this last approach, which does not technically involve an external standard. Use of physical, biochemical, or anthropometric measures to validate dietary data is problematic, since these measures are under multiple influence.[34] Block[36] notes that choice of a validation measure ultimately depends on how data will be interpreted and used, ie, what is of interest: group means, individual assessment, or distribution of individual respondents within a group or groups along a high-low spectrum.

Many factors affect the validity of diet intake as measured by tools such as the 24-hour recall and food frequency questionnaire. Examples are: failure of the respondent to remember foods eaten or amounts consumed; respondent characteristics that predispose to underreporting or overreporting; respondent's answering to please the interviewer; and respondent disinterest.[1] Errors in validity also can occur due to interviewer error or lack of training, or due to errors in the nutrient database used.[1]

Memory (or recall) is a major factor influencing the validity of responses obtained by retrospective dietary methods such as the 24-hour recall and the food frequency questionnaire.[44] Some people will not or cannot report foods consumed; some cannot remember portion sizes accurately; some may report food consumption that has not occurred. Some reports also indicate that factors such as current dietary intake and value placed on a food may also influence recall.[44]

As mentioned earlier, the validity of the 24-hour recall has been the subject of several investigations. In 1952, Young et al,[45] comparing the 24-hour recall, the seven-day diet record, and the dietary history, concluded that the 24-hour recall and seven-day diet record were comparable in terms of measuring group dietary intakes. Karvetti and Knuts[46] conclude that the 24-hour recall had a higher validity with group use, as opposed to individual use. Several studies in various population groups report that responses on 24-hour recalls tend to exhibit a "flat slope syndrome".[47-50] The term *flat slope syndrome* is used to describe the tendency to underestimate high consumption and overestimate low consumption.[46] Validity of the 24-hour recall with specified population groups has been a fertile area of research, with the elderly[48,51] and children[49,52-56] being of special concern.

The food frequency questionnaire also has been the subject of validity studies. Samet et al[57] in 1984 concluded that in large-scale studies, food frequency questionnaire results are valid when used to establish relative nutrient intakes for subject groups. Earlier in the same year, Chu and colleagues[58] reached the same conclusion, but pointed out that adjunct quantitative measures are needed to analyze individual diets and may be important in cohort studies measuring incidence of chronic disease. Mullen et al[59] also voice caution about the validity of the food frequency questionnaire with regard to estimating individual nutrient intake. Their study involving college students found that it is not a useful tool for some who misestimate their intake.

When food frequency questionnaire validity has been assessed through comparison with diet records, food frequencies have fared well. Willett and associates[60] found an overall mean correlation coefficient of 0.60 when comparing 18 nutrient intakes measured by both dietary record and food frequency. Margetts et al[61] administered a food frequency questionnaire three years after completion of a 24-hour diet record and found a correlation of 0.60 for calories and 0.34 for vitamin A. These researchers concluded that the food frequency questionnaires could substitute for diet records in large epidemiologic investigations. Krall and Dwyer[62] studied food frequency questionnaires kept by subjects admitted to a metabolic unit where known food quantities and types were given. They found that in using the food frequency questionnaire, some food items consumed were not reported. They postulated that questionnaire wording may have played a part since nonreported items were not specified by the questionnaire, but had to be designated by the respondent in "other" categories. Overall, they found that food frequency questionnaires were prone to underestimation of actual nutrient consumption.

Krall and Dwyer also had subjects complete three-day diaries and found that these too underestimated intake, especially for vitamin A and calories.[62] This finding implies that assessing validity by comparing a diet record and a food frequency may be comparing two measures that tend to underestimate actual or true intake values, and therefore may be ascribing greater validity to these methodologies than exists in fact.

Validity studies of the food frequency questionnaire instrument frequently target specific populations, assess intake of a particular nutrient or nutrients, or both. Musgrave et al,[63] for example, compared calcium intakes estimated from four-day records with those estimated through a food frequency questionnaire administered to 26 women. The correlation was found to be r = 0.73 in the winter and r = 0.84 for the summer. The Musgrave food frequency questionnaire was designed to include good sources of calcium defined by content and frequency of use. Blom and associates[64] studied the validity of the food frequency questionnaire with a specific population group, children aged 2 to 16 years. Validity was assessed through comparison of data obtained from seven-day diet records. Although agreement was "fairly good," these researchers found that sensitivity of the food frequency questionnaire was low—ie, it had a high probability of failure to identify intake extremes.

Although the use of biochemical measures to assess the validity of dietary measure is controversial, the technique has been used in validity research with the food frequency questionnaire. Roidt et al,[65] for example, correlated food frequency questionnaire intake estimates of retinol, beta-carotene, total carotenoids, and total vitamin A; serum retinol, alpha-carotenoids, and total vitamin A; and serum retinol, alpha-carotene, and beta-carotene. Only weak associations were found due to a variety of confounding factors. The weak results of this study lend credence to assertions that biochemical measures should not be used in diet validity assessments. Romieu and colleagues[66] suggest an empirical weighting system as a method of validity assessment utilizing both dietary and biochemical data. Under this system, weights would be calculated using a multiple regression model, with biochemical measures as dependent variables and foods as independent variables. A person's nutrient intake would be calculated by multiplying food amounts by the appropriate regression coefficients. It is suggested that results could be applied to other population samples.

Table 7.1
***Response Formats Frequently
Used in Professional
Questionnaire Design***

Interval (ordered and equal ranks)

Examples:
- Temperature scale with all degrees above and below zero
- Monetary scale showing monetary excesses and deficits

Ratio (interval measure with set zero point)

Examples:
- Weight scale
- Course grade scale

Nominal (nonnumerical, non-overlapping responses)

Examples:
- Male, female
- Fruit, vegetable, meat

Ordinal (rank-ordered responses with directional meaning)

Examples:
- Excellent–Good–Fair–Poor
- Agree–Disagree
- Always–Most of the time–Some of the time–Rarely or Never
- Regularly–Often–Seldom–Never
- Approve–Disapprove
- Favor–Oppose
- Too many–Not enough–About right
- Too much–Too little–About the right amount
- Better–Worse–About the same
- More likely–Less likely–No difference

Adapted from Sheatsley PB. Questionnaire construction and item writing. In: Rossi PH, Wright JD, Anderson AB, eds. *Handbook of Survey Research.* Orlando, Fla: Academic Press Inc; 1983: 195–230; and Bailey KD. *Methods of Social Research.* New York, NY: Free Press, Macmillan Publishing Co Inc; 1978.

Figure 7.1
Nominal response formats.

Vertical placement

Please indicate your sex (gender):

○ Male
○ Female

Horizontal placement

Please indicate your sex (gender):

○ Male   ○ Female

Note: Vertical placement is usually preferred since it facilitates the respondent's marking the intended response.

Adapted from Berdie DR, Anderson JF, Niebuhr MA. *Questionnaires: Design and Use.* Metuchen, NJ: Scarecrow Press Inc; 1986.

Descriptive Research

SUMMARY

Dietitians frequently use questionnaires as research instruments. The questionnaire process involves conceptualization, design and construction, pretesting, administration, analysis and reporting of results, and utilization of results to affect knowledge and/or action. The questionnaire is a product of survey design. Ideally, it contains questions that are valid and reliable and is constructed and administered in such a way as to induce high response rates. Finally, the questionnaire should obtain results that provide accurate information about the population studied.

Acknowledgments

The work of the following people in the preparation this manuscript is acknowledged and appreciated: Barbara Brand, of Gator Typing Services; Theresa Haefner; and Colleen Seale, of Reference Library West, University of Florida.

References

1. Berdie DR, Anderson JF, Niebuhr MA. *Questionnaires: Design and Use.* Metuchen, NJ: Scarecrow Press, Inc; 1986.
2. Sheatsley PB. Questionnaire construction and item writing. In: Rossi PH, Wright JD, Anderson AB, eds. *Handbook of Survey Research.* Orlando, Fla: Academic Press Inc; 1983;195–230.
3. McClendon MJ, O'Brien DJ. Question-order effects on the determinants of subjective well-being. *Public Opinion Quart.* 1988;52:351–364.
4. Bailey KD. *Methods of Social Research.* New York, NY: Free Press, Macmillan Publishing Co Inc; 1978.
5. O'Brien T, Dugdale V. Questionnaire administration by computer. *J Market Res Soc.* 1978;20:228–237.
6. Newstead PR. Paper versus online presentation of subjective questionnaires. *Int J Man-Machine Studies.* 1985;23:231–247.
7. *Pretesting Health Communications: Methods, Examples, and Resources for Improving Health Messages and Materials.* Rev ed. Bethesda, Md: US Dept of Health and Human Services, Public Health Service, National Institutes of Health, National Cancer Institute; 1982. NIH publication 83-1493.
8. McLaughlin GH. SMOG grading—a new readability formula. *J Reading.* 1969;12:639–646.
9. Gunning R. The fog index after twenty years. *J Business Communication.* 1968;6:3–13.
10. Lorge I. The Lorge and Flesch readability formulae: a correction. *School and Society.* 1948;67:141–142.
11. Taylor WL. Cloze procedure: a new tool for measuring readability. *Journalism Quart.* 1953;30:415–432.
12. Heidel JJ, Glazer-Waldman HR, Parker HJ, Hopkins KM. Readability and writing style analysis of allied health professional journals. *J Allied Health.* 1991;29:25-37.
13. Payne SL. *The Art of Asking Questions.* Princeton, NJ: Princeton University Press; 1951.
14. Geer JG: What do open-ended questions measure? *Public Opinion Quart.* 1988;52:365–371.
15. Montgomery AC, Crittenden KS. Improving coding reliability for open-ended questions. *Public Opinion Quart.* 1977;41:235–243.
16. Poe GS, Seeman I, McLaughlin J, Mehl E, Dietz M. Don't know boxes in factual questions in a mail questionnaire: effects on level and quality of response. *Public Opinion Quart.* 1988;52:212–222.
17. Poikolainen K, Kärkkäinen P. Nature of questionnaire options affects estimates of alcohol intake. *J Stud Alcohol.* 1985;46:219–222.
18. Berdie DR. Questionnaire length and response rate. *J Appl Psychol.* 1973;58:278–280.

19. Karweit N, Meyers ED. Computers in survey research. In: Rossi PH, Wright JD, Anderson AB, eds. *Handbook of Survey Research.* Orlando, Fla: Academic Press Inc; 1983:379–414.
20. Dillman D. Mail and other self-administered questionnaires. In: Rossi PH, Wright JD, Anderson AB, eds. *Handbook of Survey Research.* Orlando, Fla: Academic Press Inc; 1983:359–377.
21. Fox RJ, Crask MR, Kim J. Mail survey response rate: a meta-analysis of selected techniques for inducing response. *Public Opinion Quart.* 1988;52:467–491.
22. Fuller C. Effect of anonymity on return rate and response bias in a mail survey. *J Appl Psychol.* 1974;59:292–296.
23. Hunt SD, Sparkman RD, Wilcox JB. The pretest in survey research: issues and preliminary findings. *J Marketing Res.* 1982;19:269–273.
24. Kviz FJ. Toward a standard definition of response rate. *Public Opinion Quart.* 1977;41:265–267.
25. Goyder J. Face-to-face interviews and mailed questionnaires: the net difference in response rate. *Public Opinion Quart.* 1985;49:234–252.
26. Singer E. Informed consent: consequences for response rate and response quality in social surveys. *Am Sociological Rev.* 1978;43;144–162.
27. McCrohan KF, Lowe LS. A cost/benefit approach to postage used on mail questionnaires. *J Market.* 1981;45:130–133.
28. Fowler FJ, Mangione TW. *Standardized Survey Interviewing.* Newbury Park, Calif: Sage Publications Inc; 1990;18. Applied Social Research Methods Series.
29. Frank GC, Hollatz AT, Webber LS, Berenson GS. Effect of interviewer recording practices on nutrient intake—Bogalusa Heart Study. *J Am Diet Assoc.* 1984;84:1432–1439.
30. Schucker RE. Alternative approaches to classic food consumption measurement methods: telephone interviewing and market data bases. *Am J Clin Nutr.* 1982;35:1306–1309.
31. Krantzler NJ, Mullen BJ, Schultz HG, Grivetti LE, Holden CA, Meiselman HL. Validity of telephoned diet recalls and records for assessment of individual food intake. *Am J Clin Nutr.* 1982;36:1234–1242.
32. Cronbach LJ. Test "reliability": its meaning and determination. *Psychometrika.* 1947;12:1–16.
33. Dwyer JT. Assessment of dietary intake. In: Shils ME, Young VR, eds. *Modern Nutrition in Health and Disease.* Philadelphia, Pa: Lea and Febiger; 1988: 887–905.
34. Rush D, Kristal AR. Methodologic studies during pregnancy: the reliability of the 24-hour dietary recall. *Am J Clin Nutr.* 1982;35:1259–1268.
35. Moore FE. Committee on design and analysis of studies. Epidemiology of cardio-vascular diseases methodology. *Am J Public Health.* 1960; 50(suppl):10–19.
36. Block G. A review of validations of dietary assessment methods. *Am J Epidemiol.* 1982;115:492–505.
37. Beaton GH, Milner J, Corey P, et al. Sources of variance in 24-hour dietary recall data: implications for nutritional study design and interpretation. *Am J Clin Nutr.* 1979;32:2456–2559.
38. Beaton GH, Milner J, McGuire V, Feather TE, Little JA. Source of variance in 24-hour dietary recall data: implications for nutrition study design and interpretation. Carbohydrate sources, vitamins, and minerals. *Am J Clin Nutr.* 1983;37:986–995.
39. McAvay G, Rodin J. Interindividual and intraindividual variation in repeated measures of 24-hour dietary recall in the elderly. *Appetite.* 1988;11:97–110.
40. Willett WC, Sampson L, Stampfer MJ, et al. Reproducibility and validity of a semiquantitative food frequency questionnaire. *Am J Epidemiol.* 1985;122:51–65.
41. Pietinen P, Hartman AM, Haapa E, et al. Reproducibility and validity of dietary assessment instruments. I. A self-administered food use questionnaire with a portion size picture booklet. *Am J Epidemiol.* 1988;128:655–666.
42. Pietinen P, Hartman AM, Haapa E, et al. Reproducibility and validity of dietary assessment instruments. II. A qualitative food frequency questionnaire. *Am J Epidemiol.* 1988;128:667–676.
43. Smith-Barbaro P, Darby L, Reddy BS. Reproducibility and accuracy of a food frequency questionnaire used for diet intervention studies. *Nutr Res.* 1982;2:249–261.

44. Dwyer JT, Krall EA, Coleman KA. The problem of memory in nutritional epidemiology research. *J Am Diet Assoc.* 1987;87:1509–1512.

45. Young CM, Hagan GC, Tucker RE, Foster WD. A comparison of dietary study methods. II. Dietary history vs seven-day record vs 24-hour recall. *J Am Diet Assoc.* 1952;28:218–221.

46. Karvetti R-L, Knuts L-R. Validity of the 24-hour recall. *J Am Diet Assoc.* 1985;85:1437–1442.

47. Linusson EE, Sanjur D, Erickson EC. Validating the 24-hour recall method as a dietary survey tool. *Arch Latinoam Nutr.* 1974;24:277–294.

48. Madden JP, Goodman SJ, Guthrie HA. Validity of the 24-hour recall. *J Am Diet Assoc.* 1976;68:143–147.

49. Carter RL, Sharbaugh CO, Stapell CA. Reliability and validity of the 24-hour recall. Analysis and data from a pediatric population. *J Am Diet Assoc.* 1981;79:542–547.

50. Gersovitz M, Madden JP, Smiciklas-Wright H. Validity of the 24-hour dietary recall and seven-day record for group comparisons. *J Am Diet Assoc.* 1978;73:48–55.

51. Fanelli, MT, Stevenhagen KH. Consistency of energy and nutrient intakes for older adults: 24-hour recall vs 1-day food record. *J Am Diet Assoc.* 1986;86:665–667.

52. Emmons L, Hayes M. Accuracy of 24-hour recalls of young children. *J Am Diet Assoc.* 1973;62:409–415.

53. Frank GC, Berenson GS, Schilling PE, Moore MC. Adapting the 24-hour recall for epidemiologic studies of school children. *J Am Diet Assoc.* 1977;71:26–31.

54. Kiesges RC, Kiesges LM, Brown G, Frank GC. Validation of the 24-hour recall in preschool children. *J Am Diet Assoc.* 1987;87:1383–1385.

55. Horst CH, Obermann-DeBoer GL, Kromhout D. Validity of the 24-hour recall method in infancy: the Leiden Pre-School Children Study. *Int J Epidemiol.* 1988;17:217–221.

56. Emmons L, Hayes M. Accuracy of 24-hour recalls of young children. *J Am Diet Assoc.* 1973;62:409–415.

57. Samet JM, Humble CO, Skipper BE. Alternatives in the collection and analysis of food frequency interview data. *Am J Epidemiol.* 1984;120:572–581.

58. Chu SY, Kolonel LN, Hankin JH, Lee J. A comparison of frequency and quantitative dietary methods for epidemiologic studies of diet and disease. *Am J Epidemiol.* 1984;119:323–334.

59. Mullen BJ, Krantzler NJ, Grivetti LE, Schultz HG, Meiselman HL. The validity of a food frequency questionnaire for the determination of individual food intake. *Am J Clin Nutr.* 1984;39:136–143.

60. Willett WC, Reynolds RD, Cottrell-Hoehner S, Sampson L, Browne ML. Validation of a semiquantitative food frequency questionnaire: comparison with a 1-year diet record. *J Am Diet Assoc.* 1987;87:43–47.

61. Margetts BM, Cade JE, Osmond C. Comparison of a food frequency questionnaire with a diet record. *Int J Epidemiol.* 1989;18:868–873.

62. Krall EA, Dwyer JT. Validity of a food frequency questionnaire and a food diary in a short-term recall situation. *J Am Diet Assoc.* 1987;87:1374–1377.

63. Musgrave KO, Giambalvo L, Leclerc HL, Cook RA, Rosen CJ. Validation of a quantitative food frequency questionnaire for rapid assessment of dietary calcium intake. *J Am Diet Assoc.* 1989;89:1484–1488.

64. Blom L, Lundmark K, Dahlquist G, Persson LA. Estimating children's eating habits—validity of a questionnaire compared to a 7-day record. *Acta Paediatr Scand.* 1989;78:858–864.

65. Roidt L, White E, Goodman GE, et al. Association of food frequency questionnaire estimates of vitamin A intake with serum vitamin A levels. *Am J Epidemiol.* 1988;128:645–654.

66. Romieu I, Stampfer MJ, Stryker WS, et al. Food predictors of plasma beta-carotene and alpha-tocopherol: validation of a food frequency questionnaire. *Am J Epidemiol.* 1990;131:864–876.

PART 4
ANALYTICAL
RESEARCH

Analytical research, through observational and experimental designs, permits evaluation of hypotheses and assessment of cause and effect (chapter 8). Observational analytical research encompasses case-control and cohort–follow-up studies. Experimental analytical research, including clinical trials, allow cause and effect to be examined.

Observational research designs generate measures of association (ie, relative risk and odds ratios) and measures of effect (ie, attributable risk). Relative risk is calculated from cohort studies and odds ratios from case-control studies. Attributable risk indicates public health impact or effect on the population.

Experimental analytical research designs involve investigator-controlled intervention(s). Well-designed and carefully conducted clinical trials provide strong scientific evidence of causal relationships. Chapter 8 discusses issues important in designing clinical trials to ensure that the statistical power is sufficient to detect differences between the study groups (see also chapter 20) and that the data generated are generalizable (see also chapter 2).

Chapter 9 provides practical guidelines for designing and conducting clinical trials and suggests techniques for effective and ethical recruitment, screening, and retention of human subjects. The researcher is obligated to secure approval from the institutional review board as well as voluntary consent from all subjects before initiating the clinical trial (see also chapter 2). In addition, chapter 9 provides recommendations for assessing food composition (see also chapter 11) and developing data collection forms. Pilot tests are strongly endorsed. Future research is needed to construct efficient strategies for subject recruitment and retention, to devise objective methods for assessing compliance, and to expand food formulations suitable for controlled diets.

The importance of future research to clarify the associations between diet and chronic disease was addressed in a 1989 report on diet and health by the National Research Council of the National Academy of Sciences. Seven research topics were expressed:
• Identifying foods and dietary factors that alter risk of chronic disease and determining mechanisms of action

- Improving methods for collecting and assessing data on dietary exposures to foods and altered risk of chronic diseases
- Identifying markers of exposure and early indicators of risk
- Quantifying adverse and beneficial effects of diet and determining optimal range of intake of macro and micro dietary constituents
- Assessing the potential for reduction of chronic disease risk through clinical trials
- Incorporating knowledge of diet and chronic disease to public health programs
- Expanding molecular and cellular nutrition research

Research needed to address the above areas will rely on descriptive and analytical research designs discussed in chapters 4 through 9, and research techniques presented in chapters 10 through 19.

ERM, Editor

8. EPIDEMIOLOGIC ANALYTICAL RESEARCH

Bettylou Sherry, PhD, RD

Epidemiology seeks to describe the distribution of disease and explain associations between causative or associated factors and disease. Endeavors to identify causative factors for a disease evolve into the development of preventive and treatment strategies. This process follows a sequence of description, explanation, and control. Descriptive and analytical studies provide a perspective to a biological process that cannot be gleaned from using only laboratory experiments.

Epidemiologic descriptive research, as discussed in chapter 6, is the reporting of the natural course of events, with particular emphasis on persons, place, and time. Quantifying correlations between these variables is also a part of descriptive epidemiology. Descriptive studies generate hypotheses that can be tested by analytical research methods. Hypotheses testing, or explanation, is the goal of analytical research. Analytical research encompasses both observational and experimental studies. Observational studies include cohort and case-control (or case-referent) designs. Clinical trials are types of experimental studies. In analytical research, the investigator structures the study in such a way that groups of individuals who are exposed and not exposed to a potential risk factor can be compared for outcome. Alternatively, the investigator provides an intervention in one study group and compares their outcome to that of a group that does not receive intervention.

Leaf and Weber,[1] in their review article on the cardiovascular effects of n-3 fatty acids, provide a useful example of how different research designs are used in the process of gaining an understanding of disease causation, prevention, and treatment. Kromann and Green[2] used survey data to describe the difference between Danes and Eskimos in age-adjusted mortality from heart attacks. Other researchers[3,4] demonstrated, by using dietary intake and food composition analysis, that the difference in the diets of the two groups was the composition of the fat. In the next phase, clinical trials evaluating the effect of ω-3 fatty acids on triglyceride concentrations demonstrated a reduction of the substance.[5,6] The mechanisms for this change were then documented in laboratory research.[7-9]

The goal in selecting a study design is to make the choice that will provide the most information and the most accurate results, given the state of knowledge about the subject and the feasibility of the research project. This chapter discusses analytical research. Explanations of the epidemiologic measures of association and effect used in observational studies are outlined. Observational and experimental study designs are described; their uses and considerations in

Supported in part by grant MCJ 009043 from the Department of Health and Human Services.

implementing these designs are discussed in addition to the advantages and limitations of each of these approaches to research. A summary of the designs, uses, strengths, and limitations can be found at the end of the chapter.

MEASURES OF ASSOCIATION AND EFFECT

Association

Two goals in analytical research are to assess whether an association exists between exposure and disease, and to assess the strength of that association. In practice, these goals are expressed in terms of the probability of developing a disease when exposed, compared with the probability when not exposed. *Relative risk* and the *odds ratio* are the measures used to define these associations and the choice of their use is dependent upon the design of the research.

Relative risk, sometimes referred to as *risk ratio* or *relative rate*, is used in a cohort study. It is calculated by dividing the cumulative incidence of disease in those exposed to the variable of interest by the cumulative incidence in those not exposed to that variable:

$$\text{Relative risk} = \frac{\text{Cumulative incidence in the exposed*}}{\text{Cumulative incidence in the unexposed}}$$

For example, if the cumulative incidence in the exposed were 120/100 000 and 40/100 000 in the unexposed, the relative risk due to exposure would be 3.0. Cumulative incidence is the number of new cases of a disease occurring within a population of known size within a specific time period (usually one year). The advantage of this measure is that it is based on population data for the denominators in the calculation of the two incidence rates used in the equation. This means that the results are applicable to populations of similar composition.

Unfortunately, data are not always available to calculate relative risk. In a case-control study, the populations at risk are not determined, so there are no appropriate denominators from which incidence rates can be calculated. However, it is possible to estimate relative risk in these studies if: the controls are randomly selected from the population and are, therefore, representative of the population of interest; the case group includes all of the cases of the disease of interest in the geographic area of study and, thus, is representative of the population; and if the disease is rare (usually less than 5% of the population). This estimation of relative risk is called the *odds ratio*. It is calculated according to the following formula:

$$\text{Odds ratio} = \frac{ad}{bc}$$

where

		Cases	Controls
Risk factor	+	a	b
(Exposure)	−	c	d

*An approximation to the relative risk is the rate ratio:
$$\text{Rate ratio} = \frac{\text{Incidence density for the exposed}}{\text{Incidence density for the unexposed}}$$

In a rare disease, b approximates a + b and d approximates c + d, so the formula for estimating relative risk (RR) can be shortened as follows:

$$RR = \frac{\text{Cumulative incidence in exposed}}{\text{Cumulative incidence in unexposed}} = \frac{\dfrac{a}{a+b}}{\dfrac{c}{c+d}} = \frac{\dfrac{a}{b}}{\dfrac{c}{d}} = \frac{ad}{bc}$$

In a matched case-control study in which the controls are individually matched to the cases, the odds ratio is calculated by dividing the number of pairs in which the case has the risk factor and the control does not by the number of pairs in which the case does not have the risk factor and the control does:

$$\text{Odds ratio} = \frac{b}{c}$$

where

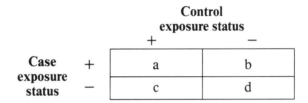

		Control exposure status	
		+	−
Case exposure status	+	a	b
	−	c	d

Both relative risk and the odds ratio quantify the magnitude of the association between exposure to a risk factor and disease. The stronger this association, the more likely the association is to be a causal relationship. However, other studies examining biological processes must be used to prove causation.

A few biases are commonly associated with these measures. Relative risk may be influenced by the length of time over which it is calculated. For example, the risk for one year may be different from that of 20 years. Sometimes rates of disease are inferred from case-control studies; however, this should not be done unless the study is population-based. A case-control study also does not permit calculation of the rate at which the disease develops based on exposure to the risk factor.

Effect

It is useful to examine the public health effect of exposure to a risk factor, provided that the association between the risk factor and disease represents a causal relationship. The measurements used to evaluate this impact are *attributable risk* and *population attributable risk.*

Attributable risk (AR), or risk difference, a concept developed by Levin[10] is defined as:

AR = Cumulative incidence in the exposed
− cumulative incidence in the unexposed

Attributable risk is calculated as the difference between the rate of disease among persons exposed and the rate of disease among persons not exposed.

The attributable risk is, therefore, simply the excess disease occurrence associated with the exposure (risk factor). It is also possible to calculate attributable risk in case-control studies; Hennekens and Buring[11] offer a clear description of the appropriate procedures.

Another measure of the effect of exposure on development of disease of public health importance is population attributable risk (PAR):

$$PAR = \text{Cumulative incidence in the population}$$
$$- \text{cumulative incidence in the unexposed}$$

PAR estimates the rate of disease in a population that could be eliminated if exposure to the risk factor of interest were avoided. This measure is frequently converted to a percentage and referred to as PAR percent. This is calculated as

$$PAR\% = \frac{\text{Population attributable risk}}{\text{Cumulative incidence in the population}} \times 100$$

PAR% estimates the proportion of disease in a population that could be eliminated if exposure to the risk factor were eliminated. For example, analysis of data from the Framingham Heart Study showed that 50% of the population studied had cholesterol concentrations between 5.68 and 8.01 mmol/L, and 75% of the excess deaths from coronary heart disease (CHD) occurred within this group.[12] Only 5% of the study population had cholesterol concentrations greater than 8.01 mmol/L, yet 15% of the excess deaths from CHD occurred within this group. Because such a large proportion of the population has cholesterol concentrations between 5.68 and 8.01 mmol/L, it would be the primary group to target for intervention from a public health standpoint, even though the group at the highest risk of excess death from CHD have cholesterol concentrations greater than 8.01 mmol/L.

Hennekens and Buring[11] offer descriptions of how to estimate PAR and PAR% in cohort and case-control studies.

Considerations for Use

Measures of association and effect have important differences. Measures of association—relative risk and the odds ratio—estimate the strength of the association between a risk factor and a disease. A strong association increases the likelihood that the risk factor is causal. In contrast, measures of effect—attributable risk and population attributable risk—measure the public health impact of exposure on frequency of disease. These latter measures are useful for planning public health policy.

Two potential sources of bias require consideration in calculating measures of association and effect. Confounding factors and effect modifiers can significantly distort the results of a study. Briefly, a confounding factor is a variable that affects both exposure and outcome in a study, but this variable is not an intermediate in the causal pathway between exposure and outcome. Common confounders include age, gender, and race. An effect modifier is a variable that influences the impact of exposure on the health outcome. For example, exercise can influence the effect of a diet high in saturated fat on the development of cardiovascular disease. For a more comprehensive discussion of how to consider confounding factors and effect modification in data analysis, see chapter 21.

OBSERVATIONAL STUDIES

Case-Control Studies

In a case-control design, the subjects are selected according to whether they have a disease; that is, the cases have the disease, the controls do not. The investigator ascertains their exposure to certain risk factors at some prior time and evaluates whether there is an association between the risk factor and the disease or health outcome of interest. A risk factor is a variable that increases the likelihood of the development of a disease. For example, sodium intake is a risk factor for hypertension.

Case-control studies can be used to evaluate more than one risk factor at a time; in addition, they are relatively cheap and useful for studying rare diseases such as metabolic disorders. Case-control studies are used to generate hypotheses of associations between potential risk or causative factors and a disease. The biological explanations for these hypotheses then can be tested in laboratory experiments or clinical trials. For example, much of the initial work documenting associations between diet and cancer evolved from case-control study designs.

Issues of design. The primary issues in planning a case-control study include case selection, control selection, ascertainment of disease and exposure status, statistical power, and assessment of the validity of the study by examining the influence of confounding factors and bias.

Case selection requires three basic strategic decisions before considering the potential sources of cases. First, the disease under study must be precisely defined; specific diagnostic and clinical criteria must be specified in advance. Only one disease should be studied at a time because risk factors may vary significantly, although symptoms may be similar.

The second strategic decision is whether the study should have population-based cases to make it possible to generalize the results, or whether it should focus on only a specific type of case, such as a certain age or gender group or those from one or two institutions. Large, population-based studies, in which cases are selected from the general population, avoid the selection bias that can occur if only one source of cases is used, and they provide a more complete representation of a disease. Although it is important to be able to generalize the results, valid information is a much more basic issue. Often it is more difficult to obtain complete and accurate information in a population-based study. For this reason, population-based case-control studies are used only in circumstances in which it is possible to evaluate or ascertain all cases occurring in the population. This circumstance is rare; however, the possibility does exist in large institutions or organizations such as health maintenance organizations.

The third important decision is whether to use incident or prevalent cases. Incident cases would include only new cases of disease that occurred during the study period, whereas prevalent cases would include new cases as well as cases identified prior to the initiation of the study. In general, it is better to use incident cases to eliminate the bias from duration of exposure. If the risk factor is not affected by duration, as is the case with congenital malformations or a specific blood type, prevalent cases may be used.

Once these decisions have been made, it is time to consider the source of cases. For a population-based study, all cases can be included, or, if that is not feasible, a random sample of cases can be selected. Hospital records, disease registries, and the records of physicians with a related medical specialty are all potential sources of specific case groups. The disease status of the cases can be obtained from death certificates, physicians' records, hospital records, case registries, and microbiology and pathology laboratory records.

Selection of an appropriate control group is perhaps the most challenging task in designing a case-control study. The best controls have the same characteristics as the cases, but lack the disease. It is essential to have data of comparable quality and completeness for both cases and controls. Controls are normally selected from the general population, the same institutions whence the cases were obtained, or from socially similar groups such as siblings, friends, or neighbors.

If controls are selected from the general population, they can be identified by visiting households, examining voter registries, or randomly dialed telephone numbers. Selection of controls can be a time-consuming and costly process, and the quality of the information obtained may not be as accurate or complete as it is for the cases. Moreover, a low response rate or reliance on only a certain type of volunteer may bias the results.

Special groups of siblings, friends, or neighbors are usually cooperative, healthy persons. However, if the risk factor under study is similar for both the cases and controls because they have similar life-styles, the effect of the risk factor will be underestimated.

Hospital or institution-based control groups are often used because they are readily available in sufficient numbers. Because hospital-based controls are not healthy people they are more likely to be aware of their past, and this can help reduce recall bias. However, using hospital patients as controls presents several disadvantages. Because they are ill, they are not representative of the general population. Hospital patients smoke more, use more oral contraceptives, and drink more alcohol than other people[13-15]; these practices could bias the results, if any were included as the risk factors of study. In connection with the control of bias, the decision has to be made as to which diseases are to be included as sources of controls. The risk factors under study must not be associated with any of the diseases selected, and no diseases that would affect the exposure to a risk factor under study should be included.

Multiple control groups sometimes are used to increase statistical power in a study. This tactic allows measurement of different effects of exposure in different groups of controls, which is helpful in understanding the range of effects of a risk factor. It also identifies the risk factors of greatest public health concern.

Another strategy to ensure that the cases and controls are similar in basic important ways (except for the risk factor under study) is matching. Variables commonly matched are age, gender, race, and socioecomomic status. For example, when age is a matching variable, the control would be required to be within an age range, eg, for infants, ± 1 month might be used if immune response were a factor of interest.

Once the cases and controls have been selected and the disease status of the cases has been confirmed, exposure status should be determined. Exposure should be clearly defined: it may mean "ever exposed," "currently exposed," or "previously exposed." The biology of the disease process must be considered and the most reasonable choice selected.

Exposure status is usually obtained from direct interviews or questionnaires sent by mail. To prevent extra probing for information from the cases, the interviewers or persons who extract information from medical records should not know whether a study participant is a case or a control for the hypothesis being tested.

Issues of analysis and interpretation. The cases and controls are compared to determine if the cases are more likely to have been exposed to the risk factors of interest. The odds ratio is calculated; if the study is population-based or the disease under study is rare, the odds ratio is an approximation of the relative risk.

Validity and bias must be considered when interpreting the results of a case-control study. Validity can be assessed by determining whether the interview instrument accurately assessed exposure, whether the study had adequate statistical power, whether bias was avoided, and whether confounding was examined and controlled.

Sample size calculations will have been done a priori. However, new hypotheses sometimes are generated during the analysis phase of a study. It is important to note in the discussion of these new hypotheses that there may not have been sufficient subjects in the study to provide adequate statistical power to be confident that this result has not occurred by chance.[16] Confidence intervals can be used to assist in interpretation. If they are wide or include 0 or 1, depending on the hypothesis, the association between the risk factor of study and outcome is unlikely to be a strong one.

Selection bias due to low or unequal response rates can be a problem in case-control studies. Another selection bias exists when public knowledge about certain risk factors has resulted in a change of habits in certain population groups. Observation bias results from poor recall or errors in information. This bias can result in either random or differential misclassification. Random misclassification, which occurs on average to the same degree among the cases and controls, leads to a reduction in the estimate of risk. Differential misclassification, which occurs unequally in the case and control groups, results in either an exaggerated or inappropriately low estimate of risk.[16]

Strengths and limitations. Case-control studies are relatively inexpensive and can be conducted within a short period of time. Several potential risk factors can be evaluated in a single study. This is a good design for evaluating diseases that are rare and those with a long latency period.

Limitations include susceptibility to selection and recall bias. Because of the retrospective nature of this design, it may not be feasible to establish the temporal sequence between exposure and disease. It is not possible to calculate rates of disease through this design unless the study is population-based. Finally, in the case of rare exposures, a case-control design is not an efficient approach unless a factor is found to be strongly associated with a disease.

Cohort Studies

A cohort study is one that has group(s) of subjects of known exposure status who are monitored over time to assess health consequences of exposure(s). At the beginning of a cohort study the study group(s) are defined by their exposure to a potential risk factor for a disease or health problem among participants who are still free of disease. The groups then are observed for the development of disease or health problem within a predetermined period. Sometimes there is no comparison group; one cohort is surveyed at baseline and monitored over time for health consequences. Monitoring the group(s) makes it possible to assess a wide range of health consequences as a result of exposure to a presumed risk factor.

Cohort studies are the design of choice for studying common diseases and rare exposures, or for assessing the multiple health effects of one or more exposures. A cohort study frequently evolves after an initial hypothesis has been generated from a case-control study. A cohort design would be useful, for example, to assess the chronic effects of a diet high in saturated fat on cardiovascular disease. This design is most frequently used in epidemiologic studies of nutrition and occupational health. The salient design principle of a cohort study is that an appropriate temporal sequence exists between the risk factor and the health consequences. That is, exposure to the risk factor must occur prior to the development of the health consequence.

Types of cohort studies. A cohort study can be prospective, retrospective, or ambidirectional in terms of the recording process for data collection. In a prospective study, exposure to the risk factor may have already occurred, but the health consequence definitely has not occurred. In a retrospective cohort study, both exposure to the risk factor and the health outcome have occurred. Both prospective and retrospective data are collected for an ambidirectional cohort study. If adequate funds are available, a prospective design is preferred. This approach is likely to provide the most accurate exposure information because it uses current records or interview data for documentation of exposure. There is also the opportunity to obtain current information on potential confounding factors and effect modifiers for all of the study participants. Careful advance planning that includes identifying feasible methods for obtaining accurate information about exposure status, potential confounding variables, and effect modifiers helps ensure that complete information will be available for all participants. Occupational or medical records, measurements, and interviews are the primary sources of information.

In contrast, in a retrospective cohort study, existing records must be used as the primary sources of data. A retrospective design is used when time for the study is short, funds are limited, or if the health consequences develop after a long latency period. In this instance the latency period will have occurred prior to the beginning of the study. Employee records, union records, or hospital records can be accurate sources of exposure information. One advantage of using these records is that classification of exposure is not biased because it was made prior to the formulation of the hypothesis. However, these records frequently are not complete for all study participants, and information on potential confounding factors is not available. Direct interview may not be a useful alternative because it may not be possible to obtain unbiased information about potential confounding factors from the participants. Subjects may not give accurate information either because of stigma about exposure or because they may have some preconceived ideas about the effect of exposure. One technique for solving these problems is to use data from diverse sources and compare the consistency and accuracy of the information.

Another potential design is a nested case-control design within a cohort study, which can reduce both cost and duration of the study. A nested design is accomplished by obtaining exposure data on all participants at the beginning of a cohort study and observing the subjects until enough cases develop the outcome of interest (eg, atherosclerosis, cancer) to provide adequate statistical power to detect a difference between the diseased and healthy subjects as related to exposure to the risk factor. An example might be to look at specific measures of school performance in children who were exposed to different levels of iron deficiency.

Issues of study design. Selection of the cohorts requires careful thought and planning. Clear definitions of the cohorts are important. One technique for avoiding misclassification (placing the exposed in the nonexposed group or vice versa) within the cohorts is to use a rigorous definition of exposure. Exposure status may be based on exposure at one moment or over a period. Stratifying for different levels of exposure status may need to be considered in the planning stages. Changes of exposure over time require adjustment in the data analysis. For common exposures, the exposed cohort can be selected from the general population. Use of a special group in which exposure is clustered is preferred for rarer exposures.

The unexposed comparison group or cohort should be similar to the exposed group in all respects except exposure to the potential risk factor. Sometimes vital statistics for the general population or a population-based sample of people are used as a comparison group; this practice is reasonable as long as only a small proportion of the general population is likely to have been exposed to the exposure under study. The disadvantage of using a sample group selected from the general population as a comparison group is that they may differ from the study cohort in some important respects such as smoking, age, or gender. One way to construct a control group from the general population is to use existing data such as national, state, or local mortality or morbidity rates as the comparison for rates found in the cohort of the exposed.

Health outcome status should be determined for both the exposed and unexposed study participants. If the outcome is fatal, a death certificate may be used; however, the recording of cause-specific death on the certificate is not necessarily accurate. If the health consequence is not fatal, medical records or disease registries may be used to ascertain outcome status. Another strategy is to conduct periodic medical examinations as part of the study protocol when a prospective design is used.

Loss to observation (lost to follow-up) can be a major source of bias in the study results, especially if the study is protracted. Such loss may result from exposure, such as moving to continue a job, resulting in a change in exposure, or from the health consequence, such as stopping work due to illness. Thus, loss to observation can significantly affect the results of a study. Constant monitoring required to avert attrition is sometimes the major expense of a cohort study. Three approaches used to avoid these high costs are: use of a retrospective design; use of a nested case-control design; or use of intermediate markers.

Issues of analysis and interpretation. The conclusions of a cohort study are based on a comparison of cumulative incidence of the outcome measure in the exposed and the unexposed groups. The results may be applied to other similar populations.

Validity of the results should be assessed by consideration of the possible effects of chance, confounding, effect modification, and bias. Selection bias occurs when exposure is misclassified. For example, if vitamin A intake is being assessed and grapefruit is a major component of the diet, it would be important to know whether the grapefruit were pink or white because pink has a much higher content of vitamin A. A subject could be placed in the wrong exposure group if it were not known which type of grapefruit he or she consumes. Random misclassification reduces the magnitude of difference between the rates of the two study groups. If the misclassification is differential, not random (eg, some of the exposed were not exposed or vice versa), the cumulative incidence of the health consequence in the exposed group is decreased, resulting in a reduced effect of exposure on the outcome variable.

A second major source of bias is nonresponse. To assess the possible effect of nonresponse, the participants and nonparticipants can be compared on all variables of interest, including exposure status. Although data will be incomplete on nonparticipants, some baseline information usually can be found in employee records, medical charts, and so forth. This will provide at least a "best" estimate of differences between the participants and nonparticipants. Nonresponse bias usually does not affect validity, but it may limit the general applicability of the results.

Attrition of the cohort can be a third source of bias. The extent of attrition should be documented by calculating the proportion of the subjects who were lost. To avert loss to follow-up, major efforts should be made by researchers to keep the participants in the study. Developing a good rapport between the subjects and the investigators is beneficial; sometimes monetary incentives are used. If subjects are lost, efforts should be made to contact them either by telephone or mail.

Strengths and limitations.   Cohort studies have many advantages. They can reveal an appropriate temporal relationship between a risk factor and a health outcome resulting from exposure. They can evaluate the effect of rare exposures on several potential health consequences. Such studies permit the calculation of incidence rates of the health consequence in both the exposed and unexposed cohorts. Prospective cohort studies are especially useful because the exposure status of the participants can be accurately assessed; it can be documented initially and monitored during the study.

The primary limitations of cohort studies are that they are expensive and time-consuming. Selection bias, inadequate records on exposure status or potential confounding variables, and nonresponse, as well as loss of participants during observation can significantly distort the results.

EXPERIMENTAL STUDIES

Clinical Trials

The clinical trial embodies an effort to maintain the methodologic rigor of a laboratory experiment to the clinical practice of medicine. A clinical trial is a research design that has a study group and a control group. Subjects of similar characteristics are randomly assigned to one of the two groups. The study group receives the intervention of interest, the control group receives nothing or a placebo. Both groups are then monitored for predetermined outcomes and side effects. Clinical trials are used primarily to assess dietary intervention; nutrition education intervention programs; or the therapeutic efficacy of medications, procedures, or vaccines. Documentation of the efficacy of an intervention is needed to evaluate its impact on health care. For example, the effect of coffee brewed by filtering or boiling on cholesterol levels was assessed by clinical trial. Filtered coffee had no effect, but boiled coffee increased serum cholesterol concentrations 10% above baseline levels.[17]

General considerations. Some general considerations for the use of a clinical trial are feasibility, generalizability, and the power of a study to detect a difference between the two groups of interest.

Feasibility. Ethics, cost, and public use of a measure or intervention may mean that it is not acceptable or worthwhile to conduct a clinical trial. For a clinical trial to be ethical, the intervention and nonintervention alternatives must be equally desirable choices. A potentially dangerous or ineffective treatment must not be an option; neither is it ethical to withhold an effective treatment from participants. In these situations, data regarding the efficacy of an intervention must be derived from laboratory experiments, or clinical trials must be stopped early if a new treatment is either dangerous or highly effective in comparison with placebos or standard treatment.

The high costs per subject and administrative costs may limit the feasibility of a clinical trial. If the costs are deemed to be greater than the benefits, it may not be possible to obtain funding. The cost per participant should be minimized without curtailing the ability of a trial to assess the differences between the experimental and control groups.

One technique used to cut costs and increase efficiency is to test more than one hypothesis in one study. The most common approach is to use a 2×2 factorial design, although a larger scale design can be used. The concept is described schematically in *Figure 8-1*.

Figure 8.1
Schematic drawing of a 2 × 2 factorial design.

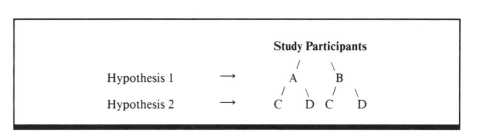

In this type of design structure, the subjects are first randomized into two treatment groups (the exposed and unexposed) and then further randomized to test a second hypothesis. For example, the initial hypothesis of interest might be to test the effect of a cholesterol-lowering drug in a group of men with high cholesterol concentrations. The men would be initially randomized into the A and B groups designated. The second hypothesis might be to test whether this drug is influenced by a high-fiber diet. To examine this issue, the A and B groups would be again randomized into C and D groups. The C group would be given a high-fiber diet and the D group given a diet with the average amount of fiber consumed by a group of men in the same age and socioeconomic status. To ensure validity in the results, adequate sample size for appropriate statistical power, confounding, and effect modification need to be considered when a matrix such as this is used.

Acceptance of some measure by the general population may make it difficult to evaluate the effectiveness of any intervention program. The Multiple Risk Factor Intervention Trial (MRFIT) study is a good example of such a situation.[18] During the course of that clinical trial, the general public reduced their dietary intake of cholesterol, and thereby made evaluation of an intervention program to reduce cholesterol intake difficult. This type of problem would reduce the magnitude of difference in cholesterol intakes between the two groups and, therefore, require a larger sample size than originally planned to provide the same statistical power.

A current example of a similar situation is the need to evaluate whether the use of vitamins before conception can prevent neural tube defects. However, the high level of vitamin use among women may make it impossible to find a large enough group of women who do not take vitamins. In addition, women who do not take vitamins may not be representative of the general population; they may be at a higher risk for a poor diet or be at greater medical risk during pregnancy.

The MRFIT and vitamin studies are examples of studies that may need to be conducted in a geographic area where these health promotional measures have not been adopted. Other alternatives are to use animal data from laboratory experiments or a case-control study design. A case-control design would make use of cases (with neural tube defects) and controls (without such defects) of similar gender and socioeconomic status as the cases. The researchers would look backward in time to discern whether mothers of both groups had similar intakes of vitamins in the preconception period.

Generalizable results.   Clinical trials are designed with the hope that the results apply to other populations. Relevant study participants and valid results are both important to permit the generalization of the results of a study. Selecting study subjects who are relevant to the study question—eg, of the appropriate age, health status, or disease status—is a basic requirement. For example, it would not make sense to use young adults as subjects for testing a short-term intervention assessment of a diuretic to be used in end-stage emphysema patients. Older persons with late-stage emphysema and without renal complications would be appropriate subjects.

Accurate data are required for the results of a study to be valid and thus generalizable. To ensure study compliance and accurate information, a subset of a relevant group of potential study participants sometimes is selected for enrollment. For example, homeless women would not be appropriate subjects in which to evaluate the effect of calcium supplementation during menopause because it would be difficult at best to keep in contact with them. In contrast, nurses or female employees of a large corporation would be easy to follow.

Power and bias.   The initial concern in sample selection is to have enough participants to ensure adequate statistical power for detecting a difference between the study groups. Power is the ability of a statistical test to reject a null hypothesis when it is false. The null hypothesis to be tested in a study specifies that there is no association between exposure and disease. For example, in a clinical trial to test the effectiveness of a nutrition intervention on serum cholesterol, the null hypothesis would be that there would be no difference in the intervention and control groups in their cholesterol concentrations after the intervention. Power is calculated on the basis of the sample size, the magnitude of difference that is to be detected, and the variability of the measure being examined (see chapter 20).

Design considerations can be helpful in ensuring a study will be able to detect a difference. Clear, measurable outcomes eliminate confusion regarding end points. Mortality, morbidity, weight gain, an increase in the rate of wound healing, or specified changes in hematologic indices such as transthyretin (prealbumin) are all good choices. In contrast, hunger is difficult to assess, due to the lack of a clear definition.

Eliminating bias is another important factor. Bias is a distortion of the results caused by some factor other than those under study. In other words, bias masks the true relationship between the factors under study and outcome of interest. Maintaining a high level of participation during a study avoids response bias. For example, if the sickest subjects are lost to follow-up, only the healthiest subjects are left to participate. This creates the possibility that a valuable treatment would not be found effective because it is being evaluated in only the healthiest of subjects.

A second type of bias is the possibility that some factor other than the intervention could cause the outcome to be attributed to the intervention. This is confounding. An example might be the confounding influence of infection on transthyretin (prealbumin) concentrations. Infection tends to decrease dietary intake, which can lead to a reduction in transthyretin. Infection alone also will cause a decrease in transthyretin concentrations. Thus, infection as well as diet are influencing serum concentrations of transthyretin.

Effect modification can impose bias. An effect modifier is a variable that is not related to exposure but is related to outcome. The classic, nonnutritional example is the role of asbestos exposure in modifying the effect of smoking on the development of lung cancer. Asbestos exposure alone can lead to lung cancer. When it is combined with exposure to smoking, it increases the likelihood of the development of lung cancer in smokers.

Another type of bias is differences in subjects and their controls in ways other than their exposure status. For example, the subjects might be older than the controls; age could affect cardiac performance, pulmonary function, or metabolism. Therefore, differences between the two groups could be due to age, not the intervention under study. Randomization or matching subjects on important influencing variables minimize this bias.

Issues of design. Once a hypothesis has been developed and issues of feasibility, generalizability, and ability of a study to detect a difference have been resolved, the mechanics need to be addressed.

In a clinical trial, the investigator selects the exposure status of the subjects. This contrasts with the procedure used for observational studies, in which exposure status is predetermined by circumstances specific to the study subjects. In a clinical trial, exposure status is based on the goal of the research instead of the needs or circumstances of the study participant.

Allocation of the participants to the study groups is an important step. This should be done once the group of eligible subjects has been determined within the referent population. Sometimes, when the group of eligible subjects is very large, only a selected proportion, eg, a 10% sample of 10 000, is needed to provide an adequate sample size for the hypothesis in question. Once the proportion of eligibles to be included has been determined by the sample size calculations, potential enrollees should be randomly selected, told about the study, and asked to sign a human subjects consent form to enroll them formally in the study. Those who are not willing to be involved in the study are referred to as nonparticipants. The allocation process for the participants should proceed as shown in *Figure 8.2.*

```
                    Reference population
                   /                    \
          Eligible group            Ineligible group
         /              \
   Participants      Non-participants
  /            \
Treatment group  Placebo group
```

Random assignment increases the likelihood that differences in outcome between the study groups are due to exposure status or to chance. This system, on average, ensures that the two groups are evenly distributed on all known and unknown variables, except for the one that is being studied. It is best to use a randomization process based on a random numbers table. Allocating subjects by alternating them can lead to susceptibility bias.[19] For example, if two subjects appear at the same time to join a study, the enroller may subconsciously assign the apparently more dependable subject to the treatment group. It is sometimes important to be able to stratify random groups of subjects by variables such as gender or age. In this case, a system called *blocking* is used. The subjects are first classified by gender or age and then randomized to the treatment or placebo group.

Whenever possible, a double-blind randomization process should be used. Double-blind assignment means that neither the subject nor the investigator knows to which exposure group the subject has been assigned. This technique reduces the possibility that those who interview the subjects will interpret measurements or symptoms and modify their impressions according to whether a subject is in the treatment or the placebo group. Double-blind assignment is used when the intervention can easily be masked, such as when a pill or an injection is used. However, when the intervention is obvious, such as with a nutrition education program, it is not feasible to use a double-blind protocol; however, the initial randomization can be blinded, which helps eliminate bias.

Attaining a high response rate—ie, having a high proportion of the eligible subjects selected to participate in the study—is required for the results to be applicable to the population of interest. First, a high response rate is needed to provide the estimated sample size necessary to test the hypothesis of interest. Second, it ensures a representative sample of the group under study. The representativeness of the sample can be assessed by comparing the participants and nonparticipants for the variables that are being assessed. In addition to the variables related to exposure and disease, age, gender, race, education, and socioeconomic indicators are important indices to compare because they may affect both exposure and outcome. If major differences are found, then the results can only be generalized to populations with characteristics similar to those who participated in the study. For clarification, the population of interest may mean the whole population, or a specific group that would be relevant to a study. For example, if the effect of a low-sodium regimen on hypertension is being studied, the results should be applied only to people with hypertension.

A study needs to have a high level of compliance. Deviation from the study protocol may affect the results. The most common types of noncompliance include subjects withdrawing, forgetting to follow the protocol, or being lost to follow-up. Usually the extent of noncompliance is related directly to the complexity and length of a study. Compliance should be assessed routinely at specified intervals during a study. This is done by examining the response rate, adherence to protocol (eg, by means of a biochemical marker in a medication such as riboflavin, which is excreted in the urine and indicates whether a subject is taking the medication; or attendance in nutrition education programs), completeness of data, and whether the data appear to be within a realistic range. The statistical power of a study is decreased if subjects are lost. Some techniques of increasing compliance include: frequent contacts between the participants and administrators of the study, use of monetary incentives, free medical care, and protocols that are reasonable for participants to follow.

Another consideration is establishing stopping rules before the beginning of a trial. This is best done in advance by consultation with a statistician. Because the welfare of the participants must be protected, a study should be stopped if the proposed treatment has significant negative or positive effects. Side effects should be monitored as well. Monitoring the data periodically is the best way to assess whether there is a strong statistical association between treatment and an effect. In a double-blind study, this is done by a special safety and data monitoring board composed of people who are not otherwise involved with the study and selected by the researchers. The board members have access to the codes identifying who is receiving the treatment of interest and the placebo so that they can assess the effects. Adequate statistical power should be used as one basis for stopping rules; another is minimizing risk to the participants. For example, investigators in the Stroke Prevention in Atrial Fibrillation Study were asked by the Safety Monitoring Committee to discontinue the placebo arm of their investigation because preliminary data indicated an 81% reduction in risk for ischemic stroke or systemic embolism in the arm that received warfarin.[20] Obviously, the treatment with warfarin had a significant benefit.

Issues of analysis. Analysis in a clinical trial involves making comparisons of outcome in the two groups of subjects. Differences in proportions, means, or medians are commonly used. Differences in changes over time can also be the focus of analysis.

Bias can significantly influence the results of a study, and its role must be examined in the analysis. First, data for all subjects who have participated in the study should be included in the analysis, even if they have dropped out or if data for all variables being studied are not available. Inclusion of all subjects is the basis for and the value of randomization. When data for only those who complete the study are used, the question of whether treatment is of benefit cannot be evaluated because the sample size will be smaller, thus reducing statistical power. Moreover, the subjects who completed the study may be different from those who did not. There may also be differences in characteristics of the participants in the intervention and control groups who did not complete the study. Post hoc analysis of response of subgroups is not appropriate because these secondary questions were not incorporated into the original study design. Levels of statistical significance of differences between the subgroups therefore cannot be accurately assessed.

In summary, when subjects are lost during follow-up or data are incomplete, the goal of the research is compromised. In addition to this bias, the biases discussed previously in relation to enhancing the ability of a study to detect a difference should also be examined. Confounding factors need to be considered and effect modification needs to be assessed.

Strengths and limitations. The primary strength of a clinical trial is that the variables and conditions can be controlled somewhat as in a laboratory experiment. Secondly, the trial can be conducted in a setting similar to the natural situation where the question of interest would be applied.

The major limitation of a clinical trial is its feasibility. Ethics, high costs, and public use of a measure or intervention may prevent this study design from being used. Clinical trials also require close monitoring, and several institutions may be required to procure adequate sample sizes. Avoiding error or bias when more than one study site is used requires meticulous attention to detail during the planning and data collection period to ensure that the same procedures are followed at each site. Quality control checks such as standardizing anthropometric measurement techniques before and at predesignated intervals during the study are essential for attaining high-quality data consistently at all sites. Periodic meetings of members from all sites are useful strategies for discussing progress and problems that arise during a study.

SUMMARY

Analytical research comprises both intervention and observation studies. Observational studies are cohort or case-control in design. Subjects in cohort studies are grouped on the basis of their exposure to a risk factor and observed for outcome. In case-control studies, the investigator groups the cases and controls on the basis of outcome status and then looks backward in time to ascertain exposure to risk factors. Intervention studies or clinical trials offer more control of variables, yet may be unfeasible because of ethics or cost. The uses, strengths, and limitations of these studies are summarized in *Table 8.1*.

Table 8.1
Summary of Analytical Research Designs, Uses, Strengths, and Limitations

Designs	Uses	Strengths	Limitations
Observational			
Case-control	Evaluate multiple risk factors from one outcome / Good for rare diseases	Free-living situation / Low cost / Short duration	Bias
Cohort	Evaluate multiple outcomes from one exposure	Free-living situation / Correct temporal sequence	Cost / Bias / Duration
Intervention (experimental)			
Clinical trial	Evaluate treatment, vaccine efficacy	Partially controlled conditions / Cause and effect relationship observed	Ethics / Cost

Measures of association and effect are used to summarize the results in observational studies. Measures of association (relative risk and odds ratio) estimate the strength of association between a risk factor and a disease, whereas measures of effect (attributable risk and population attributable risk) assess the public health impact of exposure on the frequency of disease.

The role of bias, confounding, effect modification, and chance all must be considered in the analysis of analytical research.

In addition to determining whether a risk factor is associated with a disease, as has been the goal in this chapter, it is important to consider additional criteria to ascertain whether a factor is causally related to a disease. Susser[21] translated Koch's postulates for accepting an organism as the causative agent of a disease. These have been adapted into the following criteria that are used to establish the likelihood of whether an agent is causal:

- Strength of the association—the greater the relative risk when the proposed causal factor is present, the greater the likelihood of a causal relationship
- Dose-response relationship—increasing levels of exposure would be expected to cause an increase in rates of disease
- Consistency of association—refers to obtaining a similar rate of disease in different populations and in different studies when the causal factor is present
- Temporally correct association—the proposed causal factor must be present before the development of the health consequence or disease, and the necessary induction and latency period must be present
- Specificity of the association—the disease or health outcome of interest must be associated only with the potential causal factor under study
- Biologic plausibility—reasonable biologic evidence that the proposed causal factor could result in the disease or outcome of interest

In conclusion, analytical research is used to clarify associations between risk factors and disease. The study question determines the research design to be used. Once associations are established, risk factors must be assessed in more detail to determine whether they are causal.

References

1. Leaf A, Weber PC. Cardiovascular effects of n-3 fatty acids. *N Engl J Med.* 1988;318:549.
2. Kromann N, Green A. Epidemiological studies in the Upernavik district, Greenland: incidence of some chronic diseases 1950–1974. *Acta Med Scand.* 1980;208:401.
3. Bang HO, Dyerberg J, Hjorne N. The composition of food consumed by Greenland Eskimos. *Acta Med Scand.* 1976;200:69.
4. Dyerberg J, Bang HO, Hjorne N. Fatty acid composition of the plasma lipids in Greenland Eskimos. *Am J Clin Nutr.* 1975;28:958.
5. Harris WS, Connor WE, Inkeles SB, Illingworth DR. Dietary omega-3 fatty acids prevent carbohydrate-induced hypertriglyceridemia. *Met.* 1984;33:1016.
6. Nestel PJ, Connor WE, Reardon MF, et al. Suppression by diets rich in fish oil of very low density lipoprotein production in man. *J Clin Invest.* 1984;74:82.
7. Yang Y-T, Williams MA. Comparison of C_{18}-, C_{20}-, C_{22}- unsaturated fatty acids in reducing fatty acid synthesis in isolated rat hepatocytes. *Biochim Biophys Acta.* 1978;531:133.
8. Wong SH, Nestel PJ, Trimble RP, et al. The adaptive effects of dietary fish and safflower oil on lipid and lipoprotein metabolism in perfused rat liver. *Biochim Biophys Acta.* 1984;792:103.
9. Wong S, Reardon M, Nestel P. Reduced triglyceride formation from long chain polyenoic fatty acids in rat hepatocytes. *Met.* 1985;43:900.
10. Levin ML. The occurrence of lung cancer in man. *Acta Univ Int Contra Cancrum.* 1953;19:53.
11. Hennekens CH, Buring JE; Mayrent SL, ed. *Epidemiology in Medicine.* Boston, Mass: Little Brown and Co; 1987:89–96.
12. Kannel WB, Gordon T, eds. Some characteristics related to the incidence of cardiovascular disease and death, The Framingham Study. 16-year followup. Washington, DC: US Government Printing Office; 1970. WHO Expert Committee, Prevention of Coronary Heart Disease. Copenhagen, Denmark; 1982. WHO Technical Report Series no. 678.

13. Bonham GS. *Use habits of cigarettes, coffee, aspirin and sleeping pills, United States, 1976. Data from the National Health Survey, no. 131.* Washington, DC: US Government Printing Office; 1979. DHEW publication PHS 80-1559. Vital and Health Statistics series 10.

14. McIntosh ID. Alcohol-related disabilities in general hospital patients: a critical assessment of the evidence. *Int J Addict.* 1982;17:609.

15. West DW, Schuman KL, Lyon JL, et al. Differences in risk estimations from a hospital and a population-based case-control study. *Int J Epidemiol.* 1984;13:235.

16. Hennekens CH, Buring JE; Mayrent SL, ed. *Epidemiology in Medicine.* Boston, Mass: Little Brown and Co; 1987:148.

17. Bak AAA, Grobbee DE. The effect on serum cholesterol levels of coffee brewed by filtering or boiling. *N Engl J Med.* 1989;321:1432.

18. MRFIT (Multiple Risk Factor Intervention Trial) Research Group. Multiple risk factor intervention trial: risk factor changes and mortality results. *JAMA.* 1982;248:1465.

19. Feinstein A. Epidemiologic analysis of causation: the unlearned scientific lessons of randomized trials. *J Clin Epidemiol.* 1989;42:481.

20. Stroke Prevention in Atrial Fibrillation Study Group Investigators. Special report: preliminary report of the stroke prevention in atrial fibrillation study. *N Engl J Med.* 1990;322:863.

21. Susser M. *Causal Thinking in the Health Sciences. Concepts and Strategies in Epidemiology.* New York, NY: Oxford University Press; 1973.

Further Reading

Altman DG, Dore CJ. Randomization and baseline comparisons in clinical trials. *Lancet.* 1990;335:149.

Armitage P. Inference and decision in clinical trials. *J Clin Epidemiol.* 1989;42:293.

Esdaile JM, Horwitz RI. Observational studies of cause-effect relationships: an analysis of methodologic problems as illustrated by the conflicting data for the role of oral contraceptive in the etiology of rheumatoid arthritis. *J Chron Dis.* 1986;39:841.

Feinstein A. Models, methods, and goals. *J Clin Epidemiol.* 1989;42:301.

Feinstein A. Scientific standards in epidemiologic studies of the menace of daily life. *Science.* 1988;242:1257.

Flanders WD, O'Brien TR. Inappropriate comparisons of incidence and prevalence in epidemiologic research. *Am J Public Health.* 1989;79:1301.

Hennekens CH, Buring JE; Mayrent SL, ed. *Epidemiology in Medicine.* Boston, Mass: Little Brown and Co; 1987.

Mausner JS, Kramer S. *Mausner and Bahn: Epidemiology—An Introductory Text.* 2nd ed. Philadelphia, Pa: WB Saunders Co; 1985.

Miettinen OS. Unlearned lessons from clinical trials: a duality of outlooks. *J Clin Epidemiol.* 1989;42:499.

Pocock SJ, Hughes MD, Lee RJ. Statistical problems in the reporting of clinical trials: a survey of three medical journals. *N Engl J Med.* 1987;317:426.

Rothman KJ. *Modern Epidemiology.* Boston, Mass; Little Brown and Co; 1986.

Sackett DL. Inference and decision at the bedside. *J Clin Epidemiol.* 1989;42:309.

9. DESIGNING AND MANAGING A SMALL CLINICAL TRIAL

Barbara H. Dennis, PhD, RD, and P. M. Kris-Etherton, PhD, RD

INTRODUCTION

A clinical trial is a well-controlled study designed to address a question of relevance to human health. In a clinical trial, the investigator has control over the assignment of subjects to one or more treatment and comparison or control groups.[1] The small clinical trial is an efficient means for examining many nutritional questions related to the effect of dietary components on metabolic parameters and health outcomes. For the purposes of this chapter, a small clinical trial is defined as an intervention study carried out at a single site in which dietary modification is the independent or predictive variable. Whether in a hospital inpatient facility or academic research setting, dietitians play a key role in designing and implementing such studies. This chapter explores issues involved in designing a small clinical trial utilizing techniques and methods covered in detail elsewhere in this volume.

Designing a clinical trial involves a series of steps that specify exactly why, how, and with whom the study will be carried out, and how the results will be interpreted. This process culminates in the study protocol (*Table 9.1*). The protocol contains all the necessary information for carrying out the study. It is the written agreement between the investigator, the participant, and the scientific community[2] and forms the basis for informed consent and institutional review board decisions on human subject safety. In the following sections, each element of the protocol is discussed in detail.

Table 9.1
Protocol for a Small Clinical Trial

Introduction
- Justification

Objectives

Hypotheses

Study design and duration

Subject selection
- Inclusion and exclusion criteria
- Recruitment
- Screening procedures

Diet
- Precisely defined menu(s)

Study procedures
- Sample size
- Randomization
- Monitoring, compliance, retention, termination
- Measurements, methods

Statistical statement
- Data variables
- Data collection
- Analyses

Justification for the Study

The first step in planning a clinical trial is to identify and document the need for the study. What currently unavailable information will such a study yield, and why is the information important? Various sources provide information on important and timely nutrition research needs. Agencies of the Public Health Service, the US Department of Agriculture, and the Census Bureau frequently publish statistical reports for national and specialized populations. In addition, similar information is often available at the state level in health departments (see Appendix). Workshop proceedings and task force reports such as the *Surgeon General's Report on Nutrition and Health*[3] and the National Academy of Science publication, *Diet and Health*[4] identify research needs. *The National Institutes of Health Guide for Grants and Contracts*, published weekly, identifies specific research topics of interest to particular institutes. Once the need for a clinical trial has been identified, a thorough literature review will establish the extent of knowledge and activity in the area and provide information about promising ideas for further research.

Resources

The next step is to assess resources needed to carry out the study. This often involves obtaining the approval of the Institution Review Board and top level administrative support for the study. What resources are needed for the proposed study? Feeding studies require facilities for food storage, preparation, serving, and clean-up. Location, accessibility, and ambiance of the feeding site are important factors in recruitment and retention of study participants. Most studies involve some clinical and/or biochemical measurements, which may be as simple as measuring body weight and skinfold thickness, or more complex, involving biochemical analysis of body fluids, tissue, and so forth. Resources must be available for carrying out these measurements either directly or through contractual arrangements with other laboratories with established quality assurance procedures.

Budget

The development of a budget that covers all costs of the study is essential. While the actual cost depends on the design, scope, and duration of the study, some general guidelines can be given. The major budget categories are personnel, supplies, and equipment. In most cases, a specified percentage of the direct cost of the project must be added to cover overhead. The business officer of the sponsoring institution supplies this information. Rather than designating specific personnel, the following are functional considerations. Certain persons may assume several responsibilities, which should be identified and incorporated into their job descriptions.

Senior professional staff have responsibility for scientific decisions and control of the budget. They also have an important role in compliance and building morale over the long haul. Consistent day-to-day management by a professional is also necessary to supervise the kitchen, laboratory, and data collection. Technical personnel are needed for food preparation, preparation of food aliquots for analysis, and clinical, anthropometric, and laboratory measurements. Statistical assistance is essential during the design and analysis phases of the study. Both statistical and computer capabilities are required to manage and analyze the data. Specialized software may be needed for certain aspects of the study, such as nutrient calculations. Clerical activities include preparation of recruitment materials, forms, communication, scheduling of potential recruits, and preparation of reports. General purpose office equipment may need to be leased or purchased to meet the clerical demands of the study.

The most costly supply item is likely to be the food for the study. Laboratory supplies may be incorporated in the fees charged by the laboratory if these measurements are contracted out. Forms, duplicating costs, and participant incentives are other supply costs. Miscellaneous costs to consider include monetary incentives, transportation, and parking for participants, social activities, closeout costs (celebration), and computer costs.

STUDY DESIGN

The objectives of the study should be clearly defined at the outset. Objectives are statements of the research question the study is designed to answer. They determine the design and duration of the study, selection of subjects, and statistical analysis of the results.

A hypothesis is an assertion that an association between two or more variables or a difference between two or more groups exists in the larger population of interest.[5] The statistical test is performed on the null statement, ie, no association exists.

The clinical trial should be designed to answer one major question. The primary question is the one on which the sample size estimate is based and the one that is emphasized in the reporting. Multiple hypotheses increase the number of statistical tests that are required. This can reduce the power of the study (the probability of rejecting the null hypothesis if it is false) by increasing the number of statistically significant findings that can occur by chance alone.[2]

STUDY SUBJECTS

Results from human studies are frequently difficult to interpret because of the heterogeneity in human populations and the variability in free living conditions. Therefore, a concerted effort must be made to control for these factors in the design of a small clinical trial, beginning with the subject selection criteria. Controlling as many potential confounding factors as possible in the selection process may limit the generalizability of the results, but it makes interpretation of the results easier. Random assignment into treatment and control groups also eliminates many sources of bias. Subjects should be well-defined in terms of the parameters relative to the study, such as age, sex, body weight, and health status. For example, if the objective of the study is to determine the effect of diet composition on weight loss, subjects should meet similar body mass criteria. It would also be important to control for physical activity and conditioning: marathon runners should not be grouped with sedentary people. Other potential confounding variables in a study of this type might include smoking status, fat distribution pattern, and duration of excess weight. Outcome variables delineated in the study objectives and their possible confounding factors form the basis for making decisions with respect to defining the study sample.

Recruitment

Recruiting subjects for a clinical study or trial is a task that can range from being relatively easy to being very difficult. Many factors, such as the number of subjects required, exclusion criteria for participation in the study, study requirements, length of participation, subject remuneration, and perceived benefits to subjects, affect the recruitment process. Recruiting a sufficient number of subjects is essential for the power of the study. Doing it expeditiously controls the cost of the study. Problems that investigators typically encounter include overly optimistic recruitment goals and the lack of well-defined and realistic recruitment strategies. With effective planning however, recruiting problems can be avoided.

Recruitment begins with a well-defined and organized plan containing realistic short-term and long-term goals. Accordingly, the number of subjects needed and the time frame for recruitment has to be clearly defined. (See chapter 20 for discussion of sample size calculation.) Since initial recruitment goals may be unrealistic and often are not met, a contingency plan should be ready for immediate implementation. Staff responsibilities for recruitment should be clearly defined and effectively coordinated. Irrespective of the size of the recruitment staff, its members should possess certain personality traits such as perseverance, flexibility, endurance, and commitment. Staff members have to be scheduled to contact potential subjects at convenient times (ie, evenings and weekends). A small pilot program is very useful and highly recommended to identify and resolve weaknesses in the recruitment effort.

Eligibility

Subject eligibility criteria range from broad to very specific, depending on numerous factors, including the research question(s), cost, and time frame of the study. Narrow eligibility criteria and a large required number of study subjects increase recruitment efforts. Conversely, recruitment efforts are simplified when eligibility criteria are broad and/or when few subjects are needed. Communicating eligibility criteria in advance to potential subjects streamlines recruitment efforts. Common eligibility criteria include age, gender, weight, physical activity, cigarette smoking, and health status. In addition, potential subjects must accept the conditions of the study, including randomization to either the nontreatment control or intervention group, dietary controls imposed by the study test procedures, and collection of specimens, eg, blood, urine, or feces.

Subject Sources

Subject recruitment depends on effective advertising. Numerous strategies are useful. For example, newspaper advertisements that appear in different sections, including the classified ads, usually reach a large audience, as do other mass media strategies, such as radio and television. Some radio and television stations advertise a study as a public service message. Occasionally, newspaper writers feature a story about a planned study and include important recruitment information. To initiate this approach, the investigator can contact science or health editors at the newspaper. Announcements posted on bulletin boards in the community and physicians' offices are another effective recruitment strategy, as are announcements to community groups and classes. Mailing lists, which may be obtained from various individuals or groups, allow potential subjects to be contacted personally. Word-of-mouth recruitment also can be effective, especially if done by people who have served as experimental subjects. Hospital patients also may be a source of potential subjects.

Incentives

Incentives are important for recruitment and participation in screening activities that are required before enrolling subjects in the study. Monetary incentives can be effective, though other types of incentives also encourage participation in the screening procedures. Examples of low-cost nutrition-related incentives include: dietary assessment analysis, a nutrition counseling session, a chronic disease risk profile, a calorie counter, and recipes. Other low-cost incentives include: prizes, T-shirts, cosmetics, movie and raffle tickets, coupons, and gift certificates. The primary purpose of incentives is to facilitate participant recruitment. Accordingly, incentives should be age- and gender-specific, and they should be appropriate for the time and effort required to participate in the screening process. Incentives should not be so grand that they encourage people with no intention of serving as study subjects to participate in the screening process, and they should not imply or be perceived as coercion. Negative implications of incentives include selection bias and a lack of subject commitment to the study.

A distinction should be made between incentives for recruitment and incentives for retention. Incentives may be given periodically throughout the study, but the bulk should be reserved for those who successfully complete the study.

Screening

Screening ensures that participants meet eligibility criteria and are able to comply with the requirements of the study. This process does not bias the results of the study, since subjects are randomly allocated to treatment and control groups. In fact, a rigorous screening process may be critical to the success of the study. In addition to ensuring that potential subjects meet eligibility criteria, screening provides an opportunity to evaluate subjective data, such as attitude, behavior, interest, commitment, maturity, and so forth, which are important attributes in retaining participants and maintaining compliance.

The complexity of the screening process depends on the specificity of the subject exclusion criteria. Some studies require only a simple questionnaire, whereas others may require anthropometric, dietary, and laboratory data, as well as information on life-style practices, such as smoking and exercise behavior, and a medical examination to rule out underlying disease. It is particularly important that the screening process not prompt subjects to make any behavior changes prior to the initiation of the study. The interval between screening and the commencement of the study should be minimized.

Various strategies can be utilized to screen prospective subjects. These include questionnaires that can be mailed or completed by the recruitment team, telephone interviews, personal interviews, group meetings, and sessions in which data (eg, laboratory, psychosocial, dietary) are collected. In some instances, it may be necessary to have subjects attend more than one screening session.

Informed Consent

Federal law mandates that all people who elect to participate in a scientific study give their written consent. They also have the right to withdraw from the study at any time. In addition, their anonymity must be guaranteed. Before consenting to participate, subjects must be informed of the objectives, potential treatments, and all inherent risks of the study (*Table 9.2*). This information can be presented without biasing the study. When implemented appropriately, subjects' confidence is strengthened.

Table 9.2
Sample Consent Form

This is to certify that I, _____, agree to participate as a volunteer in a scientific investigation as part of the nutrition research program of (name of institution) under the supervision of _____.

The investigation and my part in the investigation have been defined and fully explained to me by _____, and I understand his/her explanation. A copy of the procedures of this investigation and a description of any risks and discomforts has been provided to me and has been discussed in detail with me.

I have been given an opportunity to ask whatever questions I have had, and all such questions have been answered satisfactorily.

I understand that I am free to deny any answers to specific items or questions in interviews or questionnaires.

I understand that any data or answers to questions will remain confidential with regard to my identity.

I understand that in the event of physical injury resulting from this investigation, neither financial compensation nor free medical treatment is provided for such a physical injury, and that further information on this policy is available from _____.

I certify that, to the best of my knowledge and belief, I have no physical or mental illness or weakness that would increase the risk to me of participation in this investigation.

I further understand that I am free to withdraw my consent and terminate my participation at any time.

_____	_____
Date	Subject's Signature
_____	_____
Date	Investigator's Signature
_____	_____
Date	Investigator's Signature
_____	
Date	
	_____
	Witness

STUDY PLAN

The study plan includes the timetable, randomization procedures, management plan, and methods for measuring all the variables collected in the study. This document is often referred to as the manual of operations, or procedure manual. If the study is carried out in an existing clinical research unit that is staffed with trained personnel, many of the general procedures governing controlled dietary studies already should be in place; only those procedures that are specific to the study need to be documented.

Randomization

Random assignment of subjects to either treatment or control group is a key feature of clinical trials. Through the random assignment procedure, any one subject has an equal probability of being assigned to either treatment or control group. The assignment should be blinded to the investigators. Double-blind assignment, in which neither subject nor investigator knows the assignment is preferable; however, it is often difficult to blind a dietary modification to the experimental subjects. Random assignment ensures that unmeasured, potentially confounding variables do not bias the study results. Techniques for randomly assigning subjects are available.[2]

STUDY PROCEDURES

Study procedures are the detailed specifications for carrying out the protocol.

Forms

The design and use of forms is the core of operationalizing the study. Forms serve various purposes and several functions may be combined in a single form.

- *Data forms.* Data forms encompass questionnaires, laboratory, and clinical forms. They comprise the record of the data that are collected, and thus control the scope of the data analysis. Unlike medical records and other narrative-type documents, standard forms impose structure and help ensure completeness, consistency, and comparability of all data collected throughout the study. Therefore, considerable thought must be given to their development and testing during the planning phase. It is often useful to construct dummy tables of data that will be needed for analysis and interpretation of the results and then relate them back to the data collection form(s).
- *Administrative forms.* Other forms are used in the management of the study. These include food inventories, menu calculations, food preparation instructions, and work schedules. A study flow sheet is valuable for ensuring complete data collection on all subjects.
- *Quality assurance forms.* Quality assurance forms include those used to certify that the correct food was received and consumed by the participant, records of dietary adjustments, adverse reactions, and protocol deviations, such as failure to consume the prescribed diet.

General guidelines for forms are depicted in *Table 9.3*, designated as SLIPPS. For more information on designing forms, the reader is referred to references 6 through 9.

The Dietary Intervention

Two critical factors in the design of the dietary intervention are control of the composition of the diet, and compliance with the diet. These in turn are directly related to the objectives and hypotheses of the study. Consider the following situations:

Investigator A wishes to test the effect of prescribing oat bran supplements on serum cholesterol levels. A protocol is formulated in which the control group of participants follows their regular diet and the intervention group is given oat bran supplements with instructions and recipes for using them. Both groups keep records of their food intake at intervals specified by the investigator. Serum cholesterol level and body weight are measured at baseline and at regular intervals during the study. At the conclusion of the study, the investigator finds that the mean cholesterol level of the intervention group is 0.13 mmol/L lower than the control group, a statistically significant difference. The intervention group also reported eating less total fat and more carbohydrate

Space
- Appropriate format and space to facilitate data collection

Logic
- Questions presented in logical sequence
- Consistent response codes

Instruction
- Printed on forms when possible
- Units and decimals printed on forms

Parsimony
- Collect only as much data as necessary
- Each item should have a specific purpose

Pretest
- Field test and revise before the trial

Security
- Duplicate copies of electronic back-up for data forms
- Confidentiality assurance system

than the control group. Both groups maintained their weight. What does the investigator conclude? The investigator concludes that *prescribing* oat bran results in lowering serum cholesterol in a group with the characteristics of the intervention group. The investigator does *not* conclude that oat bran lowers serum cholesterol. The investigator also cannot conclude that prescribing oat bran causes people to eat less fat and, hence, lower their cholesterol, because there is no way of knowing the accuracy of the reported intake during the course of the trial.

Investigator B, however, wishes to determine the effect of oat bran supplements on serum cholesterol levels. A protocol is designed in which a specified amount of oat bran is incorporated into a diet of fixed composition. The foods for both control and intervention groups are prepared and served in a special location. The calorie content of the diets is adjusted to maintain body weight. Subjects eat all their meals in this location. At the end of the trial, the investigator observes that the mean serum cholesterol level in the intervention group is not statistically different from that of the control group. The investigator concludes that oat bran does not lower serum cholesterol in people with characteristics similar to those of the study subjects.

Both investigators have made valid conclusions with respect to oat bran, but the research questions were quite different. In the case of A, the strategy of intervention (ie, prescription of oat bran) was being tested, whereas in case B, the metabolic effect of oat bran was being tested. Case B required a much greater degree of dietary control and compliance than case A.

The Experimental Diet

There is no perfect dietary intervention study. Design of the intervention has to take into account a number of tradeoffs. As shown in *Table 9.4*, the greater the dietary control, the more costly the study and the less attractive to potential subjects. Formula diets or synthetic mixtures provide the greatest degree of consistency, since each mouthful swallowed has the same composition. However, the relevance of the results to those that would be obtained with natural foods is limited. Again, the objectives of the study must be clearly formulated and, if necessary, revised to meet the limitations imposed by feasibility and reality. Once this is done, the investigator can decide whether the attainable objectives justify doing the study. At the other end of the scale, studies that are more feasible, in terms of cost and recruitment, are more difficult to interpret because the results are confounded by issues of compliance and variability in dietary composition.

A more detailed classification system for various degrees of dietary control in clinical research has been described by St. Jeor and Bryan.[10] *Table 9.5* defines clinical research diets and describes conditions for their use.

Determining the Composition of the Diet

Once the dietary prescription has been determined, the next step is to calculate the composition of the diet. Factors that need to be considered in addition to the composition are the distribution of nutrients over the day, variability in the nutrient composition of foods that will be used in the diet, palatability, and stability. Again, there are tradeoffs. Palatability is related to variety, and variety increases nutrient variability. For example, the composition of an egg is related to the size and the relative proportions of white and yolk, as well as feed and season. Purchasing all the eggs needed for a study, homogenizing them, weighing out individual portions, and freezing them for future use would provide the best control of variability, but it would be monotonous for the participant. Likewise, canned or frozen foods from a single packing lot would be more uniform than fresh foods purchased daily. In addition, there is less nutrient variability in a three-day versus a seven-day cycle menu. This level of precision is required to define specific effects of a dietary factor on an outcome variable. The level of precision needed depends again on the objectives of the study. For example, a study of the effects of fat and cholesterol on lipoprotein metabolism would require greater control of those nutrients and less control of variation in vitamins and minerals. By contrast, studies involving heat-labile vitamins would require greater attention to controlling food sources and preparation techniques.

Table 9.4
Degrees of Dietary Control

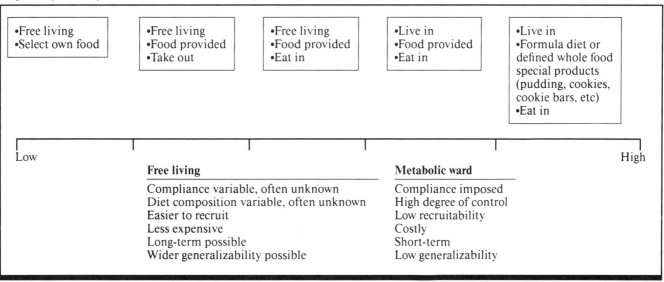

Table 9.5
*Clinical Research
Diets—Definition of Terms*

Classification	Intake Calculated	Measurement of Diet	Food Source	Water Source
Estimated	Daily (after intake charted), using equivalency lists or tables of averages	Estimated in household measures	Varied	Varied
Weighed	Daily (charted sometimes before and always after intake), using standard tables	Weighed (gram scale) portions (usual or calculated)	Varied	Varied
Controlled nutrient	Daily (before and after serving to patient), using standard tables, special references, or laboratory analyses	Weighed (torsion balance), controlled portions	Varied	Controlled or varied
Constant	Before study, using analyzed laboratory data, reliable manufacturers' data and nutrient databases, USDA Handbook No. 8, or other tables and references	Weighed (torsion balance), controlled portions	Constant	Controlled or constant
Metabolic (balance)	Before study, using analyzed laboratory data, reliable manufacturers' data and nutrient databases, USDA Handbook No. 8, or other tables and references	Weighed (torsion balance), controlled portions	Constant	Constant

Adapted from St. Jeor and Bryan.[10] Used by permission.

Analytical Research

Food Preparation Procedures	Food Refusals	Laboratory Analysis of Diet	Advantages	Disadvantages	Application
Varied	Estimated	No	Closest to "free diet"; ease and speed of estimation; most accurate observational data	Least reliable nutritive data; biased by change of setting, different foods, etc	Estimate of patient's preferred intake; data to supplement dietary history
Varied or controlled	Weighed	No	Minimal inconvenience to patient; more reliable nutritive data	Increased work with some increase in accuracy of data	More accurate idea of patient's preferred intake; more reliable observational data; general test diets
Controlled or varied	Weighed, calculated, and perhaps replaced	Rarely	Flexible, food variety; offers some variety and flexibility to patient	Expensive (dietitian's time unless computer available; constant monitoring for replacements	Diets with focus on desired maximum or minimum quantity or quality of nutrients; investigative diets
Constant	Discouraged, replaced if possible; otherwise, weighed, calculated, and perhaps analyzed	Occasionally	Highly accurate; dietitian's time used more efficiently; minimal calculations	Lack of variety and flexibility; requires a research kitchen, properly trained personnel, and standardized food preparation procedures; requires trial period for acceptability	Diagnostic diets, research diets
Constant	Discouraged, replaced if possible; otherwise, weighed, calculated, and analyzed	2-3 times per menu	Most reliable data; supported by actual laboratory analyses; dietitian's time used most efficiently; minimal calculations	Requires analyses of all intake and sometimes excreta; only as accurate as collections and laboratory analyses; lack of variety and flexibility; requires research kitchen, properly trained personnel, and standardized food preparation procedures; requires trial period for acceptability	Metabolic (balance) studies only

An important consideration in planning the diet is the anticipated energy requirements of the participants. This will affect the quantity of food needed and, hence, the budget. Energy requirements can be estimated using various methods. It is important to note that these estimates are not completely accurate for individuals, and often the calorie level of subjects' diets must be adjusted. However, they are sufficient to be used as a guide for planning for groups.

Many commercial software packages are available for estimating the nutrient composition of foods and guidelines are available for evaluating them.[11] Chapter 11 discusses this issue in detail. Nutrient databases, however, are derived from average composition values, which may not reflect what is actually being consumed. For studies in free living, free food selection groups, average values may be sufficient, but as the study design moves toward greater control of the diet, the need for analytical values increases. A good plan is to analyze aliquots of the calculated diets and to make adjustments, if necessary, before the study is started. Aliquots should then be collected and analyzed periodically throughout the study. *Table 9.6* gives instructions for preparing a diet aliquot for nutrient analysis.

Selection of a Food Analysis Laboratory

The most important criterion in selecting an analytical laboratory is the assurance of quality analyses. Inaccurate results at any price are not a bargain. Quality assurance relates to the overall concept by which the accuracy of analytical results generated by a laboratory is assured. This concept encompasses sampling, sample handling, storage, preservation methods, including validation, quality control procedures (to obtain valid and reliable results), skills of personnel, calibration of equipment, documentation of performance, reporting of results, and adequacy of the laboratory facilities.

Quality control includes such laboratory activities as the maintenance of calibration curves, and quality control charts and running recovery studies. Also important is a commitment to performing replication analyses, participation in proficiency testing, and use of certified standards.[13]

Professional organizations such as the American Oil Chemists' Society (AOCS)[14] and the Association of Official Analytical Chemists (AOAC)[15] are a valuable resource for information about nutrient analysis of foods. For example, the AOCS examination board provides a list of AOCS certified laboratories. For approval as a certified laboratory, there are two essential requirements: (1) The laboratory must have on staff, full time, an AOCS approved chemist, who is approved based on a reoccurring test of proficiency on samples submitted by the AOCS. (2) In addition to continuing participation in the proficiency test, the laboratory must perform at an acceptable level on 12 additional lipid analyses each year on blind samples submitted as "referee" materials by the AOCS.

Not all laboratories have proficiency in analyzing food matrices. Before selecting a laboratory, it should be established that the laboratory performs well on food matrices for the nutrients of interest in the study. Analysis of the diet is the common feature of all dietary intervention clinical trials, and hence has been discussed in detail in this chapter. Methods for measuring outcome and intervening variables, however, are specific to the objectives of the study and beyond the scope of this chapter.

Table 9.6
Preparation of Food Samples for
Chemical Analysis[12]

Selection of food

Prepare and weigh an additional serving of each food and beverage for the entire day. This should be done by selecting randomly from the portions weighed and regularly served.

Mixing and aliquoting

For a single day, preweigh and record the weight of a regular-sized kitchen blender bowl, place each meal in it, and refrigerate as the food is prepared. Remember to include milk, juice, condiments, or any other item that is part of the diet being served. Weigh the blender plus food and record the weight. Blenderize the food until it is a smooth slurry. Occasionally, the meal will be too dry to blenderize. If this should occur, water may be added until the mixture blends easily and the weight of the blender + food + water is taken and recorded. The weight of water is calculated by difference and must be subtracted from the final concentration reported for the nutrient analysis. The blended mixture will not be a true solution. For example, small pieces of spinach may be still detected by the eye. Pour the blenderized food into wide-mouthed polyethylene screw-cap bottles, leaving a little head space for freezer expansion. Label with date, sample name (number), laboratory, food composite weight, and weight of water added. Several aliquots of 50-100 mL are better to save than one or two at 250 mL because it takes a long time to thaw 250 mL samples.

Aliquoting the entire diet

To obtain an accurate estimate, you must sample your entire cycle of menus. Using a large institutional blender (Waring, 1 gal capacity, stainless steel) you can composite as many as four days at a time. Weigh the blender, add food each day, and either refrigerate until all the food is collected or freeze. Freezing poses problems because it takes a long time to thaw such a large mass. Blenderize as above. The larger blender generates a great deal of heat; so blend in short spurts, or occasionally take the blender off and cool in cold water before resuming the blending.

Many investigators have much longer cycles. Our suggestion for forming composites is to take aliquots of three or four days and combine these together by weight so there is a proportional representation of each day in the final composite. From each three or four-day slurry (these will have to be frozen and thawed for recompositing) take a 10% (or other appropriate percentage) by weight portion of well-mixed slurry and add this to an appropriate-sized blender. This weight portion should include any water added. Record on the aliquot bottles the total weight of the food for the entire menu cycle plus total amount of water added for the menu cycle and the number of days aliquoted. These are large numbers but less subject to calculational errors.

Mixing

The need for thorough mixing cannot be emphasized too much. Since these are mixtures, their consistency of concentration for the analyte in question always is problematic. The size of the aliquot you take for analysis or further compositing should be large enough to ensure an adequate representation from an imperfectly mixed slurry. The classical method for taking the aliquot was to use a 50 mL volumetric pipette and take the sample from the middle of the slurry. This method requires the use of added water to provide a slurry thin enough to pipette. We have avoided the use of water by pouring aliquots directly into sample bottles, since slurries look consistent throughout and have no foam on the top of the slurry. The use of a basting bulb may be another solution.

Retention and Compliance

Retaining subjects and maintaining compliance throughout the study are important in ensuring the success of any clinical investigation. Many potential problems can be minimized or prevented by careful planning. A formal protocol and adequate resources for retention and compliance activities should be incorporated into the planning phase. Criteria for subject dismissal must be established prior to the investigation. Many problems with subject retention, compliance, and dismissal can be avoided by meticulous screening of potential subjects to identify cooperative and committed subjects, and by providing continuous support and encouragement throughout the investigation.

Accurate measurement of compliance with the experimental protocol is important for meaningful interpretation of the treatment effects. In some studies, compliance may be an important outcome variable since the treatment effect may be biased by noncompliance. In either case, noncompliance must be accounted for this in the final data analysis. For example, if a clinical study is designed to evaluate the effects of iron supplementation on measures of iron status and one-half of the treatment group takes only 50% of their prescribed supplement, this must be quantified and considered in the data analyses. If this information were not collected, the results of the study would be flawed.

The actual assessment of compliance must consider several variables that vary as a function of the type and/or design of the investigation. In some studies, measurement of compliance may entail a very simple, straightforward approach, whereas other studies may be dependent on measuring some biological variable that requires a more complex assay (eg, platelet phospholipid fatty acids). Likewise, the sensitivity of the methods selected for assessing compliance may range from very sensitive (measuring a urinary metabolite) to relatively insensitive (subjects' self-assessment of compliance). Another consideration is whether compliance is assessed objectively or subjectively. Subjective assessment can be as simple as merely asking subjects if they are adhering to the protocol. This approach is successful when the investigators and subjects have established a friendly and trusting relationship. Often, investigators can ascertain compliance surprisingly well merely on the basis of subject attitude and behavior (eg, level of participation, punctuality, and so forth). If there is any suspicion that subjects are not complying with the experimental protocol, they should be directly confronted.

While total compliance is the goal of all studies, it is essential in metabolic studies. Not only must the subjects consume all the allotted food (and not lose any through emesis), they also must refrain from consuming any other food or substances that might bias the results of the study. However, it is seldom feasible to maintain study subjects in an enclosed, supervised environment 24 hours a day over an extended period. Therefore, proxy measures are often employed with varying degrees of sensitivity.

Once energy equilibrium has been established, body weight changes may signal compliance problems. This, however, is only a gross indicator. It would not differentiate changes in energy expenditure, nor would it detect small deviations in food intake that, nevertheless, could have a large effect if certain foods were systematically omitted or consumed outside the protocol.

When complete collection of excreta are obtained, metabolites and other substances may be measured. For example, a constant sodium intake should be reflective of a constant sodium excretion.[16] The validity of excretion as an index of intake depends, of course, on completeness of the collections. Urinary creatinine excretion is useful for detecting complete 24-hour collections on a diet of constant composition.[17] P-amino benzoic acid administered in tablet form has been used to assess completeness of urine collections,[18] and, added to food, to monitor dietary compliance.[19] A detailed description of various methods for assessing compliance is beyond the scope of this chapter. For more information, the reader is referred to Bingham.[20]

Finally, it is important to note that, human frailties and social needs being what they are, compliance is not likely ever to be perfect. It can be enhanced if overall morale is high and attempts are made to build into the protocol some free choices; for example, diet beverages that may be consumed at social gatherings.

Morale Incentives

Subject morale can wane quickly in response to various factors, including increasing length of the study and other constraints. It is essential to maintain a high level of morale throughout the study. This requires a major effort by the investigative team. The importance of time and resources devoted to this aspect should not be underestimated. Social support continuously provided by the investigators will be time well spent in the long run. Subjects need to feel valued and highly regarded by the investigators. Every effort should be made to ensure that the subjects are comfortable, happy, and feel a sense of ownership of the study. Effective techniques include sending birthday and other greeting cards, recognition of significant events, providing entertainment during the study, conducting raffles, and paying attention to details such as serving high-quality food, providing good service, and making newspapers and magazines available. In some studies, contests are appropriate motivational stimuli.

Dismissal

Criteria for subject dismissal must be clearly identified before the study begins and communicated to potential subjects. During the study, any behavior that compromises the results of the study is basis for dismissal. It is imperative that this policy be consistent, enforced, and, in general, not modified.

MANAGEMENT

After considerable planning, investigators are typically enthusiastic at the onset of the study. Sustained attention to the daily management and quality assurance of the study are essential. This becomes more challenging, especially during larger and longer-term studies in which the treatment period is lengthy, several different treatments are implemented, or subjects enter the study slowly (eg, one at a time). A strong management plan and capable investigative team are the key to avoiding problems that may be detrimental to the study.

Components of a good management plan include organization, communication, clear delineation and coverage of duties and responsibilities, contingency plans, and procedures for dealing with problems. It is also important that the management plan deal with the monitoring of the study vis-a-vis the goals of the study. Questions such as the following should be asked regularly throughout the study to ensure that the goals of the study are met.
- Have subject recruitment and retention goals been met?
- Is subject retention still acceptable?
- Have data been collected from all subjects at designated times?
- Has a comprehensive management plan been developed from a detailed study protocol and made available to the investigative team and staff?

The staff can vary in size for a clinical study or trial, depending upon the scope of the study. Regardless of the magnitude of a study, there is always a principal investigator (or co-principal investigator) who is responsible for the conduct of the study. A project director may manage the day-to-day activities of the investigation. In any clinical study, it is important for the chain of command to be established and for each staff person to report to someone. Likewise, it is important that staff persons be supervised, although some staff members may require only minimal supervision. A written work plan that includes specific goals, action plans, and a time line is useful in completing various tasks associated with the study.

Staff communication is essential for all studies. Frequent meetings at regular intervals are useful for keeping the staff informed about the progress of the study. Other effective types of communication include message and log books, newsletters, blackboards, bulletin boards, and the use of computer networks.

Committed, experienced, and enthusiastic leaders or supervisors avoid communication breakdowns by maintaining close contact with the project staff. They continually solicit information about the progress of various aspects of the study from staff members. Written reports submitted periodically and/or oral reports given at staff meetings summarizing each staff member's accomplishments facilitate communication among the project staff and achieving the goals of the study.

An often neglected but necessary consideration is planning for the unwanted but inevitable problems that are bound to happen during the course of the study. These include, but are not limited to, illness or emergency absence (staff and subjects), severe weather, mishaps in the kitchen and laboratory, lost or mislabeled samples, and noncompliance. Procedures for dealing with these situations should be thought out in advance and contingency plans developed. The timing of the study may have an adverse effect not only on recruitment but on retention and compliance if it encompasses major holidays or school breaks.

Quality Assurance

No study is better than the quality of its data.[2] The quality assurance program is a continuous process of assessment and evaluation according to predetermined criteria, feedback, and correction. A well-designed quality assurance system incorporates quality control procedures at every point in the study where information is transferred. The quality control component is part of an overall management strategy that includes written and oral progress reports, budget monitoring, and morale building among staff and participants.

Quality assurance begins with the selection of methods with the highest degree of accuracy and precision attainable. Whenever possible, standards should be used, and routine monitoring included to ensure the continued accuracy of the methods (an internal quality control system allows for reanalysis of samples at different times).

Quality assurance includes training of personnel, regular maintenance and calibration of equipment, monitoring performance of personnel and equipment, application of data editing criteria, and documentation of quality with corrective feedback throughout the collection, and processing of data. A well-trained staff is important for ensuring that data are collected and managed without bias and variability. Training, however, is only the first step; regular monitoring is also necessary. Subtle changes in the procedure over time can cause considerable drift, which could bias the results. The same is true for equipment. The tools for quality assurance are developed in the planning phase, and they include the protocol, procedure manuals, forms for data collection, and data management. Data management incorporates documentation of data quality: protocol violations, missing and spurious values. Visual inspection of completed forms, ranges for acceptable values, logic, and consistency checks are applied as the data are collected so that problems can be detected and corrected early (*Table 9.7*). Ideally, the quality assurance program prevents problems before they occur.

Table 9.7
Quality Assurance
Considerations in a Clinical
Trial

Aspect of the Study	Recommended Quality Control Procedures
Methods	Validate for accuracy Establish performance standards Provide staff feedback
Training staff and monitoring performance	Establish protocols Written procedures Performance standards Provide staff feedback
Forms	Design Pilot test
Data	Verify accuracy of data and data entry Adjudication of questionable data

Data Management

It is important to realize that even in a small clinical trial there will be a considerable amount of data collected, typically from many sources at different times. Management of this aspect of the study includes the coordination of the collection of the data, data entry, controlling access to the data, assuring the safety of the data, and monitoring quality control procedures. Although several of the project staff should be knowledgeable in these procedures, management should be the sole responsibility of one person. The data manager should possess specific training in statistics and computer science. Assuming that the data are collected according to the specified protocol, it is important then that the data must be secured against unauthorized access to protect the privacy of the subjects and against damage and loss. Data should be entered into a secure computer file, and duplicate copies of data files (both paper and computer) stored in a safe, secure place in another location.

There are different formats for storing data. The format selected should be consistent with the data analysis protocol established prior to the initiation of the major study.

PILOT STUDY

Major clinical trials benefit greatly from a pilot study, which is a scaled-down version of the larger investigation. The pilot study provides an opportunity for the staff to practice implementing the experimental procedures of the major investigation, "debug" and troubleshoot problems, identify pitfalls, and simply determine whether the clinical trial, as planned, is feasible. Staffing issues such as size, scheduling and skills can also be assessed. A pilot study is useful for evaluating subjects' potential acceptance of the experimental protocol and diet. Problem areas are identified and resolved so that the major study proceeds smoothly. Frequently, simple changes in the experimental protocol or diet (eg, substituting baked potatoes for baked sweet potatoes) will facilitate subject compliance and satisfaction with the study and/or diet. A pilot study also is beneficial in providing a perspective about the outcome of the major study. The variation in the subjects' response to the treatment can be determined so that sample size adjustments for the major study can be made. In addition, the pilot study can be used to determine the length of time required for the major study (ie, for the parameters measured to stabilize in response to the treatment).

Overall, the benefits of a pilot study are worth the effort and cost. Since every aspect of the clinical trial is implemented, most problems can be identified and resolved. A pilot study provides an excellent opportunity to ascertain whether the goals (recruitment, retention, compliance, response measurements, data collection, and analysis) of the major study are realistic and attainable.

DATA ANALYSIS AND PUBLICATION

Results of the study are obtained by subjecting the data to statistical testing of the primary and secondary hypotheses defined in the initial study design. It is important that the data analysis be done carefully, rigorously, and by individuals who are experienced and knowledgeable in statistical methodology and analysis. Issues such as deciding which subjects to include in the analysis (ie, how to deal with exclusions and withdrawals and noncompliance), deciding what to do about poor quality and missing data, subgroup analyses, and comparison of multiple variables are of critical importance in interpreting the results.[2] Analysis is part of the statistical design of the study which must be addressed during the planning phase of the study and specified in the protocol. (See chapter 21.)

Dissemination of the study findings and conclusions should be the result of any scientific inquiry. In-house publications are useful in disseminating information about the study to colleagues, staff, and other interested persons in the institution where the investigation was conducted.* Presentations at scientific meetings and submission of the study report to peer review journals provides valuable critical appraisal. Often, this leads to new insights in the interpretation of the study and new research directions. Chapter 22 provides guidance on preparing a manuscript for publication.

SUMMARY

The design and successful implementation of a small clinical trial is dependent on many factors. Foremost among these is careful planning and attention to all aspects of the clinical trial. With the study objectives and plan and procedures well-defined, a highly motivated, competent staff and cooperative subjects are essential for the successful completion of the clinical trial. Quality control procedures and data collection and analysis methods also are key aspects of the study. Collectively, careful planning of all facets is important to achieve the objectives of the clinical trial.

---

*Reporting and interpreting the results to the subjects should be done as early as feasible and certainly before they hear about it in the lay media.

APPENDIX

Sources of Data

Centers for Disease Control (CDC). *Morbidity and Mortality Weekly Report.*

CDC, PHS, DHHS. Pediatric Nutrition Surveillance System.

Food and Drug Administration (FDA), Public Health Service (PHS), Department of Health and Human Services (DHHS). Health and Diet Survey.

Gable CB. A compendium of public health data sources. *Am J Epidemiol.*1990;131:381–394.

Human Nutrition Information Service, US Department of Agriculture (USDA). Continuing Survey of Food Intakes by Individuals (CSFII).

Life Sciences Research Office, Federation of American Societies of Experimental Biology. *Assessment of the Nutritional Status of the U.S. Population Based on Data Collected in the Second National Health and Nutrition Examination Survey, 1976–1980.* Bethesda, Md: Federation of American Societies for Experimental Biology; 1984.

National Center for Health Statistics (NCHS), CDC, PHS, DHHS. Hispanic Health and Nutrition Examination Survey.

NCHS. *Health Statistics on Older Persons: United States, 1986.* DHHS publication PHS 87–1409, series 3, no. 25.

NCHS, CDC, PHS, DHHS. National Health and Nutrition Examination Survey (NHANES) II.

NCHS, CDC, PHS, DHHS. National Health Interview Survey (NHIS).

NCHS, CDC, PHS, DHHS. National Vital Statistics.

References

1. Lilienfeld AM. *Foundations of Epidemiology.* New York, NY: Oxford University Press; 1976.
2. Friedman LM, Furberg CD, DeMets DL. *Fundamentals of Clinical Trials.* 3rd ed. Littleton, Mass: PSG Publishing Co; 1985.
3. *The Surgeon General's Report on Nutrition and Health.* Washington, DC: US Dept of Health and Human Services, US Government Printing Office; 1988. DHHS publication PHS 88–50210.
4. National Research Council. *Diet and Health. Implications for Reducing Chronic Disease Risk.* Washington, DC: National Academy Press; 1989.
5. Riegelman RK. *Studying a Study and Testing a Test.* Boston, Mass: Little Brown and Co; 1981.
6. Wright P, Haybittle J. Design of forms for clinical trials (1). *Br Med J.* 1979; 2:529–530.
7. Wright P, Haybittle J. Design of forms for clinical trials (2). *Br Med J.* 1979; 2:590–592.
8. Wright P, Haybittle J. Design of forms for clinical trials (3). *Br Med J.* 1979; 2:650–651.
9. Gore SM. Assessing clinical trials—record sheets. *Br Med J.* 1981; 283:296–298.
10. St Jeor ST, Bryan GT. Clinical research diets: definition of terms. *J Am Diet Assoc.* 1973;62:47–51.
11. Byrd-Bredbenner C. Computer nutrient analysis software packages: considerations for selections. *Nutr Today.* Sept/Oct 1988.
12. Bowen PE. Personal communication; April 27, 1988.

13. Beecher G. Personal communication; 1990.
14. American Oil Chemists' Society. *Official Methods and Recommended Practices.* Champaign, Ill: American Oil Chemists' Society; 1987–1988.
15. Association of Official Analytical Chemists. *Official Methods of Analysis.* 14th ed. Arlington, Va: Association of Official Analytical Chemists Inc; 1984.
16. Schachter J, Harper PH, Radin ME, Caggiula AW, McDonald RH, Diven WF. Comparison of sodium and potassium intake with excretion. *Hypertension.* 1980; 2:695–699.
17. Jackson S. Creatinine in urine as an index of urinary excretion rate. *Health Physics.* 1966; 12:843–850.
18. Bingham S, Cummings JH. The use of 4-amino benzoic acid as a marker to validate the completeness of 24 h urine collections in man. *Clin Sci.* 1983; 64:629–635.
19. Roberts SB, Morrow FD, Evans WJ, et al. Use of P-amino benzoic acid to monitor compliance with prescribed dietary regimens during metabolic balance studies in man. *Am J Clin Nutr.* 1990; 51:485–488.
20. Bingham S. The dietary assessment of individuals; methods, accuracy, new techniques and recommendations. *CAB International.* 1987; 57:705–742.

Further Reading

Pocock SJ. *Clinical Trials: A Practical Approach.* New York, NY: John Wiley and Sons, 1983.

PART 5
KEY TECHNIQUES
USED IN RESEARCH

The techniques and applications described in chapters 10 through 19 give a wealth of information applicable to both descriptive and analytical research.

The first four chapters cover issues of dietary intake assessment and food choices. Methods used to secure these data need to be culturally sensitive and customized to the selected individuals or groups. Essential to the interpretation of these data are professionals with strong backgrounds in nutrition sciences, food composition, human behavior, and psychosocial sciences.

Dietary intake data, the subject of chapter 10, may be categorized as group data (such as national food availability data), individual data, or pooled individual data. Precision must be higher when the data are collected to characterize an individual (eg, when data are to be used to customize nutrition counseling or in correlating an individual client's intake with a serum value) than when the data will be pooled to characterize a group (eg, vegans versus omnivores). Chapter 11 delineates the wide uses of food composition data and the extensive development of databases. In using nutrient databases, researchers are cautioned to ascertain how missing values are handled: imputed, left blank, or designated as zero.

Record-based surveillance data and population surveys are discussed in chapter 12. Surveillance data are based on self-selected populations, eg, women and children participating in publicly funded nutrition and health programs. Population surveys, because of inherent sampling and design complexities, require adjustments for sample weights and design effects. Survey and surveillance data have multiple applications, including nutritional status monitoring, program planning, and market segment identification. Chapter 13 describes methods to assess sensory perceptions of foods: thresholds, perceived intensity, identification, and hedonic measures. Specific study design, setting, and individual variability of test subjects influence subject reaction. Genetically determined sensitivity to taste and odor, prior training, state of health, and smoking habits are among factors affecting intraindividual and interindividual response.

Chapter 14 reviews studies in foodservice production management and information systems that have been published in the past several decades. The studies are categorized as descriptive research and observational or experimental analytical research. Queuing, transport models, and assembly line balancing are three areas of research in foodservice that have employed descriptive and analytical research designs. Chapter 15 delineates research techniques critical to foodservice, emphasizing mathematical procedures appropriate in management, food production forecasting, cost accountability, investment decision making, and profit analysis. The bottom line is the most-read line of any account or budget; it deserves the support of quality research.

The next two chapters discuss documentation of practice and marketing. Chapter 16 compares cost-effectiveness analysis with cost-benefit analysis and presents clear examples related to the economics of practice. Researchers group benefits as direct (ie, expenditures conserved because of effective dietetic services), indirect (ie, improvements in quality of life that can be estimated in dollar terms, such as higher work attendance), and intangible (ie, quality of life improvements that cannot be translated into dollar terms). Chapter 17 distinguishes various methods of design appropriate for marketing research, including techniques to secure data relevant to the marketing components of price, product, place, and promotion. Common errors in marketing research are discussed (see also chapter 2).

Part 5 is rounded out with an elaboration of dietetic education research and meta-analysis. Dietetic education research emphasizes data collection techniques based on standardized tests, validated research-designed tests, questionnaires, interviews, and direct observation. Researchers are cautioned to minimize both halo and Hawthorne effects through research design and observer training. Chapter 19 describes the steps of meta-analysis: constructing selection inclusion criteria, making a comprehensive search of existing studies that meet the criteria, and combining and assessing the data from the qualifying studies.

The multiple techniques described in this section are resources that expand the assets of all researchers. Enjoy them and the further research they will kindle.

ERM, Editor

10. DIETARY INTAKE METHODOLOGY

Jean H. Hankin, DrPH, RD

Since the 1940s, diet has been increasingly recognized as a major determinant of health and disease during adult years. To identify the relationship of diet to coronary heart disease, cancer, and other chronic illnesses, epidemiologists and clinicians are including dietary assessment as an integral component in the design of cohort and case-control studies. Consequently, the dietitian has become a key member of the research team, responsible for selecting and implementing the dietary methods for epidemiologic and clinical studies and surveys of large population groups.

Unfortunately, there is no single dietary method suitable for all food consumption surveys or epidemiologic, nutritional status, and clinical investigations. Differences exist according to the purpose of the study, precision needed, particular population, period of interest (past or current), and available resources. This paper will review the various dietary methods and modifications, their strengths and limitations, and selected examples from the literature. The problems and methods of assessing the validity and reproducibility of these methods will also be discussed.

Dietary methods are often classified according to "group" or "individual" methods. Although dietitians have used several methods of individual assessment for dietary counseling and nutrition education, they may be less familiar with "group" methods, as well as with the application of various dietary methods for research.

GROUP DIETARY DATA

Group data may be based on national food availability (disappearance), statistics, or on household data.

Food Availability (Disappearance) Data

In the United States, the Economic Research Service (ERS) of the US Department of Agriculture (USDA) compiles annual supply and use data for major commodities disappearing into civilian consumption.[1-3] The total available food is determined from the sum of the beginning stocks, production estimates, and imports. The amount utilized during the year is the residual after subtracting food exported, purchased for the military, fed to livestock, put to non-food use, and ending stores. The civilian per capita consumption is then calculated by dividing the available quantity of each food by the estimated total civilian population. (Since the military data are available, per capita intakes for the total population may be easily determined.) These per capita intakes do not correct for food fed to pets, food waste, losses in transport and storage, food preparation losses, or spoilage, and consequently overestimate individual intakes. The nutritive value of the per capita supplies is calculated from the USDA food composition data. These statistics, sometimes called *food disappearance* data, have been estimated annually since 1909 to 1913 and are useful for agricultural and marketing research and analysis of trends in the United States.[3] However, they do not reveal differences by particular state, geographic region, or other demographic variables.

Similar data have been compiled by other countries and reported to the Food and Agriculture Organization of the United Nations (FAO), which publishes the findings periodically on food balance sheets. Their major usage is to measure the adequacy of the food supply and to assess the trends between and within countries. During recent years, a few investigators have correlated the per capita food and nutrient intakes from selected countries with incidence or mortality rates to illustrate associations of diet and disease. For example, the relationships of dietary fat and breast cancer,[4] meat and colon cancer,[4] and saturated fat and heart disease[5] reveal strong positive associations when per capita intakes are correlated with incidence or mortality rates of selected countries. Such correlations provide leads for further research. However, they do not demonstrate cause and effect or true associations for several reasons:

- We have no information on other potential determinants of the disease in these populations.
- The data include only supplies entering the trade channels (in many countries, local fish, garden vegetables, and indigenous root crops comprise a large proportion of the diet; these home-produced foods do not enter the trade channels, and thus are excluded from the national data).
- The dietary data do not represent individual intakes.
- The quality of the data may vary between countries.
- The per capita values may not relate to the persons at greatest risk of the disease. For example, per capita alcohol intakes, based on food disappearance data, do not represent the heaviest consumers. Hence, the use of these data to demonstrate an association of alcohol with breast cancer may be highly misleading.[6]

Household Food Intakes

In contrast to food availability, a closer approximation of food intakes may be derived from household estimates. The USDA has conducted periodic national surveys on household food use since 1936.[1,3,7,8] Briefly, the person responsible for food planning and preparation recalls quantitative information on the foods purchased and utilized during a one-week period. This person is contacted a week prior to the interview and asked to keep a record of purchases and menus during the next seven days. A recall is then obtained, with the aid of a detailed food list, of all foods used and brought into the household during the past week. This includes the foods consumed, along with foods discarded as garbage and fed to pet animals, and thus is most likely an overestimate of the actual intake. The nutritive value of the edible portion of the household foods is computed and the per person intakes calculated, after adjusting for meals eaten away from home and guest meals in the home.

These data are useful for determining if the nutrients available (based on meals eaten in the household) are sufficient to meet the Recommended Dietary Allowances (RDAs) of the particular household. The USDA[3] has developed a unique method of evaluating the food consumption data. The assumption is made that foods and nutrients are divided among the family members according to their age and sex and that food eaten away from home has the same nutrient value as the home food supply. To estimate the RDAs of the household, the allowances of a 25-year-old man are assumed to be 1.0 nutrition units; the equivalent units of other members are obtained by dividing each of their allowances by those of the reference man. The household food consumption data may be utilized to show the effects of income, household size, and other demographic variables on food intake, and to develop the USDA family food plans at different income levels.

Other household dietary methods have been reported in various countries. In the United Kingdom, random samples of 6500 households are asked to record their total food purchases (excluding candy, alcohol, and foods consumed away from home) for a one-week period annually.[9] The food purchasing data are used to obtain estimated average food and nutrient intakes per person in the households. The household data have been correlated with mortality data and have revealed inverse associations of regional colon cancer mortality rates with the average intakes of vegetables and the pentosan fraction of dietary fiber.[9] However, the exclusion of selected food items, reporting errors, and lack of data on individual dietary intakes limit the interpretation of these findings.

In some areas, particularly developing countries, per capita household intakes are calculated from weighed inventories of all foods on hand at the beginning and end of a one-week period. All foods brought into the household during that time are also weighed and recorded. Either a member of the household or a trained field worker completes the inventories and the log of daily purchases and preparation practices.

Household data are often utilized for economic evaluations. Although they are more satisfactory than food availability data, they do not account for age and sex differences and should not be considered measures of individual intake. Another serious limitation is the lack of information on foods and beverages consumed away from home. In many areas, this may represent one-third or more of an individual's dietary intake. Nonetheless, household data often provide leads for developing hypotheses on diet and disease that can be tested in epidemiologic studies of individuals.

INDIVIDUAL DIETARY METHODS

During the last 20 years, several papers,[10-15] reports,[16-18] and books[6,19] have been published concerning the selection of individual dietary methods for studies of large populations. Generally, these methods include the 24-hour recall (or occasionally recent recalls of three to seven days), food records or diaries, and diet histories. Some authors distinguish between diet histories and food frequencies.[6,20,21] However, similar to diet histories, food frequencies also pertain to the usual recent or past intakes of individuals and thus are considered a modification of the history.

24-Hour Recall

This technique is the most widely used dietary method in population studies. Information on all foods and estimated amounts consumed during the past 24 hours is obtained, beginning either with the present and working backward or beginning with the first food eaten the previous day and working forward. The information usually is collected in an interview with a dietitian, other health worker, or trained interviewer, but may also be obtained by telephone.[22-24] In face-to-face interviews, visual aids, such as food models, geometric models, pictures, or household measuring utensils, are often employed to help the subject estimate quantities consumed. Posner and colleagues[22] mailed subjects two-dimensional visual aids, modeled after those used in the National Health and Nutrition Examination Surveys (NHANES), for reference in telephone interviews.

Since 1965, the USDA has used the 24-hour recall, combined with two subsequent days of food records, to derive average daily individual intakes in their nationwide food consumption surveys.[3] Similarly, the National Center for

Health Statistics,[25,26] which conducts the NHANES, has used the 24-hour recall, as well as food frequencies of various food items, in their surveys of stratified national probability samples of the population.

The major strength of the 24-hour recall is its efficiency for comparing groups of people, who may differ according to age, sex, race, or other criteria. For example, 24-hour dietary recalls of random samples of four groups of Micronesians revealed differences in nutrient intakes and associations of diet with illness characteristics according to degree of westernization.[27] Similarly, 24-hour recalls among men of Japanese ancestry living in San Francisco, Hawaii, and Japan, demonstrated a stepwise increase in dietary fat intake and a similar decrease in carbohydrate intake from Japan to Hawaii to California, which paralleled the increase in coronary heart disease mortality rates among these populations.[28] USDA individual intakes, based on three-day means, have shown differences between blacks and whites, socioeconomic groups, geographic regions, and other demographic characteristics.[29] Because NHANES collects biologic, anthropometric, and physiologic measurements on subjects, the data have been useful for examining group differences in diet and various health and disease characteristics.[30]

The 24-hour recall is relatively quick and easy to administer. It places little burden on the subjects, is unlikely to alter behavior, and because of the short time interval, memory problems are usually minimal. For group data, the method has been demonstrated to be comparable to more cumbersome methods.[31] In some studies, participants are queried to determine if the diet was typical or atypical on the particular day of recall. If atypical, some investigators exclude these subjects from the analysis.[32] This reduces the sample size, but may increase the stability of the calculated mean intakes. The method is known to be labor-intensive, as nutrition professionals are generally involved directly or indirectly in the subject interviews and the review and coding of the recalls. The major limitation of the 24-hour recall relates to the daily variation in food selection. Due to the large intraindividual variability in food and nutrient intakes of most persons, a single 24-hour recall is not appropriate for estimating the usual intake of a particular subject. However, multiple 24-hour recalls, obtained on random days during a one-year interval, may provide a satisfactory picture of the usual diet. When group assessment is the objective, the interviews should be scheduled on various days of the week to account for daily variation in food choices, particularly between weekdays and weekends, as well as between weeks.

Food Records or Diaries

Food records or diaries require subjects to measure or estimate and record concurrently all foods consumed over a specified period, usually three to seven consecutive days or multiple periods within a year. Foods are weighed, measured, or estimated. The method requires good instructions, adequate demonstrations, and ideally some observations. Generally, persons who agree to participate are dedicated, highly motivated, literate subjects, and thus are most likely not representative of the general population. Although participants are asked to follow their usual dietary habits, they may modify their eating practices after a few days to reduce their workload (for example, by eating fewer mixed dishes than usual).

The most accurate method entails the weighing of all ingredients in recipes, the portion(s) selected, and any plate waste. This amount of detail is generally feasible only for persons familiar with using scales, either in food preparation or in the work setting.[6,14] It also has been used successfully among retired people who were motivated to participate in a scientific study.[33] Because weighing may be difficult for some subjects, household measuring utensils are used more frequently than scales in food record studies. In both instances, directions should be included for estimating and recording food items consumed away from home. Other methods of quantifying consumption in food records have been reported. In a validity study among multiethnic groups, Hankin and co-workers[34] gave subjects a book of photographs showing three typical portions of various foods for use in estimating amounts consumed. This method was appropriate for this study, which included males and females of five ethnic groups, many of whom were unfamiliar with household scales or measuring utensils.

A major strength of food records is that they do not rely on memory. Because of the difficulty in assessing a person's true usual intake, investigators have utilized food records as a reference or standard for validating other dietary methods that are based on recall.[11] Although food records are not necessarily error-free and have not been validated, investigators assume that they approximate the "truth." Thus, the validation is actually relative. The measured food record is assumed to have greater face validity than a recall or diet history. Food records also provide useful information for developing a diet history or food frequency questionnaire. Food items that are important contributors to the intakes of particular nutrients can be identified, along with the range of expected portion sizes for each item. In addition, records are useful for motivating participants in dietary intervention studies.[35]

Along with its strengths, this method has serious limitations as well. First, the particular period may be atypical for the subject, possibly due to illness, party meals, business obligations, or travel. Furthermore, this method would not be appropriate for people who consume almost all of their meals at restaurants. Second, as noted previously, those persons who agree to keep detailed food records may not be representative of the general population. In addition, due to its labor-intensive methodology, food records are difficult to administer in large population studies and are costly in time and personnel. Third, the method provides data only on the current diet. And fourth, food records of a single series of three to seven consecutive days most likely will not reflect the true variability in the diets of individuals.

Intraindividual Variability of Diet

Both the 24-hour recall and the food record are limited by their short time coverage. For most persons, eating patterns are characterized by large variations from day to day, week to week, and season to season. This is particularly true today with the wide choice of available foods in developed countries, and increasingly in developing countries. Food intakes during the weekend usually differ considerably from meals consumed on weekdays, and eating patterns frequently vary by season of the year. Furthermore, people are consuming more of their meals away from home, adding further variety to their diets. The large variation in daily and even weekly diets indicates that no single day or week is representative of long-term usual intakes.

Variability of diet within a population may be divided into within-person (or intraindividual) variation and between-person variation. It has been shown repeatedly that the within-person variation, which represents day-to-day differences in intake, is generally as large or larger than the between-person variation.[31,36–40] Consequently, a longer period is needed to characterize the usual diet of an individual person than the usual diet of a group of persons. Several investigators have analyzed the variability in multiple 24-hour recalls and food records and determined the number of days needed to achieve reliable estimates of average nutrient intakes of individuals.[9,31,38,40,41] For example, in a recent study among 13 males and 16 females who kept measured food records for a one-year period, Basiotis and associates[40] found that for measurement of total fat, 57 days were needed to estimate within 10% the true average individual intakes for males with 95% confidence; 71 days were needed for females. For vitamin A, 390 days were needed for the individual men and 474 days for the individual women. If the objective is to estimate group intake with precision, a smaller number of days of food records would be needed. In the Basiotis study,[40] six days were required to estimate the fat intakes of both males and females, whereas 39 and 44 days were needed to estimate the vitamin A intakes of males and females, respectively.

Other investigators have defined precision as an estimate within 20% of the true usual intake.[42] With this increased latitude, considerably fewer days would be needed for an estimate of the individual average intakes, for example, 10 to 23 days for dietary fat.[42] However, for most micronutrients, the situation is not as good. These findings indicate that the use of a short recall or food record for diet and disease studies could lead to considerable error, with misclassification in the distribution of individual intakes along a continuum.[21]

Diet Histories

For research concerning the etiology of diseases, such as cancer and heart disease, investigators seek information on the usual diet consumed during a considerable period of time. This has led to further development and use of diet histories for large population studies. Contrary to recent recalls and food records, which obtain information on food intake during specific days, diet histories attempt to determine the average or usual intake covering a fairly long time period, such as the past year or the year prior to onset of a disease. The objectives are to obtain a valid and reproducible estimate of each person's usual intake of foods, nutrients, and other diet components, rank or categorize the intakes, and test for associations of diet and disease. Precision is somewhat sacrificed to obtain data covering the longer time interval.

The first diet history was conceived by Burke,[43] who developed a subjective method that was administered by highly trained dietitians. The method included a 24-hour recall with typical variations (for example, different fruits that might be eaten at breakfast), a detailed account of the usual frequencies and quantities of an extended list of foods consumed during the last three or six months, and a measured three-day food record. From these data, the dietitians calculated the average daily intakes of calories and nutrients. This method was utilized in research concerning diet and child growth,[44,45] and subsequently modified for use in epidemiologic studies of heart disease.[46,47] It was the forerunner of the more structured diet histories in current use.

To simplify data collection and analysis and to increase objectivity, most diet histories today are based on lists of selected foods and groups of items with similar nutrient values, used interchangeably in the diet. In the past, food items were often selected to test particular hypotheses concerning diet and disease, such as vitamin A and beta-carotene with lung cancer.[48-50] More recently investigators have included sufficient foods to assess the total diet due to the uncertainty concerning the role of particular nutrients and other food components in the etiology of several chronic diseases. It also is desirable to examine interactions between nutrients and to have adequate data for reanalysis, should other dietary components be of etiologic interest in the future.

The food items selected for the diet history should be based on the study population's eating patterns. General guidelines are to choose foods that are consumed by a sizable number of persons, vary in frequency and quantity among the population, and provide significant amounts of calories, nutrients, and other dietary components of interest. Various procedures have been used for selecting the particular items. Willett et al,[51] with the assistance of a dietitian, developed an extensive list of food items for assessing total diet among a large cohort of nurses. The list was condensed after several pretests among samples of nurses, and the final group of items was derived by stepwise regression analysis. This statistical method has to be used with caution, since food items that are not necessarily sources of a particular nutrient may be selected by their association with another food item, for example, corn with cholesterol[6] or jelly with protein.[52] These situations occur because the selected foods, such as "corn" or "jelly," are consumed with items that are sources of the particular nutrients.

Others have utilized population data for selecting the particular food items. Block and colleagues[53,54] analyzed 24-hour recalls of adults who participated in the NHANES II survey. The quantitative estimates were based on three-dimensional geometric models, such as squares, circles, and thickness indicators. The investigators grouped the selected food items into meaningful categories and calculated the nutrient values of each group. Then they analyzed the data to identify the contribution of each food or food group to the average intake of calories and particular nutrients. The goal was to design a questionnaire that would yield approximately 90% of the dietary intakes of the adult US population.

An analogous procedure based on measured food records was utilized by Hankin and colleagues[13,55] to derive a diet history for use in the multiethnic population of Hawaii. Three-day measured food records were collected from representative samples of 60 to 65 males and females from the five major ethnic groups. After grouping the reported items into meaningful categories, the contributions of the items to the calorie and nutrient intakes of each ethnic group were calculated. This was a function of the nutrient content of the food, amount consumed, and frequency of use. The top-ranking foods that together contributed to more than 85% of the calorie and nutrient intakes of each ethnic group were included in the questionnaire.

Some diet histories solicit frequency data only,[51,56–58] although a convenient serving size may be listed with each item.[51] These are often called *food frequency* or *semi-quantitative food frequency questionnaires*, rather than *diet histories. Figure 10.1* illustrates Willett's self-administered semiquantitative frequency instrument, designed for a cohort study among nurses. Frequencies are obtained by checking the appropriate column showing ranges per day, week, month, or year. (In other diet histories, the interviewer or the respondent may record the particular frequency directly for each item.) With a frequency questionnaire, nutrient intakes are computed by multiplying the midpoint of the frequency interval by the nutrients in the specified portion of the food. This may be satisfactory if all the expected respondents generally consume similar amounts of the items, for example, 6 oz of meat or a half-cup of vegetables, and if amounts are highly correlated with frequencies. A problem arises if some subjects' usual portions differ markedly from those specified. Marr[10] noted that

Figure 10.1
Sample page, self-administered semiquantitative food frequency questionnaire. Courtesy Walter Willett, Harvard School of Public Health.

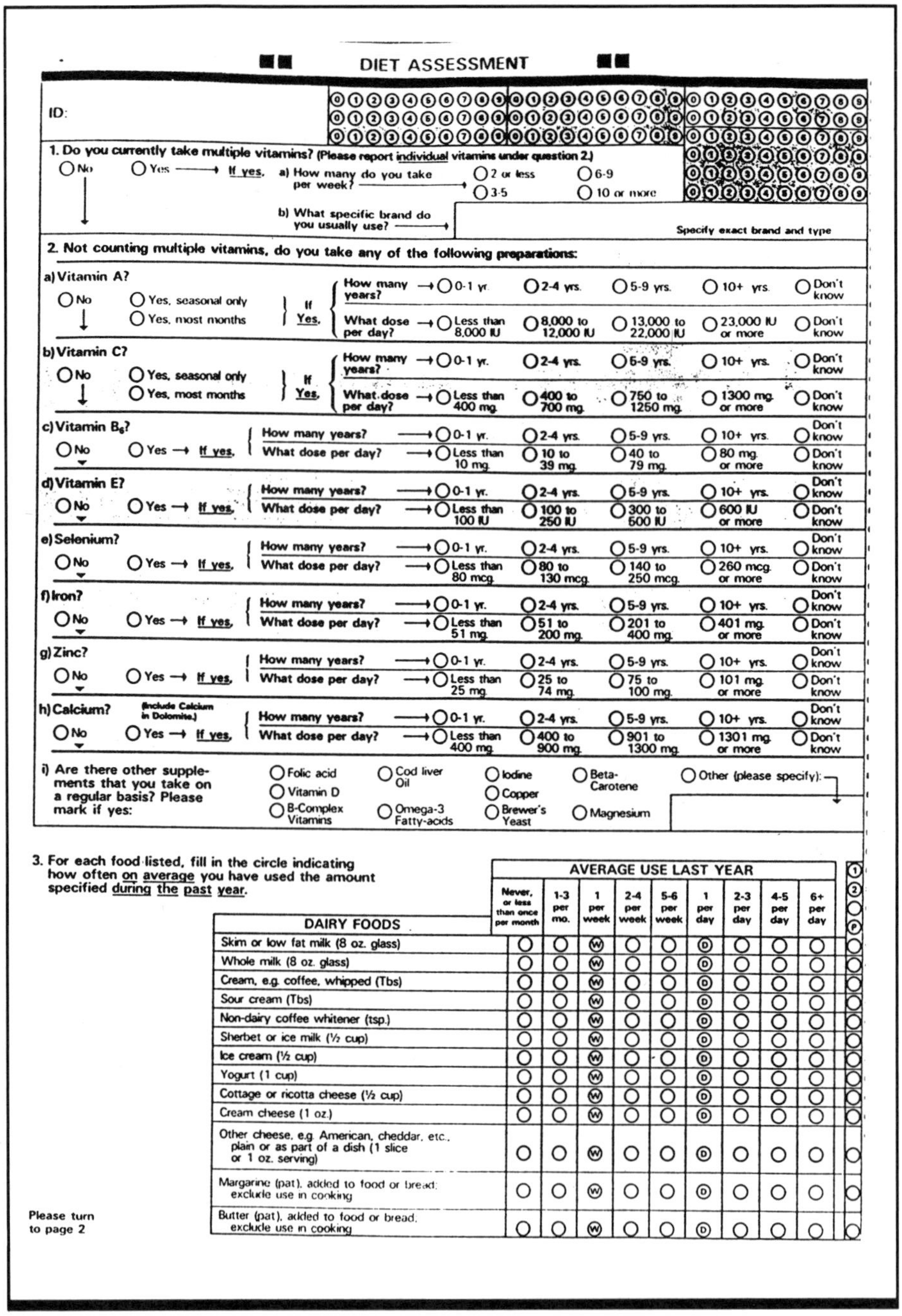

DIET ASSESSMENT

ID:

1. Do you currently take multiple vitamins? (Please report individual vitamins under question 2.)
O No   O Yes → If yes, a) How many do you take per week? → O 2 or less O 3-5 O 6-9 O 10 or more
b) What specific brand do you usually use? → Specify exact brand and type

2. Not counting multiple vitamins, do you take any of the following preparations:

a) Vitamin A? O No O Yes, seasonal only O Yes, most months — If Yes, How many years? → O 0-1 yr. O 2-4 yrs. O 5-9 yrs. O 10+ yrs. O Don't know; What dose per day? → O Less than 8,000 IU O 8,000 to 12,000 IU O 13,000 to 22,000 IU O 23,000 IU or more O Don't know

b) Vitamin C? O No O Yes, seasonal only O Yes, most months — If Yes, How many years? → O 0-1 yr. O 2-4 yrs. O 5-9 yrs. O 10+ yrs. O Don't know; What dose per day? → O Less than 400 mg O 400 to 700 mg O 750 to 1250 mg O 1300 mg or more O Don't know

c) Vitamin B_6? O No O Yes → If yes, How many years? → O 0-1 yr. O 2-4 yrs. O 5-9 yrs. O 10+ yrs. O Don't know; What dose per day? → O Less than 10 mg O 10 to 39 mg O 40 to 79 mg O 80 mg or more O Don't know

d) Vitamin E? O No O Yes → If yes, How many years? → O 0-1 yr. O 2-4 yrs. O 5-9 yrs. O 10+ yrs. O Don't know; What dose per day? → O Less than 100 IU O 100 to 250 IU O 300 to 500 IU O 600 IU or more O Don't know

e) Selenium? O No O Yes → If yes, How many years? → O 0-1 yr. O 2-4 yrs. O 5-9 yrs. O 10+ yrs. O Don't know; What dose per day? → O Less than 80 mcg O 80 to 130 mcg O 140 to 250 mcg O 260 mcg or more O Don't know

f) Iron? O No O Yes → If yes, How many years? → O 0-1 yr. O 2-4 yrs. O 5-9 yrs. O 10+ yrs. O Don't know; What dose per day? → O Less than 51 mg O 51 to 200 mg O 201 to 400 mg O 401 mg or more O Don't know

g) Zinc? O No O Yes → If yes, How many years? → O 0-1 yr. O 2-4 yrs. O 5-9 yrs. O 10+ yrs. O Don't know; What dose per day? → O Less than 25 mg O 25 to 74 mg O 75 to 100 mg O 101 mg or more O Don't know

h) Calcium? (Include Calcium in Dolomite.) O No O Yes → If yes, How many years? → O 0-1 yr. O 2-4 yrs. O 5-9 yrs. O 10+ yrs. O Don't know; What dose per day? → O Less than 400 mg O 400 to 900 mg O 901 to 1300 mg O 1301 mg or more O Don't know

i) Are there other supplements that you take on a regular basis? Please mark if yes: O Folic acid O Vitamin D O B-Complex Vitamins O Cod liver Oil O Omega-3 Fatty-acids O Iodine O Copper O Brewer's Yeast O Beta-Carotene O Magnesium O Other (please specify):

3. For each food listed, fill in the circle indicating how often on average you have used the amount specified during the past year.

DAIRY FOODS	AVERAGE USE LAST YEAR								
	Never, or less than once per month	1-3 per mo.	1 per week	2-4 per week	5-6 per week	1 per day	2-3 per day	4-5 per day	6+ per day
Skim or low fat milk (8 oz. glass)	O	O	W	O	O	D	O	O	O
Whole milk (8 oz. glass)	O	O	W	O	O	D	O	O	O
Cream, e.g. coffee, whipped (Tbs)	O	O	W	O	O	D	O	O	O
Sour cream (Tbs)	O	O	W	O	O	D	O	O	O
Non-dairy coffee whitener (tsp.)	O	O	W	O	O	D	O	O	O
Sherbet or ice milk (½ cup)	O	O	W	O	O	D	O	O	O
Ice cream (½ cup)	O	O	W	O	O	D	O	O	O
Yogurt (1 cup)	O	O	W	O	O	D	O	O	O
Cottage or ricotta cheese (½ cup)	O	O	W	O	O	D	O	O	O
Cream cheese (1 oz.)	O	O	W	O	O	D	O	O	O
Other cheese, e.g. American, cheddar, etc., plain or as part of a dish (1 slice or 1 oz. serving)	O	O	W	O	O	D	O	O	O
Margarine (pat), added to food or bread; exclude use in cooking	O	O	W	O	O	D	O	O	O
Butter (pat), added to food or bread; exclude use in cooking	O	O	W	O	O	D	O	O	O

Please turn to page 2

semiquantitative instruments could lead to a systematic bias toward either underestimation or overestimation of food and nutrient intakes; this should be considered in developing or using an existing diet history questionnaire.

The alternative procedure assumes that quantities consumed are likely to vary among the population and that more valid data will be obtained if subjects choose their own portion sizes according to their usual habits. There is support for both of these viewpoints. Samet et al[59] compared dietary data based on frequencies and standard portions with frequencies and estimated portions from the same subjects, and reported high rank order correlations of vitamin A intakes. However, the mean intakes were about 30% lower using the standard servings, as compared to the subjects' estimated amounts. Hunter and colleagues[60] found that there was large within-person variation of serving sizes in the weekly food records of 194 nurses and believed that the nurses would be unable to specify a usual portion size. These investigators concluded that frequency of eating particular foods was a greater determinant of nutrient intakes than quantity and that the use of a single serving size did not introduce a large error in the individual estimates.

On the other hand, Cummings and co-workers[61] compared the calcium intakes from seven-day records of 37 elderly women with weekly recalls from the Block questionnaire, in which subjects adjust their portions according to the specified medium serving (*Figure 10.2*). When three servings were used, the mean daily calcium intake was 637 mg, as compared with 612 mg from the records. The correlation was 0.76. When all servings were treated as medium, the mean calcium intake was 792 mg, with a correlation of 0.64 with the food records.

In analyzing data from a case-control study, Chu et al[62] compared dietary intakes obtained from a pictorial quantitative diet history with three different sets of fixed quantities used in reported studies. At the individual level, the frequency methods did not result in the same diet-disease associations that occurred with the quantitative method for any food items, food groups, or nutrients. In addition, the frequency-quantitative relationship was not consistent among the subjects for several foods, indicating that the methods were not interchangeable for assessing individual intakes.

Various techniques have been employed to help subjects estimate amounts consumed. The directions for completing Block's questionnaire (see Figure 10.2) specify that "a small portion is about one-half the medium serving size shown, or less, and a large portion is about one-and-a-half times as much, or more."[63] Pietinen and colleagues[64] developed a picture book illustrating the different portion sizes of the food items, which was distributed to subjects with the self-administered questionnaire. Geometric models, similar to those used in Canada's nationwide nutritional status survey, were used by Morgan and associates[65] in home interviews with subjects. Hankin and co-workers[13,55] used food record data from representative samples of the population to identify three modes in the distribution of serving weights for foods. The foods were weighed and photographed for use in home interviews. A sample page of the questionnaire is illustrated in *Figure 10.3*. This method is currently being modified and will be included in a mail questionnaire for a large multiethnic cohort study to be established in Southern California and Hawaii. In structured diet histories, respondents specify or circle the appropriate usual frequencies, as well as usual serving sizes, and nutrient intakes are calculated, based on both parameters.

Figure 10.2
Sample page, Health Habits and History Questionnaire, a self-administered quantitative diet history. Courtesy Gladys Block, National Cancer Institute.

	Medium Serving	Your Serving Size			How often?					OFFICE USE
FRUITS & JUICES		S	M	L	Day	Week	Month	Year	Rarely/Never	
EXAMPLE – Apples, applesauce, pears	(1) or ½ cup		✓			4				
Apples, applesauce, pears	(1) or ½ cup									11 ____
Bananas	1 medium									15 ____
Peaches, apricots (canned, frozen or dried, whole year)	(1) or ½ cup									19 ____
Peaches, apricots, nectarines (fresh, in season)	1 medium									23 ____
Cantaloupe (in season)	¼ medium									27 ____
Watermelon (in season)	1 slice									31 ____
Strawberries (fresh, in season)	½ cup									35 ____
Oranges	1 medium									39 ____
Orange juice or grapefruit juice	6 oz. glass									43 ____
Grapefruit	(½)									47 ____
Tang, Start breakfast drinks	6 oz. glass									51 ____
Other fruit juices, fortified fruit drinks	6 oz. glass									55 ____
Any other fruit, including berries, fruit cocktail	½ cup									59 ____
VEGETABLES		S	M	L	Da	Wk	Mo	Yr	Nv	
String beans, green beans	½ cup									63 ____
Peas	½ cup									67 ____
Chili with beans	¾ cup									71 ____
Other beans such as baked beans, pintos, kidney beans, limas	¾ cup									75 ____
Corn	½ cup									11 ____
Winter squash, baked squash	½ cup									15 ____
Tomatoes, tomato juice	(1) or 6 oz.									19 ____
Red chili sauce, taco sauce, salsa picante	2 Tblsp. sauce									23 ____
Broccoli	½ cup									27 ____
Cauliflower or brussel sprouts	½ cup									31 ____
Spinach (raw)	¾ cup									35 ____
Spinach (cooked)	½ cup									39 ____
Mustard greens, turnip greens, collards	½ cup									43 ____
Cole slaw, cabbage, sauerkraut	½ cup									47 ____
Carrots, or mixed vegetables containing carrots	½ cup									51 ____
Green salad	1 med. bowl									55 ____
Salad dressing, mayonnaise (including on sandwiches)	2 Tblsp.									59 ____
French fries and fried potatoes	¾ cup									63 ____
Sweet potatoes, yams	½ cup									67 ____
Other potatoes, including boiled, baked, potato salad	(1) or ½ cup									71 ____
Rice	¾ cup									75 ____
Any other vegetable, including cooked onions, summer squash	½ cup									11 ____
Butter, margarine or other fat on vegetables, potatoes, etc.	2 pats									15 ____
MEAT, FISH, POULTRY & MIXED DISHES		S	M	L	Da	Wk	Mo	Yr	Nv	
Hamburgers, cheeseburgers, meat loaf	1 medium									19 ____
Beef—steaks, roasts	4 oz.									23 ____
Beef stew or pot pie with carrots, other vegetables	1 cup									27 ____
Liver, including chicken livers	4 oz.									31 ____
Pork, including chops, roasts	2 chops or 4 oz.									35 ____
Fried chicken	2 sm. or 1 lg. piece									39 ____
Chicken or turkey, roasted, stewed or broiled	2 sm. or 1 lg. piece									43 ____
Fried fish or fish sandwich	4 oz. or 1 sand.									47 ____
Tuna fish, tuna salad, tuna casserole	½ cup									51 ____
Shell fish (shrimp, lobster, crab, oysters, etc.)	(5) ¼ cup or 3 oz.									55 ____
Other fish, broiled, baked	4 oz.									59 ____
Spaghetti, lasagna, other pasta with tomato sauce	1 cup									63 ____
Pizza	2 slices									67 ____
Mixed dishes with cheese (such as macaroni and cheese)	1 cup									71

Key Techniques

Figure 10.3
Sample page, interviewer-administered quantitative diet history. (Interviewer records portion size as A, B, or C, corresponding to photographs of small, medium, and large servings of foods, and circles the appropriate codes for items used in preparation. The same set of preparation codes is used for meats, vegetables, and salads: NO = none; BU = butter; MG = margarine; MY = mayonnaise and mayonnaise-type salad dressings; OV = oil and vinegar-type salad dressings; RO = restaurant or other unknown fat or oil; UK = unknown if fat used in preparation. Courtesy Jean Hankin, Cancer Research Center, University of Hawaii.)

IX. PORK AND HAM

1. How ofter did you eat pork and ham? How much did you eat each time? Were any of these used in the preparation at least half the time? (PREP CARD) PROBE FOR **USUAL** METHOD OF PREPARATION FOR EACH.

Item	Food Code	Freq.	Svg. Size	Preparation
1. PORK AND HAM a. Spareribs	1 17620 -- -- --	-- --	0 1 2 3 4 5 6 7 9 NO VO BU MG MY OV DD RO UK
b. Ham	2 17690 -- -- --	-- --	0 1 2 3 4 5 6 7 9 NO VO BU MG MY OV DD RO UK
c. Pork Chops	3 17170 -- -- --	-- --	0 1 2 3 4 5 6 7 9 NO VO BU MG MY OV DD RO UK
d. Kalua Pig	4 16831 -- -- --	-- --	0 1 2 3 4 5 6 7 9 NO VO BU MG MY OV DD RO UK
e. Roast	5 17160 -- -- --	-- --	0 1 2 3 4 5 6 7 9 NO VO BU MG MY OV DD RO UK
f. Chopped pork in mixed dishes (WRITE-IN)	6 -- -- --	-- --	0 1 2 3 4 5 6 7 9 NO VO BU MG MY OV DD RO UK
	6 -- -- --	-- --	0 1 2 3 4 5 6 7 9 NO VO BU MG MY OV DD RO UK
	6 -- -- --	-- --	0 1 2 3 4 5 6 7 9 NO VO BU MG MY OV DD RO UK
g. Other (WRITE-IN)	7 -- -- --	-- --	0 1 2 3 4 5 6 7 9 NO VO BU MG MY OV DD RO UK

X. BEEF AND PORK FAT

(CIRCLE "8" IF NONE OF THE MAJOR BEEF OR PORK CATEGORIES WAS REPORTED 12X PER YEAR OR MORE AND DO NOT ASK.)

When you ate beef, lamb, pork, and ham, did you eat the fat?
(CIRCLE ONE ONLY)

most of the time? 1
some of the time? 2
hardly ever? 3
DOES NOT APPLY 8

During the 1960s, Heady[66] and Hankin et al[52] proposed short dietary questionnaires in which only the frequencies of a few food items would be needed to predict the usual intakes of various nutrients. The questionnaires were easy to administer, but difficult to validate. Furthermore, the instruments omitted several foods of potential importance for diet and disease studies. Following a few trials, the limitations were apparent, and the research was discontinued.

Diet histories may be processed in two ways. If the information is obtained by personal interview, the frequency interval may be precise, for example, "three times a month", and descriptive data may be included, such as the kind of meat and vegetables in a mixed entree, along with the choice of serving size. This information requires review and coding by a nutrition professional, followed by manual data entry for the processing. The second method may be utilized in an interview or a self-administered questionnaire. The respondent chooses the appropriate frequency interval, such as "one to three times a month," for each category of foods and the usual serving size. This format can be designed for direct machine entry and is suitable for large population studies. Although some specificity is lost, the nutrient values of each category of foods will be appropriate if based on the items reported in food records or recent recalls from a representative sample of the study population. Most diet histories also include questions concerning the eating of fat on meats and skin on chicken, kinds of fats or oils used in cooking, and other eating habits. The responses are utilized for selecting the correct food codes in the computations.

The diet history is adaptable for use among various ethnic groups and is suitable for cross-cultural comparisons. Nonetheless, the method is not as precise as food records and is more affected by memory problems than the 24-hour recall. It is helpful to provide good descriptions with examples to aid the subjects, along with some visuals to help estimate amounts consumed. Generally, various studies have shown that nutrient intakes estimated with diet histories are greater than occur with 24-hour recalls or records.[34,51,64,67-71] It seems likely that the histories are closer to the truth, but this, of course, is difficult to prove.

Before using a diet history (or any method) in a research setting, the instrument should be pretested extensively among representative samples of the population.[55] Initially, the dietitian or trained interviewer should be present to identify problems needing clarification. Pretesting should be done repeatedly after each revision of the instrument. During this time, it is helpful to include a write-in section for recording other items usually eaten. This will provide further clues to improve the questionnaire, such as adding particular foods or clarifying instructions. In addition, if the questionnaire will be self-administered by mail or completed by telephone interview, trial runs should be conducted among representative samples of the study population. In some geographic areas with large migrant populations, it may be desirable to translate the instrument into other languages to ensure its comprehension. Among particular groups, such as the elderly, videotapes may be used to obtain an accurate estimate of individual intakes. Brown et al[72] recently tested this technique among elderly women living in a retirement home and showed that its accuracy was superior to the 24-hour recall.

Potential Errors of Individual Dietary Methods

It is clear that none of the individual methods is free from error. Witschi[35] classifies errors into three categories: respondent and recorder errors, interviewer and reviewer errors, and nutrient database errors. Briefly, in 24-hour recalls and diet histories, subjects may fail to recall all foods and amounts consumed. Many persons, particularly those not involved in food preparation, are not aware of the various foods eaten, such as vegetables served with entrees or ingredients in mixed dishes. They may not know what kinds of fats and oils were used, whether butter or margarine was on the table, and whether their portion of a mixed dish was one or two cups. Subjects also may want to please the interviewer and may be reluctant to admit a high consumption of alcohol or excessive amounts of sweets. In addition, some persons may believe that certain foods are "good" or "poor" for health and may exaggerate their use or non-use. Some investigators have found that large intakes tend to be underestimated, and small intakes overestimated.[73,74] This has been called the *flat slope syndrome.*

As noted previously, keeping a food record, whether weighed, measured, or estimated from photographs, is a difficult task. People may change their eating patterns to simplify the work, and consequently, the record may not be representative of the usual diet. Participants need to be convinced about the importance of their contribution to the research and the reasons for following their usual diet during the designated time periods. Because precision may decrease after a few consecutive days, Pietinen and co-workers[64,75] collected from study participants 12 two-day records, which included all days of the week during a six-month interval, for use in validating a diet history.

Interviewers conducting recalls and diet histories or instructing persons on keeping a food record need adequate training to ensure that everyone is following the established protocol. Specific guidelines and suggestions should be developed, procedures demonstrated, and several trials conducted. Dietitians or knowledgeable staff also should conduct frequent observations as well as periodic staff meetings throughout the study to maintain high quality of the data collection. Similarly, persons reviewing the completed interviews or records need standard, objective coding procedures to avoid subjective interpretation.

The food composition data are not error-free. However, the values published by the USDA are carefully selected averages from various sources and are reviewed and revised periodically.[76,77] This database is an appropriate primary resource for studies in the United States, but may need supplementation from other publications, such as Pennington,[78] Paul and Southgate,[79] commercial tables, published research papers, and laboratory analyses of local foods. For diet histories, weighted nutritive values are needed for groups of similar items. (For example, if food records or recalls from representative persons are available, the frequency and quantitative data may be used to derive the weighted values.) Also, composite dishes that are listed on the questionnaire require appropriate recipes, which may be developed from food record data. Food composition tables may include imputed values for some nutrients. There is divided opinion concerning their use, and it is likely that either inclusion or exclusion will result in some error in the estimated intakes. If used, they should be based on the analyses of similar foods and should be updated as new analytical information becomes available. Other potential unavoidable errors include changes occurring during food preparation or storage, as well as in the bioavailability of some nutrients. Although differences exist between calculated and analyzed values of food intake data,[10-14] these errors cannot be eliminated in large population studies. (For further information, see chapter 11.)

The errors in dietary methodology, along with the large random within-person variability, generally decrease the strength of the statistical association of diet with another variable, such as a biochemical measurement or disease status, providing that the errors are distributed nondifferentially among the comparison groups. This attenuation of the strength of the association often may suggest that no association exists. However, failure to identify a relationship between a dietary variable and a disease does not necessarily mean the absence of an association. For example, there has been inconsistent evidence from epidemiologic studies on the relationship of dietary fat and breast cancer.[80,81] This may be due to the homogeneity of fat intakes within populations and the substantial measurement error in dietary assessment,[82] as well as the large intraindividual variation in dietary fat intakes.[83] To illustrate, Willett and co-workers[80] examined the fat intakes among breast cancer cases and controls in their prospective cohort of nurses and found no evidence of a positive association. This could be partially attributed to the homogeneity of the fat intakes, since the highest quintile was 44% of calories from fat, and the lowest quintile was 32%. Heterogeneity might well be increased with the addition of quantitative differentiation in the questionnaire (see Figure 10.1). This does not discount the possibility that fat intake during childhood and adolescence may be more important determinants of breast cancer than diet during adulthood, but does suggest that quantitative information might well provide better discrimination of the individual fat intakes.

VALIDITY AND REPRODUCIBILITY

To promote confidence in the dietary data and the diet-disease findings, the dietary method should be tested for validity and reproducibility in a representative sample of the study population. Although it would be expedient to use a method evaluated in another population, other instruments may not be appropriate. Structured diet histories, in particular, are tailored to the eating patterns of a population. Consequently, a valid and reproducible questionnaire developed for a white population in New England most likely would not be appropriate for Asians in Hawaii or Hispanics in the southwestern United States. Several studies have been reported on the evaluation of particular dietary methods. This paper includes only a brief review to illustrate the objectives, potential methods, and general findings.

Validity

Validity is the ability of an instrument to measure what it purports to measure, such as the intake of a particular meal or day, or the usual diet consumed during the past year. Validation requires that the truth be known, which is difficult and most likely impossible to obtain among free-living persons for extended periods. However, validity for short time intervals has been assessed by surreptitiously weighing foods of persons eating in an institutional setting, and asking the subjects to recall what they ate the following day. Karvetti and Knuts[84] and Linusson et al[85] weighed one-day intakes of subjects and the following day obtained 24-hour recalls. Similarly, Madden and associates[73] and Gersovitz and co-investigators[74] weighed the noon meals of subjects 60 years or older eating at congregate meal sites and obtained recalls by interview the following day. Generally, differences between the mean intakes were not significant, but the flat slope syndrome was observed among individuals.

Key Techniques

To validate diet histories, investigators usually measure the *relative validity* of the new instrument by comparing it with a method that has evidence of greater accuracy or face validity.[6,11] The choice has generally been food records, either weighed, measured, or estimated, and collected for multiple days to reflect within-person variability; however, a more extensive interview[86] or multiple one-day recalls could be used. Because the extensive interview or 24-hour recalls and the new instrument are similar in several ways (for example, they both solicit information on frequencies and estimated quantities), the validity is likely to be overestimated, whereas comparison of the new questionnaire with food records may underestimate validity due to the inability of food records to cover the extensive within-person variability. Researchers may include comparisons of the mean nutrient intakes at the group levels. This may be satisfactory for some purposes, but not for validation of individual intakes. The appropriate criterion is the *agreement* of the two methods at the individual level. A number of studies have utilized Pearson or Spearman correlations.[34,51,64,87,88] These statistics will indicate the degree of consistency between the methods, or the ability to rank the subjects similarly, according to the distribution of the intakes. This is necessary, but not sufficient for assessing agreement, which is a measure of the interchangeability of the untested method with the method of greater face validity. Generally, the intraclass correlation coefficient (or the weighted κ statistic) is utilized to estimate agreement. Lee and colleagues[89] demonstrated that two methods may be perfectly correlated, but are interchangeable only if both methods give the same results in a particular study. In practice, most investigators include measurements of both consistency and agreement in validity studies. Values of 0.5 to 0.7 for these statistics compare favorably with several physiologic measures and are acceptable criteria for validation of the dietary method.[90]

Willett et al[51] validated a 61-item food frequency questionnaire, by comparison with four weeks of measured food intakes recorded at three-month intervals during the year. Because the record-keeping could sensitize the subjects and thus increase the accuracy of the questionnaire responses, the instrument was completed at the start and end of the year. The first administration of the questionnaire referred to the previous year and thus could underestimate the validity, whereas the second might result in an overestimate. The true relationship would likely fall between the two values. The results revealed, as expected, higher values in the comparison of the second administration of the questionnaire with the records. Pietinen and co-workers[64,75] evaluated two self-administered questionnaires among Finnish men. The first was a "food use" questionnaire that included 276 food items and the book of pictures described earlier, whereas the second was a qualitative food frequency of 44 items with no quantitative estimates. A group of 190 men of similar age kept weighed food intake records for 12 two-day periods spread evenly throughout a six-month period and completed the food use and the frequency questionnaires before and after the six-month period. Generally, as expected, the validity was higher with the second questionnaires than with the first. Also, the validity was slightly greater with the food use questionnaire which was recommended for diet and disease studies, while the qualitative instrument was suggested for monitoring compliance in intervention trials.

The quantitative photographic diet history, designed for Hawaii's multiethnic population, was validated among 262 subjects, who completed four weekly food records during the year.[34] The consistency and agreement measures indicated that the method gave reasonably accurate estimates of the usual dietary intakes of the population. Willett and associates[87] had an opportunity to test their semiquantitative questionnaire among 27 adults who recorded their food intakes for a one-year period. Thus, the reference data were more complete than is usually available. Correlations of the two data sets were generally satisfactory.

Other methods of obtaining reference data have been reported. Jain and colleagues[70] included 30 husband-wife pairs in an evaluation study. The wives maintained 30-day measured or estimated records of the husbands' diets; the quantitative diet history was administered to the men the following week. Balogh et al[91] and Yarnell and co-workers[92] compared short diet histories to weighed one-week food records. A few investigators have tested diet histories against food records kept several years in the past.[93,94] Results have been variable, which may be attributed to changes in eating patterns, as well as to memory failure.

For abbreviated questionnaires, validation has been studied by comparison with a validated, more extensive diet history. Jain and colleagues[86] compared a short, quantitative, self-administered mail questionnaire with a detailed diet history, administered by interview, among 50 randomly selected women. Correlations ranged from 0.47 to 0.60 for the nutrient intakes.

Although biological markers are not available for most nutrients, there is evidence that some biochemical measurements may be suitable for validation of dietary intakes. Bingham et al[95] obtained four-day weighed records, duplicate meals for analysis, along with 24-hour urinary and fecal excretions among 30 men in each of four Scandinavian countries. There was good agreement in the urinary and fecal nitrogen and the estimated nitrogen intake, as well as in the analyzed and calculated fat and protein intakes among the subjects. Van Staveren and associates[96] compared 19 24-hour recalls of 59 women, collected over a 2.5-year period, with fat biopsies and found good agreement of linoleic acid and the ratio of linoleic acid to saturated fat in the diet and the fat tissue. Research has also been conducted to identify biochemical markers that indicate micronutrient intakes.[6] This, of course, is difficult because the relationship between diet and serum or tissue levels is indirect. Yet, Willett's group[97] tested the validity of their semiquantitative questionnaire by comparing intake estimates with plasma carotene, retinol, and alpha-tocopherol measurements. After adjusting for age, sex, and calorie intake among the 59 subjects, the correlations were 0.35 for plasma and dietary carotene and 0.34 for plasma alpha-tocopherol and dietary vitamin E. Only a weak relationship was demonstrated between preformed vitamin A in the diet and plasma retinol.

Reproducibility

Reproducibility is the ability of the dietary method to produce the same information with the same persons on two or more occasions. In some studies, the second diet history is directed to the same time period as the first, whereas in others the history pertains to the past year, assuming that no change occurred in the interim. Reproducibility (sometimes referred to as *repeatability* or *reliability*) does not ensure that the method is valid; the same error in the instrument could be repeated with each administration. Several factors may affect the comparability of the estimates,[90] including the respondent's ability to estimate past frequency and amount consumed, a dietary change during the interval, inadequate instructions to the subjects, and error-proneness of the questionnaire. Furthermore, if there are too few frequency intervals or if portion sizes are fixed, reproducibility will probably appear higher than if the response options provided greater individualization.

In contrast to validity studies, reproducibility may easily be tested. A potential problem is that each assessment affects subsequent assessments.[35] Consequently, it would be prudent to avoid too short an interval. If the period is less than a month, subjects simply may repeat their initial responses. Similarly, if the interval is too long, a real change may have occurred. In addition, if the inquiry is directed to the time of the first interview, recall is a likely problem due to memory failure.

One of the first reproducibility studies was conducted among Framingham subjects by Dawber and colleagues.[98] The dietary method was a modification of the Burke diet history and was administered by dietitians trained in the method. Assessments were repeated among a sample at two and four-year intervals. When the respondents were classified into thirds, there was a high degree of agreement in nutrient intakes after two years. However, significant differences occurred after four years, suggesting intentional change in diet among several subjects. Correlations ranged from 0.58 to 0.92 after two years, but decreased to 0.41 to 0.84 after four years. Reshef and associates[99] also tested the reproducibility of a Burke-type interview among Israeli subjects, who were reinterviewed after an interval of 6.5 to 8.5 months. Correlations of calorie and macronutrient intakes ranged from 0.51 to 0.90.

During the 1980s, several investigators tested the reproducibility of more structured diet histories.[51,58,64,75,100,101] These studies included both self-administered instruments and interviewer-administered questionnaires, and varied according to the period of reference, using either the same interval as the original recall or the recent past, assuming no dietary change. They also differed according to the use of self-selected portions of foods or fixed serving sizes. Generally, reproducibility was higher for nutrients than for foods, for shorter intervals of a few months than for longer time spans of several years, and for standard portions than for self-selected amounts.

CONCLUSION

During recent years, there has been heightened interest in identifying the role of diet as an etiologic factor in chronic diseases, such as cancer and heart disease. As discussed, the preferable dietary method for this research is the diet history. Several studies have demonstrated that a carefully designed diet history will produce valid and reproducible estimates of the usual intakes of individuals. A structured diet history that includes representative food items to estimate the intakes of foods, nutrients, and other components, permits responses on the usual frequencies and serving sizes, and discriminates among persons in terms of their dietary intakes is the method of choice for large population studies.

It is likely that case-control studies will continue to need appropriate diet histories focusing on the food intake before onset of disease. In addition, there will be further cohort studies in which the dietary intake during a recent period, such as the past year, is relevant. In all of these investigations, the diet history should be tested for validity and reproducibility to insure the credibility of the findings.

Other group or individual dietary methods are not appropriate for estimating the usual dietary intakes of individuals. As discussed, group methods are useful for comparing per capita dietary intakes among populations, predicting agricultural and economic needs, and providing leads for research. Individual methods, such as 24-hour recalls, may be utilized for estimating and comparing the intakes of groups of people classified according to particular criteria, whereas food records are useful for validating the diet histories designed for research studies. Finally, continued research is needed to identify potential biological markers for improved validation of dietary intake methods.

References

1. Anderson SA, ed. *Guidelines for Use of Dietary Intake Data.* Washington, DC: Food and Drug Administration; 1986:16.
2. Peterkin BP, Rizek RL, Tippett KS. Nationwide food consumption survey, 1987. *Nutr Today.* 1988;23:18–24.
3. Pao EM, Sykes KE, Cypel YS. USDA Methodological Research for Large-Scale Dietary Intake Surveys, 1975–88. Washington, DC: US Dept of Agriculture; 1989. Home Economics Research Report no. 49.
4. Armstrong B, Doll R. Environmental factors and cancer incidence and mortality in different countries, with special reference to dietary practices. *Int J Cancer.* 1975;15:617–631.
5. Jolliffe N, Archer M. Statistical associations between international coronary heart disease death rates and certain environmental factors. *J Chronic Dis.* 1959;9:636–652.
6. Willett W. *Nutritional Epidemiology.* New York, NY: Oxford University Press; 1990.
7. Burk MC, Pao EM. Methodology for large-scale surveys of household and individual diets. Washington, DC: US Department of Agriculture; 1976. Home Economics Research Report no. 40.
8. Manchester AC, Farrell KR. Measurement and forecasting of food consumption by USDA. In: Food and Nutrition Board, National Research Council. *Assessing Changing Food Consumption Patterns.* Washington, DC: National Academy Press; 1981:51.
9. James WPT, Bingham SA, Cole TJ: Epidemiological assessment of dietary intake. *Nutr Cancer.* 1981;2:203–212.
10. Marr JW. Individual dietary surveys: purposes and methods. *World Rev Nutr Diet.* 1971;13:105–161.
11. Block G. A review of validations of dietary assessment methods. *Am J Epidemiol.* 1982;115:492–505.
12. Callmer E, Haraldsdottir J, Loken EB, Seppanen R, Solvoll K. Selecting a method for a dietary survey. *Naringsforskning.* 1985;29:43–52.
13. Hankin JH. 23rd Lenna Frances Cooper memorial lecture: a diet history method for research, clinical, and community use. *J Am Diet Assoc.* 1986;86:868–875.
14. Bingham SA. The dietary assessment of individuals; methods, accuracy, new techniques and recommendations. *Nutr Abst Rev.* 1987;57:705–742.
15. Lee-Han H, McGuire V, Boyd NF. A review of the methods used by studies of dietary measurement. *J Clin Epidemiol.* 1989;42:269–279.
16. Committee on Food Consumption Patterns, Food and Nutrition Board, National Research Council. *Assessing Changing Food Consumption Patterns.* Washington, DC: National Academy Press; 1981.
17. Subcommittee on Criteria for Dietary Evaluation, Food and Nutrition Board, National Research Council. *Nutrient Adequacy. Assessment Using Food Consumption Surveys.* Washington, DC: National Academy Press; 1986.
18. den Hartog AP, van Staveren WA. *Manual for Social Surveys on Food Habits and Consumption in Developing Countries.* Wageningen, Suriname: Centre for Agricultural Publishing and Documentation; 1983.
19. Cameron ME, van Staveren WA, eds. *Manual on Methodology for Food Consumption Studies.* New York, NY: Oxford University Press; 1988.
20. Sampson L. Food frequency questionnaires as a research instrument. *Clin Nutr.* 1985;5:171–178.
21. Block G. Human dietary assessment: methods and issues. *Prev Med.* 1989;18:653–660.
22. Posner BM, Borman CL, Morgan JL, Borden WS, Ohls JC. The validity of a telephone-administered 24-hour dietary recall methodology. *Am J Clin Nutr.* 1982;36:546–553.

23. Krantzler NJ, Mullen BJ, Schutz HG, Grivetti LE, Holden CA, Meiselman HL. Validity of telephoned diet recalls and records for assessment of individual food intake. *Am J Clin Nutr.* 1982;36:1234–1242.
24. Morgan KJ, Johnson SR, Rizek RL, Reese R, Stampley GL. Collection of food intake data: an evaluation of methods. *J Am Diet Assoc.* 1987;87:888–896.
25. Woteki CE. Dietary survey data: sources and limits to interpretation. *Nutr Rev.* 1986;44(suppl):204–213.
26. Welsh S. The joint nutrition monitoring evaluation committee. In: Food and Nutrition Board, National Research Council. *What Is America Eating?* Washington, DC: National Academy Press; 1986:7.
27. Hankin JH, Reed D, Labarthe D, Nichaman M, Stallones RA. Dietary and disease patterns among Micronesians. *Am J Clin Nutr.* 1970;23:346–357.
28. Kagan A, Harris BR, Winkelstein W, et al. Epidemiologic studies of coronary heart disease and stroke in Japanese men living in Japan, Hawaii, and California. Hiroshima, Japan: Atomic Bomb Casualty Commission; 1972.
29. Human Nutrition Information Service, US Department of Agriculture. *Food Consumption: Households in the United States, Spring 1977.* Washington, DC: Government Printing Office, 1982. Publication H-1.
30. Woteki C, Johnson C, Murphy R. Nutritional status of the US population: iron, vitamin C, and zinc. In: Food and Nutrition Board, National Research Council. *What Is America Eating?* Washington, DC: National Academy Press; 1986:21.
31. Beaton GH, Milner J, McGuire V, Feather TE, Little JA. Sources of variance in 24-hour dietary recall data: implications for nutrition study design and interpretation. Carbohydrate sources, vitamins, and minerals. *Am J Clin Nutr.* 1983;37:986–995.
32. Yano K, Heilbrun LK, Wasnich RD, Hankin JH, Vogel JM. The relationship between diet and bone mineral content of multiple skeletal sites in elderly Japanese-American men and women living in Hawaii. *Am J Clin Nutr.* 1985;42:877–888.
33. Garry P, Goodwin JS, Hunt WC, Hooper EM, Leonard AG. Nutritional status in a healthy elderly population: dietary and supplemental intakes. *Am J Clin Nutr.* 1982;36:319–331.
34. Hankin JH, Wilkens LR, Kolonel LN, Yoshizawa CN. Validation of a quantitative diet history method in Hawaii. *Am J Epidemiol.* 1991;133:616–628.
35. Witschi JC. Short-term dietary recall and recording methods. In: Willett W. *Nutritional Epidemiology.* New York, NY: Oxford University Press; 1990:52.
36. Hankin JH, Reynolds WE, Margen S. A short dietary method for epidemiologic studies. II. Variability of measured nutrient intakes. *Am J Clin Nutr.* 1967;20:935–945.
37. McGee D, Rhoads G, Hankin J, Yano K, Tillotson J. Within-person variability of nutrient intake in a group of Hawaiian men of Japanese ancestry. *Am J Clin Nutr.* 1982;36:657–663.
38. Hunt WC, Leonard AG, Garry PJ, Goodwin JS. Components of variance in dietary data for an elderly population. *Nutr Res.* 1983;3:433–444.
39. Sempos CT, Johnson NE, Smith EL, Gilligan C. Effects of intraindividual and interindividual variation in repeated dietary records. *Am J Epidemiol.* 1985;121:120–130.
40. Basiotis PP, Welsh SO, Cronin FJ, Kelsay JL, Mertz W. Number of days of food intake records required to estimate individual and group nutrient intakes with defined confidence. *J Nutr.* 1987;117:1638–1641.
41. Liu K, Stamler J, Dyer A, McKeever J, McKeever P. Statistical methods to assess and minimize the role of intraindividual variability in obscuring the relationship between dietary lipids and serum cholesterol. *J Chron Dis.* 1978;31:399–418.
42. Block G, Hartman AM. Dietary assessment methods. In: Moon TE, Micozzi MS. *Nutrition and Cancer Prevention. Investigating the Role of Micronutrients.* New York, NY: Marcel Dekker; 1989:159.
43. Burke BS. The dietary history as a tool in research. *J Am Diet Assoc.* 1947;23:1041–1046.
44. Reed RB, Burke BS. Collection and analysis of dietary intake data. *Am J Public Health.* 1954;44:1015–1026.
45. Beal VA. The nutritional history in longitudinal research. *J Am Diet Assoc.* 1967;51:426–432.

46. Mann GV, Pearson G, Gordon T, Dawber TR, Lyell L, Shurtleff D. Diet and cardiovascular disease in the Framingham study. I. Measurement of dietary intake. *Am J Clin Nutr.* 1962;11:200–225.

47. Paul O, Lepper MH, Phelan WH, et al. A longitudinal study of coronary heart disease. *Circulation.* 1963;28:20–31.

48. Samet JM, Skipper BJ, Humble CG, Pathak DR. Lung cancer risk and vitamin A consumption in New Mexico. *Am Rev Respir Dis.* 1985;131:198–202.

49. Ziegler RG, Mason TJ, Stemhagen A, et al. Carotenoid intake, vegetables, and the risk of lung cancer among white men in New Jersey. *Am J Epidemiol.* 1986;123:1080–1093.

50. Hankin JH. Dietary methods for estimating vitamin A and carotene intakes in epidemiologic studies of cancer. *J Can Diet Assoc.* 1987;48:219–224.

51. Willett WC, Sampson L, Stampfer MJ, et al. Reproducibility and validity of a semiquantitative food frequency questionnaire. *Am J Epidemiol.* 1985;122:51–65.

52. Hankin JH, Stallones RA, Messinger HB. A short dietary method for epidemiologic studies. III. Development of questionnaire. *Am J Epidemiol.* 1968;87:285–290.

53. Block G, Dresser CM, Hartman AM, Carroll MD. Nutrient sources in the American diet: quantitative data from the NHANES II survey. I. Vitamins and minerals. *Am J Epidemiol.* 1985;122:13–26.

54. Block G, Dresser CM, Hartman AM, Carroll MD. Nutrient sources in the American diet: quantitative data from the NHANES II survey. II. Macronutrients and fats. *Am J Epidemiol.* 1985;122:27–40.

55. Hankin JH. Development of a diet history questionnaire for studies of older persons. *Am J Clin Nutr.* 1989;50:1121–1127.

56. Stuff JE, Garza C, O'Brian Smith E, Nichols BL, Montandon CM. A comparison of dietary methods in nutritional studies. *Am J Clin Nutr.* 1983;37:300–306.

57. Gray GE, Paganini-Hill A, Ross RK, Henderson BE. Assessment of three brief methods of estimation of vitamin A and C intakes for a prospective study of cancer: comparison with dietary history. *Am J Epidemiol.* 1984;119:581–590.

58. Rohan TE, Potter JD. Retrospective assessment of dietary intake. *Am J Epidemiol.* 1984;120:876–887.

59. Samet JM, Humble CG, Skipper BE. Alternatives in the collection and analysis of food frequency interview data. *Am J Epidemiol.* 1984;120:572–581.

60. Hunter DJ, Sampson L, Stampfer MJ, Colditz GA, Rosner B, Willet, WC. Variability in portion sizes of commonly consumed foods among a population of women in the United States. *Am J Epidemiol.* 1988;127:1240–1249.

61. Cummings SR, Block G, McHenry K, Baron RB. Evaluation of two food frequency methods of measuring dietary calcium intake. *Am J Epidemiol.* 1987;126:796–802.

62. Chu SY, Kolonel LN, Hankin JH, Lee J. A comparison of frequency and quantitative dietary methods for epidemiologic studies of diet and disease. *Am J Epidemiol.* 1984;119:323–334.

63. Block G, Hartman AM, Dresser CM, Carroll MD, Gannon J, Gardner L. A data-based approach to diet questionnaire design and testing. *Am J Epidemiol.* 1986;124:453–469.

64. Pietinen P, Hartman AM, Haapa E, et al. Reproducibility and validity of dietary assessment instruments. I. A self-administered food use questionnaire with a portion size picture booklet. *Am J Epidemiol.* 1988;128:655–666.

65. Morgan RW, Jain M, Miller AB, et al. A comparison of dietary methods in epidemiologic studies. *Am J Epidemiol.* 1978;107:488–498.

66. Heady JA. Diets of bank clerks: development of a method of classifying the diets of individuals for use in epidemiological studies. *J Roy Statist Soc.* 1961;A124:336–371.

67. Young CM, Hagan GC, Tucker RE, Foster WD. A comparison of dietary study methods: II. Dietary history vs seven-day record vs twenty-four hour recall. *J Am Diet Assoc.* 1952;28:218–221.

68. Young CM, Trulson MF. Methodology for dietary studies in epidemiological surveys. II. Strengths and weaknesses of existing methods. *Am J Public Health.* 1960;50:803–814.

Key Techniques

69. Larkin FA, Metzner HL, Thompson FE, Flegal KM, Guire KE. Comparison of estimated nutrient intakes by food frequency and dietary records in adults. *J Am Diet Assoc.* 1989;89:215–223.

70. Jain M, Howe GR, Johnson KC, Miller AB. Evaluation of a diet history questionnaire for epidemiologic studies. *Am J Epidemiol.* 1980;111:212–219.

71. Young CM. Dietary methodology. In: Food and Nutrition Board, National Research Council. *Assessing Changing Food Consumption Patterns.* Washington, DC: National Academy Press; 1981:89.

72. Brown JE, Tharp TM, Dahlberg-Luby EM, et al. Videotape dietary assessment: validity, reliability, and comparison of results with 24-hour dietary recalls from elderly women in a retirement home. *J Am Diet Assoc.* 1990;90:1675–1679.

73. Madden JP, Goodman SJ, Guthrie HA. Validity of the 24-hr recall. *J Am Diet Assoc.* 1976;68:143–147.

74. Gersovitz M, Madden JP, Smickilas-Wright H. Validity of the 24-hr dietary recall and seven-day record for group comparisons. *J Am Diet Assoc.* 1978;73:48–56.

75. Pietinen P, Hartman AM, Haapa E, et al. Reproducibility and validity of dietary assessment instruments. II. A qualitative food frequency questionnaire. *Am J Epidemiol.* 1988;128:667–676.

76. United States Department of Agriculture. *Composition of Foods: Raw, Processed, Prepared.* Washington, DC: Agricultural Research Service, 1972. Data set 8-1-1.

77. United States Department of Agriculture. *Composition of Foods: Raw, Processed, Prepared.* Washington, DC: US Government Printing Office; 1976–1989. Agriculture Handbooks 8-1 to 8-21.

78. Pennington JAT. *Bowes and Church's Food Values of Portions Commonly Used.* 15th ed. Philadelphia, Pa: JB Lippincott Co; 1989.

79. Paul AA, Southgate DAT. *McCance and Widdowson's The Composition of Foods.* 4th ed. New York, NY: Elsevier/North-Holland; 1978.

80. Willett WC, Stampfer MJ, Colditz GA, Rosner BA, Hennekens CH, Speizer FE. Dietary fat and the risk of breast cancer. *N Engl J Med.* 1987;316:22–28.

81. Howe GR, Hirohata T, Hislop TG, et al. Dietary factors and risk of breast cancer: combined analysis of 12 case-control studies. *JNCI.* 1990;82:561–569.

82. Prentice RL, Pepe M, Self SG. Dietary fat and breast cancer: a quantitative assessment of the epidemiological literature and a discussion of methodological issues. *Cancer Res.* 1989;49:3147-3156.

83. Hegsted DM. Errors of measurement. *Nutr Cancer.* 1989;12:105–107.

84. Karvetti RL, Knuts LR. Validity of the 24-hour recall. *J Am Diet Assoc.* 1985;85:1437–1442.

85. Linusson EEI, Sanjur D, Erickson EC. Validating the 24-hour recall method as a dietary survey tool. *Arch Latinoam Nutr.* 1974;24:277–294.

86. Jain MG, Harrison L, Howe GR, Miller AB. Evaluation of a self-administered dietary questionnaire for use in a cohort study. *Am J Clin Nutr.* 1982;36:931–935.

87. Willett WC, Reynolds RD, Cottrell-Hoehner S, Sampson L, Browne ML. Validation of a semi-quantitative food frequency questionnaire: comparison with a 1-year diet record. *J Am Diet Assoc.* 1987;87:43–47.

88. Block G, Woods M, Potosky A, Clifford C. Validation of a self-administered diet history questionnaire using multiple diet records. *J Clin Epidemiol.* 1990;43:1327–1335.

89. Lee J, Kolonel LN, Hankin JH. On establishing the interchangeability of different dietary intake assessment methods used in studies of diet and cancer. *Nutr Cancer.* 1983;5:215–218.

90. Block G, Hartmann AM. Issues in reproducibility and validity of dietary studies. *Am J Clin Nutr.* 1989;50:1133–1138.

91. Balogh M, Medalie JH, Smith H, Groen JJ. The development of a dietary questionnaire for an ischemic heart disease survey. *Israel J Med Sci.* 1968;4:195–203.

92. Yarnell JWG, Fehily AM, Milbank JE, Sweetnam TM, Walker CL. A short dietary questionnaire for use in an epidemiological survey: comparison with weighed dietary records. *Human Nutr Appl Nutr.* 1983;37A:103–112.

93. Van Leeuwen FE, De Vet HCW, Hayes RB, Van Staveren WA, West CE, Hautvast JGAJ. An assessment of the relative validity of retrospective interviewing for measuring dietary intake. *Am J Epidemiol.* 1983;118:752–758.

94. Sobell J, Block G, Koslowe P, Tobin J, Andres R. Validation of a retrospective questionnaire assessing diet 10–15 years ago. *Am J Epidemiol.* 1989;130:173–187.

95. Bingham S, Wiggins HS, Englyst H, et al. Methods and validity of dietary assessments in four Scandinavian populations. *Nutr Cancer.* 1982;4:23–33.

96. Van Staveren WA, Deurenberg P, Katan MB, Burema J, de Groot LCPGM, Hoffmans MDAF. Validity of the fatty acid composition of subcutaneous fat tissue microbiopsies as an estimate of the long-term average fatty acid composition of the diet of separate individuals. *Am J Epidemiol.* 1986;123:455–463.

97. Willett WC, Stampfer MJ, Underwood BA, Speizer FE, Rosner B, Hennekens CH. Validation of a dietary questionnaire with plasma carotenoid and alpha-tocopherol levels. *Am J Clin Nutr.* 1983;38:631–639.

98. Dawber TR, Pearson G, Anderson P, et al. Dietary assessment in the epidemiologic study of coronary heart disease: the Framingham study. II. Reliability of measurement. *Am J Clin Nutr.* 1962;11:226–234.

99. Reshef A, Epstein LM. Reliability of a dietary questionnaire. *Am J Clin Nutr.* 1972;25:91–95.

100. Hankin JH, Nomura AMY, Lee J, Hirohata T, Kolonel LN. Reproducibility of a diet history questionnaire in a case-control study of breast cancer. *Am J Clin Nutr.* 1983;37:981–985.

101. Hankin JH, Yoshizawa CN, Kolonel LN. Reproducibility of a diet history in older men in Hawaii. *Nutr Cancer.* 1990;13:129–140.

11. DEVELOPMENT AND USE OF FOOD COMPOSITION DATA AND DATABASES

Jean A. T. Pennington, PhD, RD

Food composition databases are essential tools for assessing dietary status of patients, clients, students, and population groups; for planning and evaluating meals and diets; and for determining diet-disease relationships in clinical and epidemiologic research studies. Food composition databases may be used to assess the nutrient content of single foods or a group of similar foods for the purposes of developing food standards, formulating new food products, determining the potential use of a food in a therapeutic diet, establishing definitions for dietary claims, and determining if foods meet such claims. Databases are also used to develop nutrition education materials and programs for students and consumers.

The uses of food composition databases may be specific for some users, but may also overlap among various users. Industry uses databases for product development, nutrition labeling, and dietary claims. Grocery stores may use databases for shelf-labeling programs, and restaurants may use them to make nutrition claims about items on their menus. Hospitals and clinics use databases for diet therapy, special diet development, regular diet planning and evaluation, clinical trials, and patient counseling. Government agencies use databases to develop policies concerning nutrient fortification, food standards, label claims, and nutrient equivalents; to assess the safety and adequacy of the food supply; and to conduct epidemiologic research and clinical trials. Colleges and universities use databases for epidemiologic research, diet-disease research, and student education. Institutions with foodservices use databases for planning and evaluating meals, developing special diets, and educating patients.

In consideration of these many and varied uses of nutrient databases, this paper provides an overview of the generation, reporting, and compiling of food composition data. Special emphasis is given to the care with which these procedures should be followed and the care that should be taken in using the data because of their inherent and acquired variability and other limitations.

FOOD ANALYSTS AND ANALYSIS

Chemists in government, industry, academic, and private laboratories analyze individual or composite test samples of foods for nutrients and other substances such as pesticide residues, toxicants, heavy metals, radionuclides, and food additives. Sampling schemes and compositing (if used) should be appropriate for the intended purposes of the resulting data. For example, nationwide food sampling would involve variables different from those involved in local food sampling. The analytical methods and laboratory practices should be specific for the analytes and approved by the Association of Official Analytical Chemists.[1] Quality control procedures should include duplicate analyses, recoveries of spiked samples, and recoveries of standard reference materials.

Those responsible for food analysis should document how the foods were sampled, selected, collected, prepared, and analyzed, and how the results were verified and evaluated. Calculations, if required, should be noted (eg, protein calculated from nitrogen). Basic statistical treatment of food composition analytical data includes determination of means, standard deviations, coefficients of variation, and medians. In some cases, means may be weighted by variety, cultivar, species, market share, or year-round availability.

The distribution of the analytical data points should be evaluated; outliers should be identified and their treatment (ie, inclusion or omission from the evaluation) documented. The concentration of a nutrient in a food, as determined from many samples, may follow a normal distribution, or the distribution may be altered by legal requirements (eg, the minimum fat requirement in ice cream) or by contamination or fortification of some test samples. If bimodal or other modal distributions occur, it might be necessary to separate the samples to obtain useful data. For example, the average iron content might be 18 mg/oz for highly fortified wheat flakes, but only 4.5 mg/oz for those with lower fortification. Sampling that includes both types of cereal would reveal a bimodal distribution for iron and an overall mean that would not be useful for either type.

Nutrient composition data from the laboratory may appear in published journal papers or books; eventually they may appear in the files, hard copy, tapes, or disks of databases. Some data will remain in files and records (eg, product development or label compliance files). Nutrient data may also be published in consumer or trade literature. The data generated by and for industry may be computed and rounded (in compliance with regulations of the Food and Drug Administration [FDA] and United States Department of Agriculture [USDA]) for purposes of nutrition labeling.

When analytical nutrient data are reported, they should be accompanied by complete and appropriate food descriptions. Guidelines for describing foods, which include food group, food source, cooking method, ingredients, and so forth, have been developed.[2] Nutrients must also be adequately identified and presented in appropriate units. Nutrient data for foods are generally presented on a wet weight basis, so it must be clearly specified when a dry weight basis has been used. It is important for analysts to include the percentage of water with the other nutrients for each food. Percentage of water is absolutely essential if the values are reported on a dry weight basis. It should also be clear whether the data are presented "as purchased" or as "edible portion" and whether the foods are raw, cooked, or otherwise processed.

DATA COMPILERS AND COMPILATIONS

Many compilations of food composition data are currently available. The USDA has developed several, including the *Nutrient Database for Standard Reference*,[3] the revised and original editions of Agriculture Handbook 8,[4,5] and the nutrient database used for surveys of individual food intake.[6] Food composition databases are also produced by colleges, universities, hospitals, clinics, industry (product line databases), and private groups (eg, diet analysis programs run on personal computers). The national *Nutrient Data Bank Directory* includes 112 US and Canadian databases,[7] and the INFOODS (International Network of Food Data Systems) international directory[8] lists more than 200 databases (not including most of those in reference 7).

Features of database compilations that may distinguish one from another include availability in hard copy, tape, and/or disk, periodicity of updates, format, and type (ie, reference databases or those used for diet analysis). Some databases are updated continuously; others are updated at specific intervals. Foods in databases usually appear alphabetically or alphabetically by food group. The foods may be listed in the column beginning at the left margin, with the nutrients in rows across the page. An alternative format is one food per page with the nutrients in the left-hand margin column and the values per several serving portions in the rows. The latter format is used by the revised Agriculture Handbook 8.[4]

Compilers of food composition data are employed in some government agencies, food production companies, academia, private business, hospitals and clinics, and foodservice. Compilers should hold degrees in nutrition, dietetics, or food science and should be knowledgeable about foods, food sampling, food analysis, food descriptions, food processing, culinary terms, and cuisines.

The task of the data compiler is to gather data from many sources and then organize, evaluate, and aggregate the data into a useful compilation. Database compilers gather data from previous compilations, from industry, from scientific papers, and (in some cases) directly from the laboratory. Most databases developed in the United States have used a USDA database (eg, the *Nutrient Database for Standard Reference*[3]) as a starting point and have added data from industry and other sources to it. The compiler cannot possibly check every nutrient value for every food with regard to sampling, analytical method, number of samples, and so forth. However, any data that appear to be clearly out of line should be questioned and either verified or omitted.

Database Aggregations

Compilers often organize data into food groups (eg, desserts) and subgroups (eg, cakes, pies, cookies) and then aggregate the listings within the groups to prevent duplicates. This grouping requires that the data for foods that appear to have the same or similar name and descriptors be closely scrutinized to determine which foods and their corresponding nutrient values may be consolidated into a single food entry in the database. Aggregation from various sources requires that food descriptions be as similar as possible (eg, have the same fat content for dairy products or the same processing or preparation methods) and that nutrients have the same specificity and units of measurement (eg, international units of vitamin E are not equal to milligrams of α tocopherol).

Similarity of common nutrient values (eg, water, calories, protein, and fat) for data from several sources provides some basis for food name and data aggregation. Evaluation of major and minor nutrients might indicate that foods with slightly different names are basically the same food. Aggregation often provides more nutrients per food and uses fewer lines in the database. Data for aggregated foods may be averaged or weighted and averaged (eg, data for four brands of canned corn might be weighted and averaged by market share or averaged by number of samples from each source). The data sources and data manipulation should be documented, but it is not usually possible or desirable to publish such information with the database. This information usually remains in the files of the data compiler.

Database Checks

Some tools are available to help the compiler assess the validity and integrity of the compiled database.[9] These include checks for weights of major nutrients compared with the weight of the food, caloric sums of energy yielding nutrients compared with the caloric value of the food, and limits of nutrient concentrations in various food groups. For example, a half-cup of boiled, mashed pumpkin weighs 122 g, and the sum of the weights of the values for water, protein, fat, and carbohydrate is 121 g. The caloric value of this food is 24 kcal per half-cup, and the sum of the caloric equivalents of the protein, fat, and carbohydrate (with a correction for dietary fiber) is 25 kcal. These checks indicate data comparability.

Missing Values

Reference databases contain data gathered from available sources and generally do not contain imputed data for missing values, whereas databases used to analyze diets from food consumption surveys and studies should have as few blanks as possible. For practical purposes, some blanks may be filled in with zeros (eg, cholesterol and vitamin B_{12} for plant materials, or dietary fiber for animal-based foods). Other data may be imputed from a different form of the same food (eg, data for canned corn might be used for frozen corn with adjustment for the sodium content) or from similar foods (eg, data for pinto beans might be used for navy beans). Without these imputed values, estimates of daily intakes will be underestimated. Procedures used to impute values are found in chapter 5 of reference 10. Missing values for multi-ingredient foods may be filled in with data calculated from recipes. These calculations usually require corrections for refuse (eg, bone, shell, peel, trimmed fat), loss or gain of moisture or fat with cooking, and nutrient loss or retention with cooking. Chapter 6 of reference 10 provides information on how to estimate nutrients for multi-ingredient foods. Imputed values should be identified as such, and the processes used for imputation should be documented.

So few data are available for some nutrients, such as vitamin K and chromium, that supplemental tables are useful (in printed databases) to provide easy access to the values and prevent wasted space.

Inconsistencies

Inconsistencies in nutrient values may occur when data come from various sources. For example, one might expect higher values for vitamin C in fresh orange juice, but the aggregated data from different varieties, regions, and seasons may show somewhat higher average levels in canned or reconstituted frozen juice. Such inconsistencies may reflect differences in food storage, sampling, differences in laboratory analytical methods and techniques, and nonidentical samples.

Food Descriptions

The space allowed for a food name and its descriptive terms in a database is usually limited. The luxury of unlimited space for open-ended descriptors for analytical reports[2] is not usually allowed for databases available in hard copy, disk, or tape. Therefore, it is necessary to provide names and descriptive terms in the allotted space that will be most useful for the data user. The compiler should strive for uniformity in food names in a database by using a selected order of descriptors and standardized terms and abbreviations. For example, the compiler might use the following order: food name and descriptive terms (color, flavor, physical state, part of plant or animal, accompaniments, components), preservation or treatment methods and containers, preparation or cooking method, brand name, and serving portion. Not all of these descriptors are applicable or useful for each food. The entry for "part of the food" should also indicate if peel or seeds are present for fruits and vegetables, if fat is present on meat cuts or has been trimmed away, if rind is included or not for cheese, and so forth.

The task of identifying foods in a database becomes easier if the compiler has established the order of descriptors. An example of a format for standard descriptors in a database in which each entry occupies less than 73 spaces is illustrated in *Table 11.1*. Redundant or commonly assumed information is not included (eg, that ice cream is frozen, that frozen dinners are heated before serving, that food in a boil-in-bag container is boiled). Footnotes might be added to provide ingredients for homemade or restaurant items (eg, tuna-noodle vegetable casserole), but are not necessary for well-known items with rigid quality control (eg, Big Macs).

Table 11.1
Examples of Food Names and Descriptive Terms in a Standardized Format with Space Limitations

Food name and descriptors* (preservation/preparation; brand; serving)
Apple, red delicious w/ peel, w/o core, raw - 1 med
Beet greens, fresh, boiled - 1/2 cup
Cake, choc w/ white icing, prep from box mix, Pillsbury - 1/12 cake
Frankfurter, beef & pork, boiled - 1 frank (12/lb)
Fruit cocktail in light syrup, cnd, Del Monte - 1/2 cup
Frzn dinner, chicken, fried w/ mashed potatoes & peas - 11 oz dinner
Ground beef patty, extra lean, pan ckd, well done - 3" diameter, 1/2" high
Ice cream, vanilla w/ choc syrup - 1/2 cup w/ 2 T syrup
Lowfat milk, 2% fat w/ vit A & D, past, homo, - 8 fl oz
Milk from nonfat solids, reconstituted - 2 T solids in 8 fl oz water
Peas, green w/ cream sce, frzn, Birdseye - 1/2 cup
Salisbury steak w/ gravy, frzn boil-in-bag, Banquet - 3 oz w/ 5 T gravy
Scrambled egg w/ milk, cooked in marg - 2 large eggs w/ 1 T marg
Spaghetti in tomato sce, cnd, Campbells - 1 cup

* color, flavor, physical state, part of plant or animal, accompaniments, components.

A computerized retrieval vocabulary named Langual, which can be used with food composition and other food databases, has been developed by the Food and Drug Administration.[11] Langual allows retrieval of foods or food-related data, based on characteristics such as food type, preservation method, and container. Langual has been adapted for use in France and other countries. The concept of a master database of food descriptors has been proposed[12] to facilitate communication and exchange of data among food composition database users.

Cross-References and Food Groupings

A thorough index with cross references is needed to locate foods in a database because of the many synonyms for some foods (*Table 11.2*) and the many ways of describing and placing foods in alphabetical listings. For example, the many types and brand names of pizzas may all be listed under the heading "pizza" or they may be listed alphabetically by pizza type (eg, sausage, deep-dish deluxe, vegetarian). Even if all pizzas are listed under a main heading, the subheadings might be made according to crust type (thick, medium, thin), topping, or source (frozen, carry-out, restaurant chain). Likewise, cakes may be subcategorized by flavor (chocolate, cherry, pound, yellow) or by source (bakery, homemade, box mix, frozen, grocery store). Ready-to-eat cereals may be grouped by grain type (oat, wheat, corn) or listed alphabetically by cereal brand name (Trix, Froot Loops, Shredded Wheat). The decisions for groupings and subgroupings are made by the compiler and often depend on how many items are available under each subhead. The group and subgroup designations affect the usefulness of the compilation, and the compiler must make these decisions with care.

Table 11.2
Examples of Different Names for the Same or Similar Food for Which Cross-referencing Is Necessary

Green beans; snap beans; string beans
Pancake; hotcake; flapjack
Shake; malt; milkshake
Hamburger; ground beef; minced beef
Fries; french fries; fried potatoes; home fries; cottage fries

The use of food groups and subgroups prevents redundancy in terms (eg, repetition of the term "ready-to-eat breakfast cereal" for 150 cereals or "candy bar" for 60 different types); however, food groupings have cultural significance that might make a database more useful in its country or region of origin, but less useful internationally. Therefore, databases designed specifically for international use may need an alphabetical organizational structure or very broad food groups (eg, grains, fruits, vegetables) that reflect food source, rather than food usage (eg, breakfast cereals, snacks, beverages, desserts, entrees).

Basis of Data

It is most useful to dietitians to report the nutrient values per weight of edible portion of "as consumed" food (eg, cooked meat, popped popcorn, or apples with core removed). The weight may be per typical serving portion or per 100 grams. If a serving portion is given, it should be unambiguously described. Consistency in listing serving portions throughout the database is useful for comparative purposes (eg, 8 fl oz for milks, 6 fl oz for fruit juices, 1 oz or 1 cup for ready-to-eat breakfast cereals, 3.5 oz for meats, 0.5 cup for cooked vegetables, 0.5 cup for canned fruit, 1 oz for nuts, and 1 oz for cheese).

Food Contaminants

Some food composition database compilers have ventured into the area of food contaminants. Assessment of these substances poses special problems because "average" levels may not exist. The presence of pesticide residues, toxins, and other contaminants in foods is often a matter of chance. Experts in these areas frequently speak of the number of detections, rather than average levels, and residue levels are usually quite low. For example, an analysis of 200 samples of a food may reveal a pesticide residue in only ten of them. The average level for these ten may be measurable; however, the average for the 200 may have no significant figures. Although much work has been done on pesticides and other contaminants, it has been done to monitor the food supply (to assess safety by confirming that levels are below Acceptable Daily Intakes), rather than to provide values for databases. We may need to identify foods by different and specific variables for these substances. For example, when evaluating lead intake, one might describe foods as "tomato sauce in can with lead solder" or "tomato sauce in laminated can." Interest in data on pesticides might require

Key Techniques

descriptions such as "whole wheat flour from farms using (or not using) a specific pesticide." This might provide more useful information on the levels of these substances in foods and the risks associated with them.

DATA USER CONCERNS

Compilers of food composition data are often users, but most users are not compilers. Therefore, many users may not understand or be aware of the problems and limitations of databases. The most frequent user complaints (especially from lay users, such as students and consumers) are missing data, missing foods, and the need for serving portions different from those listed. Most often data are missing because the analyses have not been performed or the manufacturers will not release the data. Indeed, the most common shortcoming of databases is lack of availability of data for multi-ingredient foods (eg, homemade, frozen, and shelf-stable entrees and desserts; fast foods; and ethnic foods).

The most frequent user errors are selecting the wrong food (not making the best match between the food of interest and the foods listed in the database); assuming that missing values are zeros; and not adjusting serving portions (ie, assuming that the portion listed in the book is what is consumed). The challenge in using databases for food consumption surveys is matching the foods described by study participants to the foods listed in the databases (ie, selecting the best fit). This is why food descriptions are so important. Unfortunately, study participants are not always able to provide accurate food descriptions. The nutrient databases used with USDA food consumption surveys include NFS (not further specified) codes for foods that are not accurately remembered or described by study participants. The nutrient data for NFS foods may be based on other data (eg, an NFS sandwich might reflect the most commonly consumed sandwich in the survey or it might be a composite sandwich with nutrient values calculated from weighted data from other sandwiches in the database).

The selection of a nutrient database or database system for use in a dietary department, educational facility, or research clinic requires consideration of the specific needs of the user(s) and the features and limitations of the various database systems.[13] The user(s) should consider factors such as the number of foods, the nutrients included, the sources of the data, the reliability and currentness of the data, and the desired output, along with considerations for such items as initial cost, maintenance costs, and software or hardware concerns. It may be useful to talk with those who use different database systems and to ask specific questions of the database system developers. The choices are many and varied. Experimentation with database systems at exhibits and demonstrations is helpful in making decisions.

IMPLICATIONS FOR DIETITIANS

When using nutrient databases, investigators should not think of nutrient values as precise, unless they are dealing with a carefully formulated product. For example, the average vitamin C content of an orange is 80 mg; however, the actual content of each orange depends on many factors, such as season, sunlight exposure, cultivar, species, variety, time of day of picking, storage length and temperature, and ripeness at picking. Averages have variation on both sides. Most food composition tables do not have room for standard deviations, ranges, number of samples, notes, or documentation. Considering the extent of nutrient variation, investigators must not be rigid about diet recommendations for patients and clients. One food should not be recommended over another as a better or lesser source of a substance, unless the difference between them will be of practical importance in the diet.

Investigators must remember that the many causes of nutrient variation are compounded in compiled databases. Within-food variation includes variables such as genetics; environment; preservation, processing, and preparation methods; and containers or wrappings. Multi-ingredient foods have mixtures of these variables. Contributing further to nutrient variation are different analytical methods and techniques, use of various recipes to calculate nutrient values, and the compiler's aggregation of foods and nutrient values.

The uses of food composition databases should not go beyond their limitations. They may be used for multiday individual dietary assessments or one-day group assessments, but they probably should not be used to assess the dietary adequacy or deficiency of one-day diets of individual subjects, for metabolic research or balance studies, or for patients on very restricted diets. Food analysis or specific information from food manufacturers might be used for research studies or very restricted diets.

Investigators must use databases knowledgeably; they must be aware that they are not fully documented because it is impractical to do so. They should not become unduly alarmed about uneven quality (eg, more detailed description and more nutrient data for some foods than others) and inconsistencies, but they should not accept unreasonable data (ie, values that clearly appear to be out of line compared with values for similar foods). Sometimes there are reasons for apparent inconsistencies. For example, the cholesterol content of drained tuna canned in vegetable oil is less than that for tuna canned in water (*Table 11.3*). One might expect them to be the same; however, some cholesterol, which is lipid-soluble, dissolves into the vegetable oil, thereby reducing the amount in the drained tuna. The tuna in vegetable oil might appear to be a better choice for cholesterol-conscious patients; however, the cholesterol difference is probably insignificant. Tuna in water is still a better choice for patients on diets low in total fat and calories.

Table 11.3
Example of Apparent Data Inconsistency: Cholesterol Content of 3 oz of Canned, Drained White Tuna*

	Canned in oil	Canned in water	Difference
Energy (kcal)	158	116	+42
Fat (g)	6.9	2.1	+4.8
Cholesterol (mg)	26	35	−9

* Data from USDA.[4]

Those who need more information about nutrient data in a database or clarification of questionable data should contact the database compiler or the data source for confirmation:
• USDA and trade associations for data on basic and traditional foods
• USDA for data contained in the USDA reference databases
• industry representatives for data on brand-named products and some restaurant foods

A dietitian or food scientist within a company usually can supply the data or the answers needed; however, making this initial contact is not always easy. Food companies receive many requests for nutrient data and may not have the resources or appropriate personnel to respond to these requests or to provide the data as requested. The author's experience has been that only about half of written requests to industry are answered. About half of these responses are form letters prepared for consumers; the food composition data they contain are similar to nutrition label data and therefore not appropriate for databases. Thus, follow-up letters are required.

OUTLOOK

Food composition databases are improving with time. More samples analyzed by better analytical techniques and monitored by better quality control procedures produce more results and better results. This does not mean that variability decreases; it means that it is more readily measured. With more data, some outliers are more clearly identified; other values previously thought to be outlying are accepted as real. The greater the number of representative samples appropriately analyzed, the better.

With regard to current databases, efforts must continue to fill in the missing values for foods previously analyzed and to analyze foods for which data are most needed (eg, prepared entrees and restaurant foods). Work must continue to improve analytical methods, quality assurance techniques, and statistical analysis of results. Better ways of determining and expressing nutrient variability and of validating nutrient data and compiled databases must be found.

References

1. Association of Official Analytical Chemists. *Official Methods of Analysis.* 15th ed. Arlington, Va: Association of Official Analytical Chemists; 1990.
2. Truswell AS, Bateson DJ, Madafiglio KC, Pennington JAT, Rand WM. INFOODS guidelines for describing foods. *J Food Comp Anal.* In press.
3. USDA. Nutrient Data Base for Standard Reference. Hyattsville, Md. Periodic releases available from the National Technical Information Service, Springfield, Va.
4. USDA. *Composition of Foods: Raw, Processed, Prepared.* Rev. ed. Washington, DC: US Government Printing Office; 1976–1989. Agriculture Handbook 8.
5. USDA. *Composition of Foods: Raw, Processed, Prepared.* Washington, DC: US Government Printing Office; 1963. Agriculture Handbook 8.
6. USDA. Database for use with surveys of food intakes of individuals. Continuously updated. Available from the National Technical Information Service, Springfield, Va.
7. Hoover LW, ed. *Nutrient Data Bank Directory.* 7th ed. Columbia, Mo: Curators of the University of Missouri; 1988.
8. Heintze D, Klensin JC, Rand WM, eds. *International Directory of Food Composition Tables.* 2nd ed. Cambridge, Mass: Massachusetts Institute of Technology; 1988.
9. Murphy SP. Integrity checks for nutrient databases. In: Stumbo PJ, ed. *Proceedings of the Fourteenth National Nutrient Databank Conference June 19–21, 1989.* Iowa City, Ia: CBORD Group Inc; 1990: 89–91.
10. Rand WM, Pennington JAT, Murphy SP, Klensin JC. *Compiling Data for Food Composition Databases.* Tokyo, Japan: UNU Press; in press.
11. McCann A, Pennington JAT, Smith EC, Holden JM, Soergel D, Wiley RC. FDA's factored food vocabulary for food product description. *J Am Diet Assoc.* 1988; 88:336.
12. Soergel D, Pennington JAT, McCann A, Holden JM, Smith EC, Wiley RC. A network model for improving access to food and nutrition data. *J Am Diet Assoc.* In press.
13. Buzzard IM, Price KS, Warren RA. Considerations for selecting nutrient-calculation software: evaluation of the nutrient database. *Am J Clin Nutr.* 1991; 54:7–9.

12. INTERPRETATION AND UTILIZATION OF DATA FROM THE NATIONAL NUTRITION MONITORING SYSTEM

Catherine E. Woteki, PhD, RD, and Faye L. Wong, MPH, RD

The collection of surveys and surveillance activities known as the National Nutrition Monitoring System arose from the needs of federal agencies for information about per capita food and nutrient consumption, household food use, and the dietary and nutritional status of the American people. The information was needed to plan programs and to evaluate existing policies and programs. The patchwork of activities that had answered different agencies' specific questions was poorly coordinated, and as the potential usefulness of more comparable data was recognized, political pressure was brought to bear on the agencies to integrate them into a National Nutrition Monitoring System. The Food and Agriculture Act of 1977 required the Secretaries of Agriculture and of Health, Education, and Welfare to develop a plan for a national system of coordinated surveys and surveillance activities. The resulting plan established two goals for the National Nutrition Monitoring System: the creation of a mechanism for periodic review of data and reporting to the Congress on the nutritional status of the American population, and the coordination, to the fullest extent possible, of the two largest nutrition surveys.

The nutrition-related data collected by the government are designed to provide the information needed for nutrition policy and program decisions, but the collection also is a rich database for research. Frequently, these two uses of the data overlap. Government survey and surveillance data can be used for program planning and evaluation, regulatory decision making, epidemiologic research, and commercial uses. Program planners and analysts rely heavily on information about the nutritional status of the population and the identification of subgroups at risk. Program analysts use repeated cross-sectional surveys to determine whether change has occurred in certain population characteristics. Regulatory decision makers use the data to determine and document the need for regulatory actions, to design the actions, and to evaluate their effectiveness. Epidemiologic researchers use the data for both descriptive and analytical studies, and commercial companies use the data for developing marketing strategies and advertising campaigns.

For all of these purposes, the survey and surveillance data are analyzed:
- To estimate the prevalences of health and nutritional characteristics of the population and of subgroups in the population
- To produce normative values of nutrition and health status indicators in population groups
- To evaluate interrelationships among health and nutrition variables
- By repeating measurements in subsequent surveys, to monitor changes over time
- To study the etiology and natural history of disease through longitudinal studies of survey participants

The intent of this chapter is to provide an introduction to the use of these extensive data by dietitians in their own research. A brief overview is given to analytical approaches for the record-based surveillance systems and the population surveys included in the National Nutrition Monitoring System. Because several recent publications provide detailed descriptions of the data systems,[1-3] the methods used to collect the data,[4,5] as well as the methodological issues related to interpretation of dietary survey methods,[6,7] these topics are not discussed in any depth here. Rather, emphasis is given to some of the statistical issues necessary to analyze and interpret surveillance or population survey data.

Most of the activities of the National Nutrition Monitoring System can be classified into two categories: record-based surveillance systems and population surveys. The record-based systems make use of the multitude of data collected and maintained for purposes other than nutrition monitoring; for example, the systems use medical records of people receiving benefits under the Special Supplemental Food Program for Women, Infants and Children (WIC). Population surveys use statistical sampling approaches to select representative samples of US households and their residents who are then asked to answer questionnaires, keep records, or participate in physical examinations. Examples of record-based surveillance systems and population surveys are described in this section.

RECORD-BASED SURVEILLANCE SYSTEMS

The Pediatric Nutrition Surveillance System (PedNSS) and the Pregnancy Nutrition Surveillance System (PNSS) are both coordinated by the Division of Nutrition (DN), Centers for Disease Control (CDC).[8-12] These surveillance systems are program-based and collect data from a population of children and pregnant women who obtain services in publicly funded food assistance, nutrition, and health programs.

Traditionally, nutrition surveillance data are analyzed by the CDC and returned to the participating states for use in making programmatic decisions. PedNSS data are returned to the states monthly, quarterly, and annually, whereas PNSS data are returned only annually at this time. In recent years, PedNSS nutrition surveillance software has been increasingly distributed to states so that they can manage and produce their own data. PNSS software will be distributed when it becomes available. The CDC provides ongoing technical assistance, consultation, and training to states in conducting all aspects of nutrition surveillance, including the collection, processing, analysis, interpretation, and practical utilization of these data.

Nationally, PedNSS and PNSS data are used to describe the nutritional status of low-income populations of children and pregnant women and to monitor trends.[8-10,13-17] Adverse health behaviors associated with low birthweight are also monitored. Epidemiologic analyses are conducted to investigate the relationships between risk factors and birthweight outcome and to describe high-risk persons.

Pediatric Nutrition Surveillance System (PedNSS)

In 1989, more than 40 states, territories, and Indian tribes participated in the PedNSS.[9] Started in 1974,[8] this surveillance system continuously monitors selected indicators of nutritional status among low-income infants and children younger than 18 years of age. Monitored are simple indicators of nutritional status, such as short stature, underweight, overweight, anemia, and low birthweight. Routine clinical measurements such as height, weight, hematocrit, hemoglobin, and birthweight are collected. The data are rapidly edited and compared with data from the reference population to generate prevalence estimates of the nutrition problems monitored. PedNSS data are analyzed by clinic, county, and state; thus, geographic areas with higher risks are identified. Age and ethnic analyses of the statewide data also provide information on high-risk subpopulations for targeting interventions for specific nutrition problems.

Pregnancy Nutrition Surveillance System (PNSS)

During 1988, approximately 20 states, territories, and Indian tribes participated in the PNSS,[10] which was initiated in 1979.[8] Nutrition data monitored by the PNSS include pregravid underweight and overweight, and prenatal weight gain and anemia, identified from readily available clinic information.[11,12] This surveillance system was enhanced in 1987 to improve the monitoring of prenatal health behaviors that have an adverse effect on infant birthweight. In the future, it will be possible to examine the dose effect of the mother's self-reported smoking and alcohol consumption on the infant's birthweight. Age and ethnic analyses of the statewide data identify subpopulations with higher rates of nutrition problems and adverse health behaviors that should be targeted for interventions.

Factors to Consider When Analyzing Data From Surveillance Systems

The data collected by pediatric and pregnancy nutrition surveillance are subject to a number of biases that need to be considered carefully when analyzing and interpreting this information. Knowledge of the following influences on nutrition surveillance data is a key factor in the appropriate use of this information in making programmatic decisions.[9,10,18,19]

Surveillance population. Nutrition surveillance data are collected on children and pregnant women who participate in publicly funded food assistance, nutrition, or health programs. Because this is a self-selected population, the data are not representative of the nutritional status of children and pregnant women in the community-at-large (eg, city, county, state). The population used for nutrition surveillance may differ in one or more ways from those who do not participate in publicly funded programs. Factors that make them different from the general population include their meeting an income criterion for program eligibility, being at nutrition or health risk (if applicable), and having the personal initiative to participate in assistance programs. That is, motivated program participants may be different from those who are equally eligible but do not participate. The PedNSS and PNSS populations are primarily low-income and are overrepresented by racial or ethnic minority groups in comparison with the general population.

It is important to note, however, that although this bias is a major limitation of using nutrition surveillance data for some purposes (eg, for describing the nutritional status of all children in a state), the information can be representative of program participants. Program managers can use nutrition surveillance data to describe the nutritional status and behavioral risk factors of the population served when making programmatic decisions. For example, appropriate interventions can be targeted at specific subpopulations with high rates of anemia, or additional resources can be earmarked for local programs that serve a greater percentage of these children.

Program eligibility criteria. The majority of PedNSS and PNSS data originate in the WIC program. The remaining surveillance data are from the Early, Periodic, Screening, Detection, and Treatment Program (EPSDT) and the Maternal and Child Health Program (MCH). The eligibility criteria for participation in these programs can influence a state's nutrition surveillance data. For example, if a state WIC program is targeting anemic children for priority enrollment, a high rate of anemia may be found. In this case, other children in the community who are at lower nutrition risk have less opportunity for WIC enrollment; thus, the surveillance data reflect the disproportionate number of children with anemia in the WIC program and not the true rate of anemia.

On the other hand, if the state uses a very liberal cutoff for low height-for-age as an eligibility criterion for WIC recertification (eg, below 25th percentile of the growth reference), a high prevalence of short stature may result. In this case, the surveillance data reflect the disproportionate number of short children in the WIC program, rather than the true rate of this problem. Knowledge of these program enrollment criteria assists in appropriately interpreting nutrition surveillance data.

Accuracy. Nutrition surveillance data are collected in more than 4000 public health clinics throughout the country. The clinic staff has a wide range of expertise in nutrition assessment and data collection. Many potential errors can be minimized by placing a high management priority on routinely monitoring data quality and promptly correcting problems.

Calibrated equipment, periodic training for clinic staff, and daily supervision of clinic practices, including data collection, are important to the integrity of nutrition surveillance data. Consultation, training, and written procedures are available from the CDC. Computer edit programs for nutrition surveillance can also identify data problems and trace them to their clinic source for correction.

Quality assurance checks of data processing procedures are equally important. Promptness and accuracy in processing nutrition surveillance data are important for the early identification of errors, especially those that originate at the data collection level. Data processing procedures should be monitored to ensure the accurate entry of data, the application of current reference criteria in data analysis, and the use of correct formulas to generate nutrition surveillance information. Many errors in data processing can be very subtle and can easily escape detection.

Self-reported data. Certain PNSS data are self-reported, such as the woman's pregravid weight and her smoking and drinking behavior during pregnancy. The accuracy of self-reported information is another important consideration in the interpretation of nutrition surveillance data. Problems with accuracy may be caused by poor recall or by the sensitivity of the question. For example, if a pregnant woman has been told that drinking alcohol can hurt her baby, she may not truthfully report this practice to the clinic staff. The accuracy of these self-reported data has not been validated. Interviewer training on how to ask sensitive questions is essential to minimize this source of data bias.

Infant birthweight is reported by the mother in both PNSS and PedNSS. Maternal recall of infant birthweight has been validated; linking nutrition surveillance data to birth records showed the recall to be very accurate.[20]

Record volume. Calculating prevalences of nutrition problems can be more difficult when analyzing nutrition surveillance data at the local level, especially in rural areas where the clinic population is small and few records are available. The few records can cause the prevalence estimates to be unstable and to vary considerably from one point in time to another. The variance, in this case, reflects the low record volume analyzed, rather than a real change in the nutritional status of the surveillance population.

Completeness of reporting. Incomplete reporting is a potential for bias in the nutrition surveillance data in two respects. First, data need to be collected on all children and women in the participating surveillance programs to be truly representative of the population served. For example, if nutrition surveillance data are collected only in certain local clinics, the overall prevalences of nutrition problems or behavioral risk factors would not be representative of the program participants in the state.

Second, essential data elements need to be collected for each person. For example, missing information on the smoking status of pregnant women would make it difficult to interpret the prevalence of low birthweight because smoking doubles the risk of having a low birthweight infant. Thus, its influence needs to be considered in the analysis of PNSS data. As another example, missing weights would make it difficult to estimate the prevalence of underweight and overweight. Records with missing weights would need to be excluded from an analysis of weight status.

Monitoring trends. Obviously, changes over time in any of the factors previously mentioned can influence trends in the prevalence of nutrition problems. It is useful for states participating in nutrition surveillance to maintain records on changes, such as modifications in program eligibility criteria, periodic large increases in program funding, purchases of new clinic equipment, introduction of new procedures, training of staff, enhancements of computer systems, or additions of new clinic sites.

POPULATION SURVEYS

Since 1936, the federal government has conducted periodic population surveys designed to provide nutrition-related information.[1] *Tables 12.1* and *12.2* list the surveys and specialized activities contributing to the National Nutrition Monitoring System and provide a brief description of their content. All contained a cross-sectional design at baseline; two (NHANES I and NHANES III) included or will include a longitudinal follow-up; and the Continuing Survey of Food Intakes by Individuals (CSFII) 1985–1986, designed as a panel study, reinterviewed the initial sample five additional times during the year after the initial interview.

Nationwide Food Consumption Surveys

Since 1955, the design of the surveys conducted by the US Department of Agriculture (USDA) has been a stratified probability sample of the 48 conterminous states. Since 1965, data have been collected over a 12-month period to capture seasonal differences in food use.

The first nutrition survey, undertaken by the USDA in 1936–1937, obtained information about household food use from 20 466 housekeeping households. Through interviews with the person in the household who was most responsible for food purchasing and preparation, information was obtained about the quantity, source, and cost of food used during the previous seven days. These Nationwide Food Consumption Surveys (NFCS) have been

Table 12.1
Dietary and Nutrition Status
Surveys and Surveillance
Activities of National Nutrition
Monitoring System

Date	Agency*	Survey	Target US Population	Sample Selected	Number Interviewed (Response rate)	Number Examined (Response rate)
1909—annual	USDA	US Food Supply Series	NA†	≈350 foods currently	NA	NA
1936–37	USDA	Household Food Consumption Survey—Household Food Use	Housekeeping households, with husband and wife, native born, nonrelief	NR‡	20 466 households	NA
1942	USDA	Household Food Consumption Survey—Household Food Use	Housekeeping households	3060 households	2748 households	NA
1948	USDA	Household Food Consumption Survey—Household Food Use	Urban housekeeping households	5681 households	4489 households	NA
1955	USDA	Household Food Consumption Survey—Household Food Use	Civilian, housekeeping households	6792 households	6060 households	NA
1965–66	USDA	Household Food Consumption Survey—Household Food Use	Civilian, housekeeping households	18 890 households	15 112 households	NA
1965	USDA	Nationwide Food Consumption Survey—Individual Intakes	Eligible individuals residing in eligible households (all except half of persons 20–64 y)	NR	14 519 persons	NA
1968–70	DHEW	Ten State Nutrition Survey	Low-income families in 10 states	29 935 families	23 846 (80%) families 86 352 persons	40 847 (47%)
1971–74	NCHS	First National Health and Nutrition Examination Survey	Civilian, noninstitutionalized individuals, 1–74 y	28 043 persons	27 753 (99%)	20 749 (74%)
1974–75	NCHS	NHANES I Augmentation Sample	Civilian, noninstitutionalized persons, 25–74 y	4300 persons	4288 (94%)	3053 (71%)
1973—continuous	CDC	Pediatric Nutrition Surveillance System	Low-income, high-risk children, 0–17 y	5 states (in 1987, 36 states plus District of Columbia and Puerto Rico)	NA	NA
1976–80	NCHS	Second National Health and Nutrition Examination Survey	Civilian, noninstitutionalized individuals, 0.5–74 y	27 801 persons	25 286 (91%)	20 322 (73%)
1977–78	USDA	Nationwide Food Consumption Survey—Household Food Use	Civilian households	24 408 households	14 964 households	NA
1977–78	USDA	Nationwide Food Consumption Survey—Individual Intakes	Eligible individuals residing in eligible households (All except half of persons over 18 y in summer, fall, and winter)	44 169 persons	30 770 persons	NA
1977–78	USDA	Supplemental Nationwide Food Consumption Survey—Household Food Use	Civilian households in Puerto Rico, Alaska, Hawaii. Elderly adults in 48 states.	18 162 households	10 341 households	NA
1977–78	USDA	Supplemental Nationwide Food Consumption Survey—Individual Intakes	Individuals residing in eligible households	28 984 persons	21 465 persons	NA
1977–78	USDA	Low-Income Nationwide Food Consumption Survey—Household Food Use	Low-income civilian households in 48 states.	NR	4623 households	NA

(continued)

Table 12.1 (continued)
Dietary and Nutrition Status
Surveys and Surveillance
Activities of National Nutrition
Monitoring System

Date	Agency*	Survey	Target US Population	Sample Selected	Number Interviewed (Response rate)	Number Examined (Response rate)
1977–78	USDA	Low-Income Nationwide Food Consumption Survey—Individual Intakes	Individuals residing in eligible households	16 208 persons	12 847 persons	NA
1979—continuous	CDC	Pregnancy Nutrition Surveillance System	Low-income, high-risk pregnant women	13 states (in 1986, 12 states plus District of Columbia)	NA	NA
1979–80	USDA	Low-Income Nationwide Food Consumption Survey—Household Food Use	Low-income civilian households	NR	3002 households	NA
1979–80	USDA	Low-Income Nationwide Food Consumption Survey—Individual Intakes	Individuals in eligible households	NR	8492 persons	NA
1982–84	NCHS	Hispanic Health and Nutrition Examination Survey	Civilian, noninstitutionalized individuals, 0.5–74 y			
			Mexican-American (AZ, CA, CO, NM, TX)	9894 persons	8554 (87%)	7462 (75%)
			Cuban (FL)	2244 persons	1766 (79%)	1357 (61%)
			Puerto Rican (CT, NJ, NY)	3786 persons	3369 (89%)	2834 (75%)
1985–86	USDA	Continuing Survey of Food Intakes by Individuals	Women and men, 19–50 y Children, 1–5 y	4359 households	3224 households 4618 persons	NA
1985–86	USDA	Continuing Survey of Food Intakes by Individuals in Low-Income Households	Low-income, women and men, 19–50 y, children 1–5 y	3711 households	3239 households 5619 persons	NA
1987	CDC	Surveillance of Severe Pediatric Undernutrition	Low-income, high-risk children, 0–5 y	4 states	NA	
1987–88	USDA	Nationwide Food Consumption Survey—Household Food Use	Civilian households	NR		NA
1987–88	USDA	Nationwide Food Consumption Survey—Individual Intakes	Individuals residing in eligible households	NR		NA
1988–94	NCHS	Third National Health and Nutrition Examination Survey	Civilian, noninstitutionalized individuals, 2 mo+	~ 40 000 persons		
1989–96	USDA	Continuing Survey of Food Intakes by Individuals	Individuals of all ages residing in eligible households			
			All income	1500 each year		
			Low income	750 each year		

* USDA, US Department of Agriculture; DHEW, Department of Health, Education and Welfare; NCHS, National Center for Health Statistics; CDC, Centers for Disease Control.

† Not applicable.

‡ Not reported.

From Woteki CE, Fanelli-Kuczmarski MT.[1] ©1990, ILSI–Nutrition Foundation. Used by permission.

Table 12.2
Specialized activities
contributing to National
Nutrition Monitoring System

Date	Agency*	Survey	Target US Population	Sample Interviewed	Objective
1957—annual	NCHS	National Health Interview Survey	Civilian, noninstitutionalized individuals	~ 50 000 households	To collect data on personal and demographic features, incidence of acute illness and injuries, prevalence of chronic conditions and impairments, and utilization of health resources and other current health issues
		Supplemental topics:			
1984	NCHS	Aging	Persons, 55+ y	16 148 persons	To assess health status and care of elderly people
1985	NCHS	Health Promotion/ Disease Prevention	Persons, 18+ y	33 630 persons	To measure progress towards 1990 Health Objectives for the Nation
1986	NCHS	Vitamin/Mineral Supplements	Children, 2–6 y Persons, 18+ y	1877 children 1775 persons	To determine supplement usage and intake levels
1987	NCHS	Cancer Epidemiology and Control	Persons, 18+ y	~ 45 000 persons	To assess cancer risk factors
1961—annual	FDA	Total Diet Study	Specific age-sex groups	NA†	To assess levels of a variety of nutritional components and contaminants in food supply and representative diets of target population
1980	FDA	Vitamin/Mineral Supplement Intake Survey	Civilian, noninstitutionalized persons, 16+ y	2991 persons	To assess nutrient intakes from supplements and to examine characteristics of supplement users
1981–83, 1984—continuous	CDC	Behavioral Risk Factor Surveillance System	Persons, 18+ y, residing in participation states in households with telephones	23 113 persons (30 730 persons in 1986)	To assess prevalence of personal health practices related to leading causes of death
1982–84, 1986	NCHS	NHANES I Epidemiologic Followup Study	Persons examined in NHANES I, 25–75 y at baseline	12 220 persons (1982)	To examine relationship of baseline clinical, nutritional, and behavioral factors assessed in NHANES I to subsequent morbidity and mortality
1982, 1984, 1986, 1988	FDA	Health and Diet Study	Civilian, noninstitutionalized persons, 18+ y	4000 persons response rate of 70–75%	To assess public knowledge, attitudes, and practices about diet and health and public's use of information on food labels
1988–90	NCHS	National Maternal and Infant Health Survey	Reproductive-age women	20 000 vital records, 60 000 persons linked with sampled vital records	To examine factors associated with low birth weight and fetal and infant deaths

* NCHS, National Center for Health Statistics; CDC, Centers for Disease Control; FDA, Food and Drug Administration.

† Not applicable.

From Woteki CE, Fanelli-Kuczmarski MT.[1] ©1990, ILSI–Nutrition Foundation. Used by permission.

repeated at roughly ten-year intervals. Since 1965, the USDA has collected information from individual household members about the food they have eaten. The major purpose of these individual intake surveys is to determine the adequacy of food and nutrient intake by the US population by region and urbanization. Two series of surveys have been undertaken—interviews with members of households selected for the NFCS, and a CSFII initiated in 1985.

Ten-State Nutrition Survey

The first comprehensive survey to evaluate the nutritional status of a large segment of the US population was the Ten State Nutrition Survey conducted in 1968–1970. In each of ten states, a random selection of families was made from 1960 Census Bureau enumeration districts where the highest percentage of families had incomes below the poverty index. Nutritional status was assessed on the basis of dietary intakes and food patterns, dental examinations, and anthropometric and biochemical measurements. Information about factors affecting food intake, such as socioeconomic characteristics, health status, and income, was also gathered.

Health and Nutrition Examination Surveys

The importance of a reliable assessment of the nutritional status, particularly the extent of malnutrition and hunger, of the population in the United States was recognized at the 1969 White House Conference on Food, Nutrition, and Health. Subsequently, the US Department of Health and Human Services (DHHS) incorporated nutritional status assessments into its ongoing Health Examination Survey. Two National Health and Nutrition Examination Surveys have been conducted (NHANES I in 1971–1975, NHANES II in 1976–1980), a third is under way (NHANES III in 1988–1994), and a special survey of Mexican Americans, Cubans, and Puerto Ricans living in the continental United States (the Hispanic HANES), was conducted in 1982–1984. The NHANES samples were drawn from the 50 states, and the surveys were conducted in two stages: an initial interview conducted in the respondents' homes in which information was obtained about their health histories and sociodemographic characteristics, and a dietary intake assessment and physical examination conducted about two weeks later in a mobile examination center.

Although the content and specific aspects of the designs of the NFCS, CSFII, and HANES conducted in the past 20 years differ, the surveys share some common characteristics. They all used multistage probability sampling to select representative samples. They were cross-sectional and provided a snapshot of the population's characteristics at one point in time. The surveys restricted the samples to the noninstitutionalized population and excluded persons on active duty with the military.

Each of these national surveys used either a daily food consumption method or a food frequency questionnaire method to obtain information about food and nutrient intakes. The daily food consumption method used most frequently was the 24-hour recall. The USDA surveys supplemented this method with a two-day food diary to provide a better description of usual food intake patterns. The HANES used a 24-hour recall and a food frequency questionnaire to provide estimates of usual food intake. The NHANES I Epidemiologic Follow-up Study and the 1987 National Health Interview Survey relied on food frequency questionnaires exclusively. The CSFII obtained a 24-hour recall in a personal interview, and five follow-up interviews were conducted by telephone to obtain additional recalls.

Behavioral Risk Factor Surveillance System (BRFSS)

The Behavioral Risk Factor Surveillance System (BRFSS), conducted by the CDC, is designed to monitor personal risk factors for the ten leading causes of premature death in the United States.[21] The CDC has assisted participating states in using random-digit dialing telephone methods to conduct BRFSS since 1981.[22] Today, the monthly telephone interviews are conducted in most states by using computer-assisted telephone interview (CATI) technology. The BRFSS sample is selected by using a multistage cluster design based on the Waksberg method,[21] a three-step procedure for obtaining a sample. First, nonresidential clusters are eliminated from the random sample of telephone numbers selected. Second, the actual numbers called are randomly generated from the last two digits of the telephone number. And third, one adult, aged 18 years or older, is randomly selected for interview.

The BRFSS interviews are conducted following a core questionnaire developed by participating states with technical assistance from the CDC. In 1990, the core questionnaire included information on seat belt use, alcohol consumption, cigarette smoking, hypertension, exercise, preventive health practices (eg, to reduce elevated serum cholesterol), and self-reported height and weight.[23] There are additional questions on mammography and breast examination for women. In 1989, questions about weight control practices were included in the core questionnaire.[24] These questions are now offered as an optional module. In 1990, optional dietary fat and fruit and vegetable consumption modules were added to the BRFSS. More than half of the participating states have incorporated these modules into their BRFSS interview for 1990.

Nutrition-related problems monitored on the BRFSS thus include adult overweight, excess dietary fat intake, inadequate fruit and vegetable intake, weight loss practices, cholesterol screening and awareness, and hypertension.[25-28] Data from the BRFSS are used by participating states to increase public awareness about nutrition and health problems in the population, to target interventions to reduce risk factors for chronic disease, and to monitor trends. In the case of tobacco use, BRFSS data have been used successfully to support legislation that restricts cigarette smoking in public places.

Factors to Consider When Analyzing Survey Data

When analyzing survey data, one must consider whether the data are suitable for the questions being asked. This requires consideration of the design of the survey, the appropriateness of the methods used, and whether any bias has been introduced. Bias is a consistent error that can be introduced in a number of ways and can take many forms.

Sampling bias. Examples of sampling biases include frame biases and consistent sampling biases. A "frame" is the sampling list used when the listing of the sampling units in the population is too difficult or tedious. Frame biases would be caused by the use of an incomplete list, eg, the telephone book as the list from which to draw the sample for a survey of residents of Washington, DC. Such a sample would include only those households who have telephone numbers in the directory. It would therefore be biased in two directions: households without telephones would not be represented, nor would households with unlisted numbers. The sample probably would underrepresent poor households and might also underrepresent some professionals who prefer unlisted numbers.

Consistent sampling biases can be introduced by the mechanical procedures used to select units from the frame into the sample. In the telephone survey example, a consistent sampling bias could arise if the sample of telephone numbers were contacted during the hours of 9 AM to 5 PM on weekdays. It would be unlikely to find employed persons at home during these hours, and the sample would underrepresent this important segment of the residents of Washington, DC.

Sometimes decisions are made to narrow the areas covered in area probability samples to reduce the costs associated with collecting the data. These decisions can lead to noncoverage bias, that is, the failure to include elements in the sample that would properly belong in the sample. An example would be the exclusion of areas with a low Hispanic population from the Hispanic HANES that resulted in a slight underrepresentation of more affluent Hispanics in the sample.

Nonsampling bias. Nonsampling biases arise from systematic errors related to nonresponse, measurement, or data processing. Nonresponse bias results from the failure to obtain observations on some elements selected and designated for the sample. This bias occurs because people are not at home despite repeated attempts to contact them, they refuse to participate, or they may be incapacitated and unable to participate. This bias also occurs because of lost data (eg, lost interviews, laboratory accidents).

Statisticians frequently use the survey response rate as an overall indicator of the quality of a survey. When a substantial proportion of the sample selected for a survey does not participate, a potential for bias exists if the nonrespondents differ from the respondents in some systematic way. The greater the nonresponse, the greater the potential for bias.

Even when a substantial proportion of the original sample does not participate in the survey, the sample may not be biased, and studies of nonresponse bias can be performed. These types of studies have been performed for some of the national surveys.[3,30] Nonresponse bias analyses to examine whether there were systematic differences between those interviewed but not examined and the examined samples were performed for NHANES I and II and found no evidence of bias. No similar analyses have been performed for the NFCS 1977 or the CSFII 1985 one-day data, although comparisons have been made that indicate that use of sample weights will adjust demographic characteristics so that they are very similar to census estimates for the appropriate time periods. The USDA has compared data from the CSFII 1986 with data from the 1986 Current Population Survey and also conducted a follow-up of nonrespondents. They found differences that may be related to food intake patterns, particularly overestimating food stamp usage. With the exception of food stamp usage, these differences disappear when the sample weights are used.

Measurement bias refers to consistent errors arising in the interview or laboratory method used to obtain the data. In 24-hour recalls, measurement bias can be introduced through the interview methods (when probing for amounts of fat or alcoholic beverage consumption, for example), coding assumptions (rules for assigning default codes, for example), errors in the food composition data base used to estimate nutrient levels, or selection of days of the week to conduct the interviews. This type of bias has been recently reviewed.[6,7,29]

Sample weights and design effects. The statistical technique used to identify survey samples introduces complexities into the analysis of the data.[31] In area probability sampling, some trade-offs are made in the randomness of the sample to minimize the costs of the survey. The technique is multistage, and at each stage sample elements with a known probability are selected. In the NHANES, the stages of selection are defined as counties, areas within counties (called segments), households, and household members. To produce the estimates for the nation based on observations from individuals, the data for individuals must be inflated by their probability of selection, adjusted for nonresponse, and then poststratified to bring the population estimate into close agreement with the US Census Bureau estimates. To make these procedures easier for those who use the survey data, sample weights incorporating the three levels of adjustments appear on the data tapes.

Area probability samples are not simple random samples, and the assumptions of simple random sampling do not apply when hypothesis testing is performed with survey data.[31] Special computer programs are now widely available that can take into account the complex nature of the sample in the calculation of test statistics. How greatly a survey sample differs from a simple random sample is summarized in the design effect—the ratio of the variance for a statistic from a complex sample to the corresponding variance from a simple random sample of the same size. The design effect can be used to adjust estimates and statistics computed by using assumptions of simple random sampling for the complexities in the sample design.

In hypothesis testing using data from the population surveys, it is worthwhile to proceed stepwise.[31] In the long range, this approach will save computer time and will simplify the initial analyses. At the first level of analysis, the data should be explored without using the weights or design effects. Any relationships found not to be significant at this screening stage probably will not be significant when sample weights and design effects are considered. However, there are rare occasions when this may not be true, and if the hypothesis has a strong biological plausibility, it probably would be worthwhile to pursue the analysis regardless of the results at the first level of analysis. At the second level, sample weights should be used; and at the third level, both sample weights and design effects should be used, refining the analysis at each stage. All the analyses at level one can be performed with standard statistical packages.

Defining the analytic sample.   Frequently, investigators take a subsample from a larger survey sample, perform analyses on the data for the subsample, and conclude that the findings are generalizable to the US population. Whenever analyses of this type are performed, it is essential that the analytical subsample be examined for bias and that the sample weights and design effects be used in the analysis.

Determining whether a subsample is free from bias can be done by comparing the subsample with the overall sample for characteristics related to the subject of inquiry. For example, one would determine whether the distribution of income, educational attainment, cigarette smoking, and vitamin supplement usage were similar in the subsample and the overall sample when examining serum vitamin C levels. If the distributions are reasonably similar, one could conclude that the subsample does not appear to be biased on factors known to be related to serum vitamin C levels.

EXAMPLES OF ANALYSES

As discussed earlier, the data from the National Nutrition Monitoring System are put to multiple uses. This section provides examples of the five types of analyses that can be performed with the data.

Prevalence Estimates

Anemia among low-income pregnant women has been described using pregnancy nutrition surveillance data.[15] The prevalence of anemia increased during the second and third trimesters. For white and black women respectively, the prevalence of anemia was 3.5% and 12.7% during the first trimester, 6.4% and 17.8% in the second trimester, and 18.8% and 38.1% during the third trimester. Black women had a higher rate of anemia for all age groups. Early enrollment in the WIC program was associated with a lower prevalence of anemia. Based on these findings, efforts to promote earlier enrollment into public health programs, to provide iron nutrition education, and to ensure timely referrals were recommended.

The prevalence of high blood cholesterol levels among adults was determined using the guidelines of the National Cholesterol Education Program and data from the NHANES II.[32] The analysis showed that 41% of adults should have lipoprotein analysis after an initial measurement of serum total cholesterol, and 88% of them would need lipoprotein analysis. Approximately 36% of the adult population would be candidates for medical advice and intervention for high blood cholesterol levels. The implications of the analysis are that 60 million Americans 20 years of age and older are candidates for a Step 1 diet to lower blood cholesterol levels.

Normative Values

The NCHS growth curves[33] are probably the most widely used product from the National Nutrition Monitoring System. Developed in 1977 using data from the National Health Surveys, the NHANES I, and the Fels Institute, the growth curves are charts used to assess the stature and weight attainment of children from birth to 18 years. The charts showing percentile levels of stature and weight in relation to age are used widely by physicians and other health care professionals to assess growth and nutritional status.

Evaluate Interrelationships

The interrelationships among diet, nutritional status, demographic factors, environmental factors, and health can be studied using survey data. For example, data from NHANES I and NHANES II were analyzed to determine whether low dietary calcium intake was associated with hypertension.[34–38] These articles and the published correspondence[39,40] are particularly helpful to understanding the importance of sample weights, design effects, and the appropriate statistical software when performing hypothesis testing.

Monitoring Trends

Trends in the prevalence of anemia among low-income children in the United States[17] have been analyzed using pediatric nutrition surveillance data. In six states that participated consistently in the system from 1975 to 1985, a steady decline was found in the prevalence of anemia from 7.8% to 2.9%. A significant decline was found among both children seen at the screening visit and those seen at the follow-up visit, suggesting a generalized improvement in childhood iron nutrition status in the United States.

Etiology and Natural History of Disease

When longitudinal follow-up of survey participants is performed, the opportunity arises to study the etiology and natural history of disease. Studies of the association of diet with later disease experience are possible with data from the NHANES I Epidemiologic Follow-up Study. For example, the relationship between dietary fat intake and development of breast cancer ten years later was examined.[41] Using the 24-hour recall data collected in the original survey and information on breast cancer history obtained in follow-up interviews, no significant differences were found in dietary fat intake between breast cancer cases and non-cases. The findings from this prospective study do not support the hypothesis that high fat diets increase breast cancer risk.

HOW TO GET STARTED

Several resources exist for the person who wants to begin analyzing data from the National Nutrition Monitoring System. The *Directory of Federal Nutrition Monitoring Activities*[2] is an excellent place to start. For each of the nutrition surveys and surveillance activities conducted by the Federal Government, it provides a description of the purpose, target population, design, measures and control variables, as well as information on how to order data tapes and a contact person at the agency. In addition to the written references listed in this article, the agencies that collect the data often hold conferences or workshops to help acquaint researchers with the methods and resources available to them.

CONCLUSION

This chapter provides an introduction to the analysis of some representative surveys and surveillance activities conducted under the National Nutrition Monitoring System. The complexities and problems associated with the analysis of these data were discussed to assist those who want to begin such analyses, but the information is also useful to help understand the limitations of survey data and to evaluate publications using the data.

Care must be taken when analyzing the data, both from a statistical standpoint and an interpretive one. The data are largely cross-sectional in nature, and therefore it is difficult to relate nutritional measures, such as current dietary intakes to risk factors of diseases incurred over a long and/or earlier period. Frequently, the surveys lack the full complement of measures needed to evaluate a relationship of diet or nutritional status to health.

These data systems are important for policy decisions, and offer powerful research opportunities. The data have been used to evaluate nutrient fortification for the national food supply, design and evaluate food programs and nutrition education initiatives, develop growth charts that are used worldwide, design and target the National Cholesterol Education Program, and develop criteria for anemia for use in the CDC surveillance programs. Literally hundreds of analytical articles have appeared in refereed journals in the past 15 years that have relied on the survey and surveillance data.

References

1. Woteki CE, Fanelli-Kuczmarski MT. The National Nutrition Monitoring System. In: Brown ML, ed. *Present Knowledge in Nutrition*. 6th ed. Washington, DC: International Life Sciences Institute Nutrition Foundation; 1990: 415–429.
2. Interagency Committee on Nutrition Monitoring. *Nutrition Monitoring in the United States—The Directory of Federal Nutrition Monitoring Activities*. Washington, DC: Public Health Service, US Government Printing Office; 1989. DHHS publication PHS 89-1255-1.
3. Life Sciences Research Office, Federation of American Societies for Experimental Biology. *Nutrition Monitoring in the United States—An Update Report on Nutrition Monitoring*. Washington, DC: Public Health Service, US Government Printing Office; 1989. DHHS publication PHS 89-1255.
4. Woteki CE, Briefel RR, Kuczmarski R. Contributions of the National Center for Health Statistics. *Am J Clin Nutr.* 1988;47:320–328.
5. Peterkin BB, Rizek RL, Tippett KS. Nationwide Food Consumption Survey, 1987. *Nutr Today.* 1988;23:18–24.

6. Dwyer JT. Assessment of dietary intake. In: Shils ME, Young VR, eds. *Modern Nutrition in Health and Disease*. 7th ed. Philadelphia, Pa: Lea and Febiger; 1988:887–905.

7. Willett W. *Nutritional Epidemiology*. New York, NY: Oxford University Press; 1990.

8. Centers for Disease Control. *Nutrition Surveillance: Annual Summary 1983*. Atlanta, Ga: Centers for Disease Control; 1985. DHHS publication CDC 85-8295.

9. Division of Nutrition, National Center for Chronic Disease Prevention and Health Promotion. *Pediatric Nutrition Surveillance 1987, 1988 and 1989 Annual Summaries and Graphics*. Atlanta, Ga: Centers for Disease Control; unpublished.

10. Division of Nutrition, National Center for Chronic Disease Prevention and Health Promotion. *Pregnancy Nutrition Surveillance 1987 and 1988 Annual Summaries and Graphics*. Atlanta, Ga: Centers for Disease Control; unpublished.

11. Division of Nutrition, National Center for Chronic Disease Prevention and Health Promotion. *Enhanced Pregnancy Nutrition Surveillance System User's Manual*. Atlanta, Ga: Centers for Disease Control; unpublished.

12. Fichtner RR, Simmons JC, Zyrkowski CL, et al. *Monitoring Trends in Pregnancy Risks and Outcomes: The CDC Pregnancy Nutrition Surveillance System, Proceedings of the 1989 Public Health Conference on Records and Statistics*. Washington, DC: Government Printing Office: 1989. NCHS, CDC, PHS, USDHHS publication PHS 90-1214.

13. Gayle HD, Dibley MJ, Marks JS, Trowbridge FL. Malnutrition in the first two years of life. *Am J Dis Child*. 1987;141:531–534.

14. Peck RE, Marks JS, Dibley MJ, Lee S, Trowbridge FL. Birthweight and subsequent growth among Navajo children. *Public Health Rep*. 1987;102:500–507.

15. Anemia during pregnancy in low-income women—United States, 1987. *MMWR*. 1990;39:73–76,81.

16. Larsen CE, Serdula MK, Sullivan KM. Macrosomia: influence of maternal overweight among a low-income population. *Am J Obstet Gynecol*. 1990;162:490–494.

17. Yip R, Binkin NJ, Fleshood L, Trowbridge FL. Declining prevalence of anemia among low income children in the United States. *JAMA*. 1987;258:1619–1623.

18. Wong FL. Effective application and utilization of data available for program management. In: *Demystifying Data: Data Use in State and Local Public Health Nutrition Programs Measuring Achievement of the 1990 Health Promotion/Disease Prevention Objectives for the Nation*. Proceedings from the Conference of State and Territorial Public Health Nutrition Directors, May 21–24, 1985.

19. Trowbridge FL, Wong FL, Byers TE, Serdula MK. Methodological issues in nutrition surveillance. *J Nutr*. 1990;120:11s.

20. Gayle HD, Yip R, Frank MJ, Nieburg P, Binkin NJ. Validation of maternally reported birthweights among 46,637 Tennessee WIC Program participants. *Public Health Rep*. 1988;103:143.

21. Remington PL, Smith MY, Williamson DF, Anda RF, Gentry EM, Hogelin GC. Design, characteristics and usefulness of state-based behavioral risk factor surveillance: 1981–1987. *Public Health Rep*. 1988;103:336–375.

22. Office of Surveillance and Analysis, National Center for Chronic Disease Prevention and Health Promotion. *Behavioral Risk Factor Surveillance System (BRFSS) Operations Manual* (1989). Atlanta, Ga: Centers for Disease Control; unpublished.

23. Office of Surveillance and Analysis, National Center for Chronic Disease Prevention and Health Promotion. *1990 Behavioral Risk Factor Questionnaire and Optional Modules*. Atlanta, Ga: Centers for Disease Control; unpublished.

24. Office of Surveillance and Analysis, National Center for Chronic Disease Prevention and Health Promotion. *1989 Behavioral Risk Factor Questionnaire and Optional Modules*. Atlanta, Ga: Centers for Disease Control; unpublished.

25. *Chronic Disease and Health Promotion: Reprints from the MMWR 1985–1989. Vol 3: Behavioral Risk Factor Surveillance System*. Atlanta, Ga: Centers for Disease Control; 1990.

26. Weight-loss regimens among overweight adults—behavioral risk factor surveillance system, 1987. *MMWR*. 1989;38:519–520, 525–528.

27. State-specific changes in cholesterol screening and awareness—United States, 1987–1988. *MMWR*. 1990;39:304–305, 311–314.

28. Factors related to cholesterol screening and cholesterol level awareness—United States, 1989. *MMWR*. 1990;39:633–637.

29. Yetley E, Johnson C. Nutritional applications of the Health and Nutrition Examination Surveys (HANES). *Annu Rev Nutr.* 1987;7:441–463.
30. Forthofer RN. Investigation of nonresponse bias in NHANES II. *Am J Epidemiol.* 1983;117:507–515.
31. Landis JR, Lepkowski JM, Eklund SA, Stehouwer SA. *A Statistical Methodology for Analyzing Data from a Complex Survey: The First National Health and Nutrition Examination Survey.* Washington, DC: US Government Printing Office; 1982. DHHS publication 82-1366. Vital and Health Statistics series 2 no. 92.
32. Sempos C, Fulwood R, Haines C, et al. The prevalence of high blood cholesterol levels among adults in the United States. *JAMA.* 1989;262:45–52.
33. Hamill PVV, Drizd TA, Johnson CL, Reed RB, Roche AF. *NCHS Growth Curves for Children.* Washington, DC: US Government Printing Office; 1977. DHEW publication PHS 78-1650. Vital and Health Statistics series 11 no. 165.
34. Sempos C, Cooper R, Kovar MG, Johnson C, Drizd T, Yetley E. Dietary calcium and blood pressure in National Health and Nutrition Examination Surveys I and II. *Hypertension.* 1986;8:1067–1074.
35. McCarron DA, Morris CD, Henry HJ, Stanton JL. Blood pressure and nutrient intake in the United States. *Science.* 1984;224:1392–1398.
36. Harlan WR, Hull AL, Schmouder RL, Landis JR, Thompson FE, Larkin FA. Blood pressure and nutrition in adults. The National Health and Nutrition Examination Survey. *Am J Epidemiol.* 1984;120:17–28.
37. Harlan WR, Hull AL, Schmouder RL, Landis JR, Larkin FA, Thompson FE. High blood pressure in older Americans: the First National Health and Nutrition Examination Survey. *Hypertension.* 1984;6:802–809.
38. Gruchow HW, Sobocinski KA, Barboriak JJ. Alcohol, nutrient intake, and hypertension in U.S. adults. *JAMA.* 1985;253:1567–1570.
39. Morris C, McCarron DA. Dietary calcium intake in hypertension. *Hypertension.* 1987;10:350–352.
40. Sempos CT, Johnson C, Kovar MG, Cooper R, Yetley EA. Dietary calcium intake in hypertension: author's response. *Hypertension.* 1987;10:352–353.
41. Jones DY, Schatzkin A, Green SB, et al. Dietary fat and breast cancer in the National Health and Nutrition Examination Survey I epidemiologic follow-up study. *JNCI.* 1987;79:465–471.

13. SENSORY EVALUATION METHODS IN NUTRITION AND DIETETICS RESEARCH

David J. Mela, PhD

The nutrition and dietetics literature makes frequent reference to the importance of sensory perceptions in the selection and appreciation of foods, and it is commonly noted that unappealing foods or disorders of the chemical senses may impact upon nutritional status. However, whereas training in the field of nutrition usually includes some discussion of the physiology of taste and smell, sensory evaluation is a hybrid of physiology, psychology, and nutrition in which few dietitians are likely to have received formal instruction.

Sensory evaluation research methods fall into two broad, often overlapping, categories: those intended primarily to assess the sensory properties of selected foods, and those intended to evaluate individual sensory capabilities or preferences. These are often quite different matters, with correspondingly different scientific and methodologic considerations. Studies of the sensory properties of foods or food constituents have been largely the domain of food scientists and industrial product developers. These methods use human sensory panels as instruments to assess the properties of foods, discern and characterize differences among formulations, and to select appropriate ingredient mixes and processes to optimize sales or profit margins. In contrast, the sensory physiology and perceptions of individuals are of greater interest to clinicians and biomedical researchers, and they are the primary focus of the discussion that follows. This research is largely concerned with understanding the function and capacity of the senses, their role in food selection and quality of life, and identifying differences between individuals and groups with relevance to clinical or nutrition issues.

The intent of the chapter is to introduce some background concepts with regard to the chemical senses, and to offer some practical considerations and general guidelines for selection and conduct of common sensory evaluation methods in humans. No attempt has been made to create an exhaustive compendium of all methods used in the field of sensory evaluation or to discuss all of the specific procedures involved in conducting and analyzing the procedures described. Such an effort would (and does) fill volumes. Descriptions of specific issues and methods are accompanied by relevant references, and the interested reader is strongly advised to consult these original sources or one of the many excellent texts listed in the appendix.

PHYSIOLOGY AND FUNCTION OF THE CHEMICAL SENSES

Much of the fundamental knowledge of the physiology of the chemical senses is derived from research on animals, and there is a large volume of experimental animal work relating sensory processes and nutrition. However, in discussing the use and applications of sensory methodology, this chapter will focus exclusively on research with humans.

Human perceptions of "flavor" in foods are largely derived from combinations of sensations mediated via the gustatory, olfactory, and trigeminal systems. These systems are briefly characterized in *Table 13.1*.

Gustation (Taste)

The gustatory system responds only to selected water-soluble compounds (*tastants*) in the oral cavity. Taste sensations are derived from signals transduced from interactions of these compounds with specific receptors or channels in specialized epithelial cells. Like other epithelial tissues of the alimentary tract, these cells have a half-life of about 8 to 12 days and are susceptible to deterioration in association with several specific nutrient deficiencies. Clusters of these receptor cells with support tissues make up the *taste buds*, which are predominantly located in the visible papillae of the tongue.

Table 13.1
Sensory Systems Involved in
Flavor Perception

Sensory System	Sensations Mediated
Gustatory	Taste: sweet, sour, salty, bitter, others? ("umami"?)
Olfactory	Odor: unlimited number?
Trigeminal	Tactile, thermal, pain/irritation

Modified from Mela DJ, Mattes RD.[128] ©Williams and Wilkins, 1988, with permission from the publisher.

There are three distinct morphologic types of gustatory papillae. The fungiform papillae populate the anterior portions of the tongue; foliate papillae occupy slits along the posterior lateral edges of the tongue; and 8 to 12 large circumvallate papillae are located in a groove at the posterior base of the tongue. These different types of papillae vary markedly in taste bud density. While there is an average total of about 9000 taste buds on the human tongue, wide interindividual variation is observed in their number and regional distribution.[1] Functional taste buds also may be found in small numbers on the soft palate and elsewhere in the oral cavity.[2,3] Associations between the taste bud density and gustatory function of individual humans have often been hypothesized, but differences in sensory response—specifically, lower taste intensity ratings among people with fewer taste buds—has only recently been demonstrated.[4]

The predominant view is that taste is limited to mixtures of four basic qualities: sweet, sour, salty, and bitter. However, other schemes have been proposed, and the issue is not fully resolved.[5] The savory qualities of monosodium glutamate and ribonucleotides are accepted as a fifth basic taste (termed *umami*) in Japanese science and culture. There are also suggestions that the "basic" tastes may merely be easily recognized points in a continuum, or the result of limitations in semantics or cultural exposure. The lingering nature of this disagreement may stem in part from the lack of clear understanding of the biochemical mechanisms of taste; however, recent work has generated greater scientific consensus in this area.[6–8]

It is frequently stated that different tastes are perceived solely or most intensely in certain regions of the tongue; eg, sweet and salty at the front, sour on the posterior lateral edges, and bitter at the back. However, this common notion is at best an oversimplification. Most taste buds, regardless of location, appear to be receptive to multiple taste qualities and most areas of the tongue can sense all taste qualities over a wide range of concentrations.[9-11] Although it does appear that certain regions may be more sensitive to detecting or recognizing very low concentrations of particular tastes, the same or another region may be more responsive to high concentrations of the same taste.[10,12] The reasons for this are briefly described by Bartoshuk.[13]

Olfaction (Smell)

While the gustatory system appears limited to the detection of only a small number of discrete qualities, there is no apparent limit to the number of unique odors that can be discerned. Furthermore, despite numerous attempts to organize the world of odors into a limited set of categories,[14] no single odor classification scheme has ever received general endorsement. It is almost axiomatic that humans describe odors by their specific source (eg, "mold," "rose," "vomit") and the ability to do so forms the basis of many common tests of olfactory function.

Odors are elicited by small, volatile compounds that flow through the nose with inhaled and exhaled air. Although it seems obvious upon reflection, it is not commonly appreciated that the volatile flavors of foods and beverages in the mouth are largely perceived retronasally; ie, during the outward flow of odorous compounds through the nasal passageways upon exhalation. Interactions with saliva, changes in temperature, and differences in air flow all may cause food aromas to smell different when the food is actually in the mouth or swallowed than when it is sniffed.

Small patches of olfactory epithelium are found in the roof of the nasal cavity, just under the brain. Several lines of evidence indicate that the initial response to odorants occurs on the cilia projecting from receptor cells located in this region.[15] These cells are unique among neurons in that they maintain the capacity to regenerate continuously.

Recent work has begun to shed some light on the molecular events of olfaction. Theories relating structure to activity and hypothesized receptors or channels can explain some of the differences and similarities of tastants (though such schemes have shown only marginal predictive power), but schemes for categorizing or predicting the quality of odorants are less well developed.[16] The question of whether the recognition mechanism employs a galaxy of different and highly specific sites or a smaller range of more broadly tuned regions has not been resolved. It has been noted that many features of the olfactory system recognition of odorants have parallels in the immune system recognition of antigens.[16,17] Studies of individual receptor cells have found that most cells responded to many odorants, but none responded to all tested odorants, and no two cells responded identically to any subset of odorants.[18] A number of possible olfactory detection, recognition, and transduction mechanisms may be considered.[7,15,17,19]

Taste and Smell Independence and Interactions

The preceding discussion should make it abundantly clear that the peripheral taste and smell systems are completely separate and distinct in anatomy and physiology, as well as in the sensations they mediate. Nevertheless, confusions regarding the meaning and function of *taste* and *smell* are frequent, even in the scientific literature. Although the word *taste* is commonly equated with *flavor* in colloquial speech, the former technically describes only the sensations

Key Techniques

derived from the limited repertoire of the gustatory system. However, it is clearly in their volatile flavors (aroma) that many individual foods may be recognized as unique.

The different contributions of taste and smell to flavor, as well as the critical role of aroma in distinguishing foods, is easily demonstrated. With the nose pinched shut, the flavors of chicken and beef broths (or patés) may be virtually indistinguishable. Their tastes (salty and umami) are nearly identical; it is their odors that differ. Similar illustrations could be made using carbonated or fruit-flavored beverages or food purees. Pinching the nose largely stops the flow of air carrying the unique volatile flavors of foods from the oral cavity to the olfactory receptor areas. It is for this reason that, although people with colds commonly complain of a loss of taste, it is in fact their ability to smell that has been temporarily lost; the sense of taste is usually unaffected. Indeed, many, if not most, patients undergoing clinical evaluation for self-reported loss of taste and smell are diagnosed as having only loss of smell.[20]

The presence and absence of tactile experience associated with gustatory and olfactory chemoreception may largely explain the natural inclination to refer sensations of food-related aromas incorrectly to the mouth. Nothing solid contacts the olfactory epithelium, and no sensation would indicate the actual site of origin of odor sensations. But people do feel foods in the mouth, thus there appears to be a strong inclination to conclude that many odor sensations emanating from food in the mouth are partially or totally taste.[21,22] However, it is apparent that some of the associations between odor and taste are learned; hence strawberry, but not peanut butter, aromas enhance the perception of sweetness.[23]

Trigeminal System (Common Chemical Sense) and Texture Perception

Free nerve endings of the trigeminal nerve terminating close to the epithelial surfaces of the lips and oral and nasal cavities mediate tactile, thermal, nociceptive (pain) and proprioceptive (muscle/joint position) sensations.[24] While often confused with taste or smell, experiences such as the "burn" from hot peppers and ethanol, "cooling" from menthol and wintergreen, and irritation from ammonia and other vapors are, in fact, primarily mediated through this anatomically distinct sensory system. The onset, duration, and intensity of oral and nasal trigeminal stimulation may vary substantially with the source. Potency of many chemical trigeminal stimulants appears to be closely related to lipid solubility, perhaps reflecting the necessity to cross through the surface epithelial tissues to stimulate nerve endings below.[25]

Many, if not most, common odor materials combine their olfactory quality with some trigeminal stimulation, particularly at high concentrations.[26] Because many compounds that stimulate the trigeminal system also possess a distinct taste or odor quality, this adds to their perceived sensory characteristics. It is well known that people who have lost their sense of taste or smell can distinguish the presence (though not the identity) of many compounds because of their ability to stimulate the intact trigeminal system.

Although texture perception does not necessarily require a true chemical sense, it is typically discussed in the same context. The physiological basis of oral texture perception is complex and poorly understood. Free nerve endings constituting branches primarily of the trigeminal nerve sense the presence of food within the mouth and many qualities that may be attributed to the food surface. Mechanoreceptors sense the orientation and movement of food,[27] while Pacinian-type corpuscles convey sensitivity to roughness of the food surface as it crosses the oral surfaces.[28] Pain receptors may be triggered by particularly spiked surfaces or jagged edges of food fragments.

The tactile senses also discriminate between liquid and solid matter in the mouth, although the process by which lipid and aqueous material are differentiated is poorly understood. The particular melting or lubricating properties of fats may contribute to characterization of these fluid phases, while flavor appears to be less important.[29,30]

Textural qualities arising from the internal structure of the food are perceived by applying force, ie, with the tongue and palate, or the teeth. Sensory feedback from the muscle spindles transmit information about the forces applied, while touch and pressure receptors in the periodontium or palate detect the reactive forces from the food.[31] The changes in directional forces during the closing and opening of the jaw largely determine the textural qualities typically designated as hardness and toughness (elasticity, plasticity), fracturability (brittleness, crispness, crunchiness), and, to some extent, stickiness. Vibrations set up in the bony structures of the face by sudden changes in these forces convey sensations of fracture characteristics, while transmission of these vibrations to the inner ear provide auditory information augmenting that from the periodontium.[32]

Information on the relative position of the mandible and maxilla on contacting resistance from the food is interpreted to deduce the size of the food bolus or of particulate matter within it. This is likely of importance in determining grittiness, lumpiness, and similar characteristics.

An abundance of technology and machinery is available for measuring textural properties of food material such as viscosity, hardness, brittleness, elasticity, and particle size. Analysis of such properties has proved useful in monitoring product specifications, though the analytical procedures tend to be highly specific for a particular product or manufacturer. Attempts to correlate these measurements with consumer assessment of the corresponding food characteristics have met with limited success.[33] Poor correlations may be due to the use of force and speed parameters that are not within the physiological range for the textural attribute under study. However, the complexity of the sensory information on which food texture is judged renders measurement of texture by analytical means an extremely difficult problem, even if physiologically relevant parameters are included. The variations inherent between individuals in their awareness and sensitivity of any one sensation are compounded by the use of multiple sensory channels in texture assessment.

ASSESSMENT OF SENSORY PERCEPTIONS

Specific Test Measures and Methods

There is an abundance of methods for accessing information on individual sensory function or preferences, and they generally fall into one of the categories described in *Table 13.2*. Investigators new to this field will find an array of variations in the specific details and recommendations for each method as practiced by investigators at different sites. It must be recognized that many of the oft-repeated beliefs about methodologic particulars, though stated as firm convictions, may well lack any supporting proof. In essentially all sensory evaluation methods, samples under evaluation are presented in random order and the subject is blind as to their specific nature or source. However, other methodologic considerations, such as the appropriate size and number of stimuli, length and timing of sniffs or tastes, duration of test sessions, and specific rinse procedures commonly are chosen without clearly documented advantage.

Table 13.2
Common Measures in Sensory
Evaluation

Threshold	A measure of absolute sensitivity; the lowest detectable or recognizable concentration of a stimulus in a given medium
Perceived intensity	A measure of relative strengths of sensations; the relationship between physical concentration and perceived intensity of a stimulus at levels above the threshold range
Identification/recognition	A measure of the ability to associate stimuli with a commonly accepted descriptor, such as their usual or natural source; used most often for olfaction
Hedonic (preference)	A measure of the relative or absolute preference for or acceptability of a stimulus

Modified from Mela DJ, Mattes RD.[128] ©Williams and Wilkins, 1988, with permission from the publisher.

Many of the procedures described here are, in theory, equally suitable for testing taste or smell. The mode of presentation will, of course, vary between these two modalities, and a brief discussion of these issues can be found in the section on Test Stimuli.

Finally, it should be said that these procedures are largely intended and validated for use with intelligent adults. Infants and young children would require the use of specialized age-appropriate methods. Similarly, most of the procedures described herein would require modifications to ensure their validity in subjects exhibiting memory loss, dementia, or other specific mental disabilities.

Thresholds (sensitivity). Thresholds are a measure of the lower limit of ability to detect the presence of a stimulus (detection threshold) or to identify correctly its quality (recognition threshold). In effect, thresholds are a statistical phenomenon; they are an indication of the level of stimulus an individual can detect or correctly identify 50% (or other specified percentage) of the time, under particular test conditions. Bartoshuk[13] presents an excellent discussion of the practical aspects of threshold procedures, and additional methodologic details can be found in that paper and other sources.[14, 34–36]

Stimuli for classical threshold testing are almost always solutions of a single stimulus in a neutral vehicle: usually tastants in deionized water or odorants in high-quality mineral oil. In some situations it may be of interest to determine thresholds (eg, for an off-flavor or taint) in a real food product, in which case the food or other complex matrix may serve as the vehicle.

The determination of thresholds is generally time-consuming and labor-intensive and requires that the investigator begin with or gain some prior knowledge of the approximate range of threshold values likely to be encountered. Typical values for a large number of compounds in various media can be obtained from the *Compilation of Odor and Taste Threshold Values Data.*[37] Within a normal population, the range of threshold values may be quite large; it is not uncommon to observe tenfold or greater variation in thresholds for certain stimuli, particularly odorants,[38] and wider ranges may be expected if a clinical or nonhomogeneous population is examined. The actual threshold assessment procedures require preparation of a large number of stimulus solutions to span the limits of this range. For most purposes, half-log concentration steps are sufficiently spaced, as well as convenient to prepare, since they can be made by serial half dilutions of a starting stock. Thus, to determine taste recognition thresholds for sucrose, in which the anticipated median is about 1×10^{-2} mol/L, the stimuli typically would descend by half dilutions from 1.0×10^{-1} mol/L to 4.88×10^{-5} mol/L (ie, 12 steps).

There are numerous variations on several basic techniques for determination of thresholds. As practiced today, most require subjects to make a "forced choice"; ie, verbal responses of "don't know" or "not sure" are not allowed. This is largely because levels of stimuli near threshold almost always generate some level of indecision; hence there is a need to eliminate responder bias, in which subjects may differ not only in their thresholds, but also in their criteria for committing themselves to a judgment. For recognition threshold testing, it is also important to ensure that subjects are sufficiently familiar with the terminology for naming the taste or the odor qualities of interest. Misapplication of taste names, and confusion of "sour" and "bitter" in particular, has been documented,[39] and could lead to artifactually high recognition threshold values.

A common set of procedures used in threshold determination are exemplified by the "staircase" methods described by Cornsweet.[40] The basic approach in these types of tests is to present repeatedly single samples of stimuli (for recognition thresholds) or pairs of stimuli (one sample of stimulus, one sample of vehicle, for detection thresholds) at concentrations near threshold. The task is to identify the quality of the sample (recognition) or determine which sample in a pair contains the stimulus (detection). The concentration presented is decreased or increased following "reversal points," concentrations at which the subject's response changes from incorrect to correct (resulting in presentation of weaker solutions) or from correct to incorrect (resulting in presentation of stronger solutions). The mean (geometric mean for log-spaced stimuli) of reversal points from an equal number of ascending and descending series (typically three of each) is taken as the threshold. The practical deployment of this method for determination of taste recognition thresholds has been described by various authors.[10, 41–43]

In the detection threshold method of Harris and Kalmus,[44] subjects are given, simultaneously and in random arrangement, four cups containing a given concentration of tastant and four cups of the solvent (eg, deionized water). The task is to separate the cups into the tastant and water groups. From a very low starting point, the tastant concentration ascends until the task is accomplished, and this is taken as the threshold.

The method described by Stevens and associates[38] for olfactory detection threshold testing is also typical of many procedures. In this case, subjects are presented with two bottles, one odor-containing and one vehicle. The task is to identify which bottle contains the odorant. Five successive presentations of the pair are made at each concentration, starting at the lowest level and ascending. Threshold is determined as the lowest concentration at which correct responses are given to all five pairs at that and the next highest concentration.

Numerous variations and combinations of these types of methods have been employed by different investigators. The choice of one procedure over another often appears simply to reflect the personal preferences of the investigator, though more valid reasons to use certain methods may exist. There is little question that identical methods should be used if it is important to relate results, in an absolute sense, to previous studies. If there are time constraints, procedures such as that of Harris and Kalmus[44] are more rapid than the up-down staircase methods, and other rapid procedures have been proposed.[45] In most cases, the task is relatively easy for subjects to understand, though some methods may be seen as simpler. If the focus of the research is on classification or clinical evaluation of individuals (as opposed to group comparisons), then procedures with stricter measurement criteria and lower levels of chance results may be preferred. For example, in the Harris-Kalmus method,[44] the probability of selecting out four of the eight samples correctly by chance is 1 in 1680. In the method of Stevens and colleagues,[38] the chance of correctly guessing ten pairs correctly is 1 in 1024. These are both rigorous criteria, although the tests may be biased by the fact that thresholds are determined only in an ascending sequence. A change in the criteria (eg, to increase the speed) of any procedure will affect its accuracy and reliability.

Perhaps because they appear as single values in common physical units, threshold measures are often incorrectly assumed to be absolute physiologic measures. When properly performed, they can be fairly reliable;[42] however, they are also highly sensitive to the actual testing methodology. For example, small differences in the number of stimuli rated, test media, or rinse procedures between testings can lead to differing outcomes; thus, comparisons between values from different laboratories must be made cautiously. The tests are also highly subject to unintentional bias and may be influenced by many environmental as well as physiologic variables.

Great caution must be exercised in the use and interpretation of threshold measures by themselves in nutrition and dietetics research. Threshold values for specific taste stimuli appear unrelated to responses to other measures of gustatory function,[41] although odor detection thresholds have been found to be positively correlated with tests of odor recognition.[46–48] Nevertheless, subjects with isolated decrements in threshold sensitivity generally do not report a consistent feeling of loss of chemosensory function, and links between threshold measures and food selection or dietary intake are likely to be tenuous at best. Because real foods contain a variety of chemosensory stimuli at levels well above threshold and in a complex matrix, the measure of sensitivity to one or more compounds in a simple vehicle is, by itself, unlikely to be of great relevance.

Despite these liabilities, there are appropriate uses for threshold measures in assessing sensory function. They are typically among the most sensitive indices of the functionality of sensory systems, and they may be more responsive than other measures to the initial stages or moderate levels of nutrient deficits or other disease processes, including pathologies of iatrogenic origin. For food processors, knowledge of average threshold values may be used in quality control, in that the level of human sensitivity to common desirable or undesirable flavor compounds may provide guidelines against which product formulation and processing procedures may be assessed. However, for most research purposes, threshold procedures are best combined with other measures or avoided, unless there is a good theoretical reason to employ them.

Perceived Intensity. Threshold testing tells the experimentor something about sensitivity to stimuli, but nothing about the strength of the sensation they evoke. The most salient sensory responses in everyday experience result from perception of concentrations of stimuli at suprathreshold (greater than threshold) levels. Distortion or loss of chemosensory function in this range commonly affects normal perceptions of foods, and therefore it may be well argued that suprathreshold distortion or loss should be a focus of interest in nutrition-related sensory research. Sensory testing at this level generally involves an assessment of the relationships between stimulus concentration and perceived intensity.

As with threshold testing, stimuli may consist of simple solutions of a single compound in a neutral vehicle; however, real food products can also serve as a suitable matrix. The stimulus range and spacing depends on the nature of the research. In most clinical studies, stimuli are typically prepared in half-log steps, by serial half-dilution. However, they could also be spaced by a constant percentage of the stimulus material. The critical considerations are that the concentration steps are spaced evenly and equally across the range of interest. The effects of context and stimulus range can be severe, and the reader is advised to consult the literature, where excellent discussions of these points are presented.[49-51]

There has been considerable discussion within the sensory evaluation literature regarding the appropriate methods for measurement and analysis of perceived intensity, and different procedures retain their avid proponents. The lack of consensus stems from the fundamental difficulty (or, perhaps, impossibility) of quantifying human sensations. The theoretical considerations include both the underlying psychophysical "laws" that relate stimulus to sensation and the types of scales used to access this relationship. These issues are beyond the scope of the present discussion, but do bear upon it. Investigators entering this field may wish to gain a general background from the literature.[52-57] Practical information on measurement of perceived intensity is available in most references on sensory evaluation, but the reader is advised to begin by consulting some suggested sources.[14,35,36,58-60]

For many sensory systems, the relationship between sensory intensity and stimulus concentration is perhaps best modelled as a power function of the form:

(Equation 1) $$I = kC^{\beta}$$

where I is perceived intensity, k is a proportionality constant, C is physical concentration, and β is an exponent characteristic of the stimulus, subject population, and test conditions. If one takes the log of both sides of the power function, the result is:

(Equation 2) $$\log I = \log k + \beta(\log C)$$

which describes a straight line of slope β when the log of the perceived intensity (log I) is plotted against the log of the stimulus concentrations (log C), as in *Figure 13.1.*

The approximate range of values of β are generally a function of the stimuli tested. When β is greater than 1, perceived intensity more than doubles with a doubling of physical stimulus concentration. This is a property shared by many painful stimuli, eg, electric shocks. The value of β is generally found to be

Figure 13.1
Three different patterns of abnormal sensory response. A, a relatively constant decrement in perceived intensity at all concentrations; B, an elevated threshold with normal perceived intensity; and C, a change in the stimulus-intensity relationship reflected as relative decrement in perceived intensity at higher concentrations. Modified from Bartoshuk LM, Gent J, Catalanotto FA, Goodspeed RB.[61]

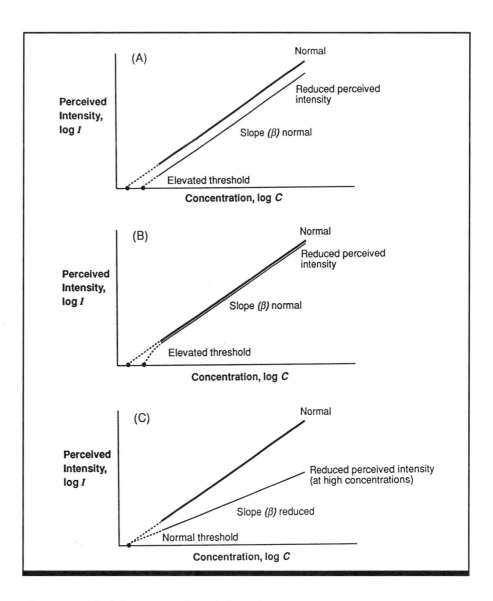

close to or slightly greater than 1 for substances such as sucrose and NaCl. When β is less than 1, perceived intensity increases at a rate proportionally lower than the increases in physical stimulus concentrations. This tends to be the case for many bitter and sour tastants and for most odorants. Both k and β may be of interest from a clinical standpoint, and are not necessarily related to each other or to thresholds (see Figure 13.1). A change in perceived intensity at all concentrations would be reflected by a difference in the value of k (see Figure 13.1, A). Relative changes in perception of intensity at the high or low range, or the general characteristics of the stimulus-intensity relationship are reflected by changes in β (see Figure 13.1, C).

Magnitude estimation. Determination of β for any stimulus, or differences in perceived intensity (k and β) among individuals or groups typically makes use of the method of magnitude estimation. Clear, practical guidance to the use of the method is given by Bartoshuk and Marks[62] and by Moskowitz.[58] In magnitude estimation, subjects basically assign their own numerical values to stimuli in proportion to the intensity of the sensation they perceive. For example, a stimulus perceived to be half as intense as one rated 16 would be assigned an intensity rating of 8. Compared with line or category scales, this type of scaling procedure has several theoretical and practical benefits. It avoids so-called end effects, in which the range of response is limited by the scale itself and by the common hesitancy to use extreme response categories. No assumptions must be made about the relationships between verbal descriptors, category spacing, and numerical assignment. Since the subject response is, in theory, on a ratio scale with a true zero and true proportionality, mathematical treatments and statistical handling of the data are facilitated. As noted above, transformation of the power function by taking the logarithm of both magnitude estimates and stimulus concentration generates a function in the form of equation 2. Magnitude estimation data are usually treated by such log-normalization,[63] which should enable them to meet the assumptions for classical linear regression and analysis of variance (ANOVA) hypothesis testing.

There is a large array of options for the collection and analysis of magnitude estimation data, and their use varies substantially between investigators. Some problems result from the inherent difficulty of the task. For the data in any test session to be valid, the subjects always must relate each sample to those that preceded it, and they must do so in a consistent manner. One means used to improve performance is the repeated presentation of a standard calibrating stimulus or modulus, to which each subject assigns an initial rating and compares all other samples. However, this may distort the shape and nature of the stimulus-response curve, particularly if the standard is not from the mid-range of intensity. Another major practical problem results from individual or group differences in absolute number usage, since the range and actual magnitude of the numbers are generally unrestricted. For example, subject A may rate all stimuli in the range of 1 to 12, while subject B may elect to use the range 20 to 300. From these numbers alone, the investigator cannot conclude that subject A and B differ in their perceptions of intensity. One method of controlling for this is the additional inclusion of a reference stimulus with an assigned intensity. However, forcing all responses onto an identical number range in this manner may not be at all appropriate, as it has the effect of making the constant k identical for all subjects. In addition, this may alter the responses of subjects for whom the value assigned to the reference and the resulting numerical range are felt to be intuitively inappropriate.

Numerous other inventive approaches to these problems in magnitude estimation have been employed by various investigators.[14] A prominent solution is the procedure of cross-modal matching.[64,65] This uses individual responses to a second sensory modality to normalize idiosyncrasies in number usage in the modality of interest (eg, ratings of loudness of tones used to normalize taste intensity ratings). While cross-modal matching is commonly used and theoretically correct, it can also be cumbersome and unsatisfying in actual practice.

A final issue that has never been fully resolved regards the handling of zeroes in magnitude estimation. By definition, 0 values, equivalent to "no sensation," should not occur in response to suprathreshold stimuli, but in reality 0 may be given as a response. The geometric mean is frequently identified as the preferred averaging method, and data are typically log-transformed and plotted on log-log axes. Neither of these procedures is suited to data containing nonpositive values. Some investigators prohibit subjects from assigning zeroes or remove them from analyses, whereas others may substitute an arbitrary, very low number or a value predicted for that individual by a regression equation using the ratings assigned to the higher stimulus concentrations. In the opinion of this author, prohibiting 0 ratings or arbitrarily assigning them low values would seem to sacrifice validity for efficiency. This particular difficulty is representative of the lack of consensus on general handling of magnitude estimation data, as described previously and by Lawless.[66] Nevertheless, it should be noted that if a particular experimental situation generates a large number of 0 ratings, then the stimulus concentration range simply could be extending too low for that subject population.

Compelling cases have been presented for and against the use of magnitude estimation procedures.[66-68] There can be many difficulties in using magnitude estimation, as noted, and many occasions when other techniques offer distinct advantages.

Category scaling. The most common alternative to magnitude estimation of intensity is some form of line (also called *visual analogue* or *graphic scaling*) or category scale. These scales are inherently easy to design and use, simple to explain, and require minimal data handling. However, these types of instruments have several theoretical problems. Categories are not equally spaced intervals, and they do not have the mathematical properties of ratio scales. The following nine-point scale can be used to illustrate these problems.

0 = none

1 = extremely weak

2 = weak

3 = weak to moderate

4 = moderate

5 = moderate to strong

6 = strong

7 = very strong

8 = extremely strong

It cannot be assumed that the one category distance between 1 ("extremely weak") and 2 ("weak") is perceptually equivalent to the distance between from 6 ("strong") to 7 ("very strong"). Indeed, research addressing this point shows that such distances are rarely equal. Also, a rating of "strong" (6) cannot be said to be twice the perceived intensity of "weak to moderate" (3). Line scales share similar limitations in mathematical properties and interpretation. End-effects are also a commonly mentioned criticism of these scales, describing subjects' reluctance to make responses near the upper and lower end points. Moskowitz,[14] and Riskey[51] present excellent discussions of these and other issues related to implementation of category and line scales. Despite the potential complications, it is common to enter this type of data directly into standard parametric statistical procedures, and this appears to be a satisfactory practice.

In terms of general results and response characteristics, several studies indicate that magnitude estimation and category scales are similar, though one method may have certain advantages in particular circumstances.[66,69-72] Giovanni and Pangborn[69] rightly conclude that no method can be proved superior without a clear external standard by which it can be judged. Nevertheless, the recent work of Lawless[66] and Lawless and Malone[71,72] provide evidence to support the growing number of investigators who have begun to reject the theoretical benefits of magnitude estimation in favor of the tangible advantages of category and line scales.

It is the opinion of this author that for many nutrition studies in which group comparisons are the focus, category and line scales are wholly suitable and easy to implement. However, in studies that require derivation of accurate (ie, absolute, externally valid) values of the power function variables, such as in clinical classification of individuals with regard to chemosensory function, magnitude estimation is clearly the standard method. Although semi-log transformation of category and line scales (ie, log C versus I) generally produces a linear response curve, the slopes are rarely accorded great importance. This fact may change, as it is not clear that the results are substantially different or less valid than those derived from the more elaborate magnitude estimation procedures. The practical differences between category and line scales themselves are not pronounced, provided the category scale has gradations which enable subjects to make sufficiently fine distinctions.

The appropriate use of different scaling procedures and corrections for the way in which subjects use scaling systems is critical to proper interpretation of data, particularly when contrasting the responses of individual subjects or groups with different demographic or psychological profiles. Even when category scales are used, it is advisable to assess ratings for an unrelated stimulus to ensure that no underlying bias in number or category usage exists.

The methods just described all consider intensity at a single time point after exposure. In reality, however, perceptions of chemosensory stimuli have a temporal component. That is, there is a time lag between exposure and sensation, a rise in intensity to some peak, and then a decay to extinction. The sequence may take only a few seconds or several minutes, depending upon the stimulus and sample matrix. A number of different methods for assessing time-intensity (T-I) responses have been used, and Lee and Pangborn[73] present an excellent discussion of these techniques and their applications. With increasing availability of computerized data collection and improved statistical methodology for analysis of T-I curves, use of this technique is likely to expand. In particular, the recent development of improved methods for averaging and comparing group curves[74] could stimulate exploitation of this technique in biomedical research.

Identification tests. Identification tests differ from threshold and suprathreshold assessments in that they are used to evaluate whether the quality or "meaning" of the sensation is normal. For the taste system, this problem may be identified subjectively, or by recognition threshold testing with compounds representative of the four basic taste categories. However, identification tests as such are not common in taste testing because of the limited number of possible response options. As previously noted, odors do not generalize into a small number of well-established descriptive classifications, and are most commonly described by the specific objects or conditions with which they are associated.

The unique, well-recognized odors of familiar objects and foods provide a basis for the use of odor recognition tasks as a common method to investigate olfactory function.[75-77] In these tests, subjects sniff familiar odors at fixed intensities and identify the common source of each from a provided list of possibilities. The presentation of such a list is critical to the validity of the procedure, as humans are notoriously poor at attaching the correct name to even very familiar odors without some sort of guidance, a common occurrence known as the "tip of the nose" phenomenon.[75] Without the list, the limiting factors in performance may be semantics and memory, rather than olfaction. A typical test might include such commonly recognized odors as gasoline, smoke, rose, coffee, lemon, and others common in food and the environment. In practice, with specific clinical populations such as the neurologically impaired, some type of control for memory loss and other generalized cognitive dysfunctions must accompany this procedure.

Odor recognition and threshold tests have been found to correlate well, with the former possibly superior in reliability and sensitivity.[46–48] In addition, different versions of recognition tests performed at different laboratories have been found to correlate extremely closely.[47,48,77] At least one of these tests, the University of Pennsylvania Smell Identification Test (UPSIT)[76] has come into widespread clinical use. This may be largely because it consists of a convenient, rapidly administered booklet of microencapsulated odors that is readily available in a commercial form. But the test is also supported by a very large database indicating its sensitivity and reliability in a variety of clinical populations. However, similar tests, such as that described by Cain and associates[46] are easily and inexpensively set up and conducted in a research setting, and share comparable, if less well-publicized performance attributes. Schiffman[78] described a test based on identification of blended real foods.

It appears that humans are poor at distinguishing the number or identity of individual components within simple mixtures containing more than two to three odors.[79,80] Whereas combinations of a pair of different but complex odors may sometimes be easily recognized as such (eg, fresh paint and grilled meat), other complex combinations may be perceived as a "single" odor (eg, walnut flavor is derived from at least 51 volatile compounds, none of which smell like walnut).[81] Perhaps complicating this further is the fact that the perceived quality of a single odorant may change with its intensity.[82]

Hedonic measures.   Hedonic measures access feelings of liking and disliking for chemosensory stimuli. While threshold sensitivity, perceived intensity, and recognition define, in many ways, the physiologic capabilities of chemosensory systems, exposure to chemosensory stimuli also introduces a powerful affective component. In contrast to the other measures, hedonic measures for selected stimuli are not generally used as specific indicators of chemosensory disorders (exceptions being when people experience a persistent unpleasant taste or smell, or when highly preferred foods consistently take on an undesirable flavor), but represent another dimension of sensory response.

Whereas the test stimuli for determining thresholds or intensity functions are usually purified substances (eg, a single tastant or odorant by itself in a neutral medium), stimuli for hedonic tests often (or should) include samples of real or modified foods varying in their content of one or more compounds of primary interest (eg, salt or pepper levels in soup) or in their method of processing. The goal in hedonic testing in nutrition-oriented research is usually to compare chemosensory or food preferences among individuals or populations, or to assess relationships to energy balance or nutrient utilization. This is considerably different from similar work in food processing, in which the objective is product optimization. However, in both cases, a number of independent indicators of relative or absolute preference could be employed. The following discussion focuses on laboratory sensory evaluation, but measures of "liking" could be derived from laboratory or home consumption trials, surveys of preference or preferred frequency of consumption of food items, habitual dietary intake, or combinations of these.

While the different approaches each offer certain advantages, laboratory hedonic testing can reveal: the shape of the relationship between concentration of a stimulus and preference, the stimulus concentration or sample most preferred, and the degree of liking of any given level of stimulus. These results then can be used to compare or categorize populations and to assess the effect of time or specific treatments on individual preferences.

The most common methods of assessing sensory preference in biomedical research are based on the nine-point hedonic category scale ("dislike extremely" to "like extremely") developed by Peryam and Pilgrim.[83] This scale, typically in its original form, is still extensively employed, and has been applied to simple solutions, real foods, and verbal descriptors of foods. A similar scale, also in common use and having some possible advantages, particularly for real food stimuli, is the nine-point Food Action Rating (FACT) scale ("I would eat this only if I were starving" to "I would eat this every opportunity I had").[84] Drewnowski and colleagues[85–87] have described an innovative application of the nine-point hedonic scale to more complex stimuli in biomedical research. In this approach, mixtures of two different components are evaluated on hedonic and intensity category scales, and responses are analyzed by a multivariate statistical technique (response surface method) to identify interactions and maxima for both intensity and hedonics.

If the intent of an experiment is to determine the most preferred level of a stimulus, it is important to ensure that that optimal point can be identified unambiguously. This means that the concentrations employed must span a range on both sides of the optimum, such that an inverted-U- (or inverted-V-) shaped curve with a clear peak is produced. If the resultant curve unimodally rises (or declines), a most preferred level really cannot be determined, although other types of comparisons are still possible. A practical problem with these nine-point scales is that individual responses often bear little resemblance to the mean. Even when group data may indeed generate an inverted-U curve and clear maxima, these procedures may fail to allow identification of the stimulus most preferred by individual subjects. It is not at all uncommon for individuals to generate monotonic, flat, or saddle-shaped (ie, lower in the middle than at the ends) curves. This individual variation can be turned to advantage if the investigator has a priori rules for classifying subjects into response categories. However, it can render procedures such as correlations with hedonic maxima impossible.

There are several alternatives to category scaling. "Relative-to-ideal" ratings combine intensity and hedonic ratings on an end-point and midpoint-anchored line scale. The task is for subjects to rate the intensity of a quality (eg, saltiness) from too low (eg, "not nearly salty enough") to too high (eg, "much too salty") with the midpoint identified as ideal (eg, "just right").[88] The advantage to this method is that the individual hedonic maxima are more easily identified, and the slope of the line can be used to examine individual sensitivity to deviations from ideal. Disadvantages to this method stem from the fact that it requires rating on a single, specific sensory attribute. It therefore may prove unsatisfactory when overall liking is a function of less distinct sensations or a more complex combination of attributes, particularly if their salience differs among subjects.

Ranking methods, in which subjects compare two or more stimuli and order them for preference, also may be used. These procedures have the advantage of allowing rapid and ostensibly unambiguous identification of a most preferred sample. However, they allow determination only of relative preference, not absolute liking, and the options for statistical hypothesis testing on this type of data are limited.

A final method, suitable for some compounds in liquid media, allows subjects to mix samples containing high and low concentrations of stimulus to generate the most preferred concentration, which is then analyzed by physical or chemical methods. A number of factors affecting performance of this task have been evaluated,[89] and the procedure described by Mattes and Mela[90] appears to produce an unbiased estimate of most preferred concentration for individual subjects. The method is rapid, conceptually simple, and reliable; however, it is only useful for a very limited number of types of materials, must be performed carefully to avoid bias, and generates only a single point measure of relative preference.

Hedonic measures bear closer associations with actual dietary intakes than assessments of sensory function.[91] Hence, several issues relevant to the role of hedonic evaluations in nutrition research warrant some mention here. First, as noted in the later section on Test Stimuli, preferences for a given level of a chemosensory stimulus in one medium (or food matrix) does not necessarily generalize to others. Second, it is clear that the types of sensory evaluation measures described here access only one dimension of food acceptance. Other laboratory tests, such as actual consumption, may reveal other information about acceptability that may or may not coincide with sensory testing.[92] Simple extrapolation from sensory data to food preferences or selection or overall dietary intake, without actually measuring these, must be viewed as inappropriate. Finally, Meiselman[93] and Schutz[94] argue for acceptance testing under more realistic conditions. Although laboratory testing situations allow a great deal of control, they also may restrict the expression of behaviors and affect exhibited in more common eating circumstances, leading to highly reliable, but invalid and irrelevant results.

A note on statistical treatment of data. Most of the sensory measures described above are commonly treated by classical parametric hypothesis testing (eg, t-tests, linear regression, and ANOVA). However, threshold and perceived intensity data typically deviate substantially from normality and may exhibit high interindividual variation and non-homogeneity of variance. Other procedures yield ordinal data. Parametric statistics are not the most powerful or appropriate method in such instances, and it is the author's belief that nonparametric statistics should be considered for these data whenever possible.

A point that is not often appreciated is that parametric indicators of variance (eg, standard deviation, SD) can be inappropriate descriptors of this type of data because they describe and graphically depict normality when generated from highly skewed data, and they can lead to illogical interpretations for highly variable biological data (eg, a mean $\pm$ SD of 2 ± 3 implies confidence intervals with negative lower bounds). Alternatives include selected transformations (eg, log transformations) and the underused but logical nonparametric descriptors, the median and interquartile range. The latter simply indicates the range that encompasses the middle 50% of responses, one-quarter of all responses falling above the upper limit of this range, and one-quarter falling below its lower limit. If the data are skewed, the spread of data on one side of the median is greater than on the other, and the interquartile range reflects this. In addition, regardless of the variability in the data, the interval can only include obtainable responses.

Multivariate statistical techniques have been employed extensively in the characterization of foods for product development and processing, and a variety of novel methodologies are available.[95,96] Multivariate analyses also may be applied to biomedical research, both to characterize individuals and groups and to understand the underlying structure of sensory perceptions.[87,97] Use of these techniques in nutrition-related research may be expected to increase, particularly as the field moves toward greater use of more complex stimuli.

Research Facilities and Equipment for Sensory Testing

The space, room layout, and resources required to conduct sensory tests vary widely, depending on the methodology employed, the subject population, and the concomitant need for other (eg, clinical) measures. At one extreme, sensory data are collected in highly specialized taste panel facilities with multiple test booths fitted with running water, cuspidors for rinsing and expectorating, on-line computerized data capture and analysis systems, and laboratory bench and kitchen preparation and analysis facilities nearby. At the other extreme, sensory testing may be conducted in "hall tests" (eg, in shopping malls or stores), in the home, or at the bedside of clinical patients, where little, if any, specialized equipment may be employed. Research institutions with an active sensory evaluation component generally have some type of purpose-built laboratory arrangement. New entrants into this area of investigation generally find that commonly existing "wet lab" benches are poorly suited for many types of sensory assessments.

For laboratory-based sensory measurements, control of the room environment is crucial. Access to a source of consistent, high-quality (deionized or distilled) water is important. Tap water is not suitable for preparation of controlled stimuli, particularly simple taste solutions. The temperature and humidity must be comfortable, the test room should be isolated from outside noise and other distractions, and it should be possible to erect some sort of visual barriers so that individual test subjects cannot see one another, the observer or technician, the preparation areas, or the source or number of test stimuli while formulating their responses. Control of extraneous odors is imperative, and personnel should be aware of the possible influence of colognes, shampoos, and other unintended personal odors. It should go without saying that smoking should be prohibited at all times in the sensory testing area. For many types of olfactory testing, additional portable or room ventilation may be needed to remove test odors continuously.

Lighting is not a critical consideration for many types of tests, particularly if testing involves simple solutions that do not differ in appearance. For hedonic judgments of real foods, appropriate, high-quality illumination should be available.[98,99] If appearance is not an intended variable and the appearance of samples may influence judgments, dimmed or filtered (especially red/blue) lighting should be made available. In this case, it is advisable to ascertain that the desired effect of the masking definitely has been achieved. For example, differences in viscosity or surface reflectance of solutions or foods may still be apparent under filtered light. Colored sample vessels may be of additional value in some instances.

Test Stimuli and Presentation

The selection of appropriate test stimuli may be one of the most crucial and difficult decisions made in studies of sensory evaluation. In some cases, the choice of stimuli may be relatively straightforward, such as when comparing a new formulation to an existing product. In other cases, selection of appropriate stimuli may be difficult, particularly in food acceptance and nutrition research in which it may be of interest to relate a sensory measure to some aspect of food consumption or dietary habits.

Until recently, sensory evaluation in biomedical research had relied largely on purified compounds in a simple vehicle. This is probably still suitable for threshold and intensity testing, with the recognition that their relevance to perceptions of real foods is uncertain. It is increasingly understood that hedonic evaluation of these types of preparations may be irrelevant, particularly if the results are to be interpreted in relation to dietary preferences.

It is generally presumed that more complex stimuli should have greater dietary relevance, although it is more difficult to control all aspects of flavor and composition in real food samples. Recent studies with fat-containing stimuli highlight some of these problems.[100] In the case of fats, the constituent of interest performs multiple sensory functions, making it difficult to assess independently the importance of each. Furthermore, the ability to discriminate fat content in various foods may be quite different, and preferences for fat content are poorly correlated among different foods.[101,102] This latter point should serve as a caution against overgeneralizing results from a single stimulus type.

The number of stimuli, rinse procedures, and preferred mode of presentation are not well established, though some general guidelines can be given. For all tests involving taste and smell, particularly threshold testing, adaptation phenomena can be responsible for anomalous results.[103] Constant or frequent exposure to stimuli can diminish or eliminate sensation by effectively raising the "background" against which a stimulus is judged. On the other hand, the existence of sensory "fatigue," while frequently mentioned, has not been proved. It seems unlikely that the sensory apparatus should suffer from true decline or loss of physiologic function with use; however, there is little question that subjects may begin to suffer from mental fatigue, loss of concentration, and perhaps metabolic changes affecting perception (particularly if stimuli are swallowed). In general, presentation of stimuli can be self-paced, at a rate of up to one sample per minute or more for simple tasks. One or two thorough mouth-rinsings with deionized water between samples should be sufficient, although more aggressive procedures should be adapted for extremely strong or lingering stimuli.

Presentation, handling, and duration of evaluation of stimuli are not standardized across laboratories, but should be constant within a study. Liquid taste stimuli typically are presented in approximately 10 mL volumes in medicine cups, although droppers, filter paper, constant flow, and many other modes of presentation have been used for certain purposes. Presentation of olfactory stimuli is more problematic. Berglund and associates[104] present an extensive discussion of some of the more elaborate methods for controlling delivery of odorants. However, simpler methods, such as simply placing odorants into a plastic squeeze bottle,[46,105] appear to be suitable for most research purposes in which absolute control of stimulus flow is not critical.

The decision as to whether samples should be swallowed or expectorated may depend on several factors. Although this author is unaware of any definitive studies examining the issue, Kelly and Heymann[106] found no effect of ingestion versus expectoration on difference thresholds (sensitivity to differences between samples), though ingestion of samples was associated with less variability in the data. Bartoshuk and colleagues[107] and Mattes and Mela[90] also observed no significant procedural differences on sweetness intensity and preferences, respectively. For real foods, swallowing would seem to be more appropriate, as it allows for the airflow patterns and interactions needed to produce a normal flavor profile, as well as being more relevant to normal eating experiences. There is some indication that sensory responses to swallowed stimuli may show stronger relationships with dietary habits.[90] However, the continuous consumption of material during a sensory evaluation session may produce some shift in response. For example, Rolls and colleagues[108] have delineated the phenomenon of "sensory-specific satiety," in which the hedonic ratings of foods decline with consumption, as a function of specific sensory properties. While this appears to be true even in very low energy foods, postingestive factors may also affect perceptions of foods.

Test Subjects

The subject populations and the types of screening instrument employed obviously differ with the purpose of the study. To be able to assess the potential for unanticipated variations in chemosensory function, subject screening should consider, in addition to normal demographic and nutritional assessment data, items such as those described in *Table 13.3*.

Table 13.3
Typical Screening Data for Participants in Sensory Evaluation Studies

---

Anthropometric data
Age, height, weight, body composition (if possible).

State of dentition
Decayed teeth and dentures are sometimes associated with persistent odors or tastes.

Presence of colds, influenza, sinus conditions, nasal polyps
Because these conditions can reduce nasal patency, olfactory function may be diminished or lost.

Existence of allergies and food sensitivities
This information can be critical if testing involves use of real foods or complex ingredients.

Use of medications
A large number of medications have been associated with altered chemosensory function.[109,110]

Smoking
Studies of smoking and chemosensory function have had equivocal results, despite popular belief to the contrary. However, recent work has identified a substantial dose-related effect of present and past smoking on olfactory function.[111]

The metabolic state of subjects may also have some influence on responses. Testing in the fasted state, as opposed to the fed state, does not appear to have a substantial effect on threshold or intensity, but it may, in some cases, influence hedonic ratings for selected stimuli.[85, 112-115]

Researcher should be aware of the very wide innate variability in human sensory responsiveness to many chemical stimuli.[116] Genetic differences may be a significant underlying basis for differing perceptions of everyday sensory experiences: Many of the compounds known to produce wide variation differences in response are components of foods and environmental odors.

One well-characterized interindividual difference in sensory function is the genetically determined sensitivity to the taste of compounds such as phenylthiocarbamide (PTC). These compounds have been of particular nutritional interest, as they are goitrogens, naturally occurring in selected cruciferous vegetables. "Tasters" perceive weak concentrations of PTC as intensely bitter, while "nontasters" generally perceive no taste at all, except at very high tastant concentrations. The proportion of tasters has been found to vary from 60% to almost 100% among different racial and ethnic groups,[117] as shown in *Table 13.4*. Tasters also appear to demonstrate differences in the perception of several unrelated bitter and possibly some sweet tastants also. Similar extreme variation in taste perceptions of other compounds, such as mannose, creatine, and sodium benzoate have also been described, but are not as well documented.

Table 13.4
Ability to Taste
Phenylthiocarbamide among
Selected Populations

Population	% PTC "Tasters"
Northern European	69
Spanish and Portuguese	76
Japanese	93
Black African	97
Brazilian Indian	99

Data from Allison and Blumberg.[117] Modified from Mela DJ, Mattes RD.[128]
©Williams and Wilkins, 1988, with permission from the publisher.

Specific anosmias (inability to smell a particular compound) have been described for a large number of odorants, with the percent of population not able to smell a given odor found to range from 3% for the sweaty odor of isovaleric acid to about 90% for the medicinal odor of iodocresol (*Table 13.5*). The latter was discovered during development of a commercial cake mix, when a small percentage of taste panelists consistently reported a strong, unpalatable off-flavor, to the great consternation of the technical flavor experts who were all anosmic to the offending compound.[119] As with PTC, sensitivity to several of these odorous compounds is believed to be genetically determined in part, though other factors can be involved. Androstenone presents an outstanding example of this complexity in individual variation in the chemical senses. The compound is perceived as offensively sweaty or urine-like by about 35% of adults, subtle and perhaps somewhat pleasant by about 15%, and not at all detected by the remaining 50%.[105] In addition, there is a loss of ability to detect the odor during puberty, particularly among males.[120] Finally, about half of the anosmic group can become sensitive to the smell with repeated exposure.[121]

Table 13.5
Prevalence of Selected Specific
Anosmias in Humans

Odorant	Characteristic Odor	Estimated % of Humans Insensitive to Odor
Iodocresol	Medicinal	90
Androstenone	Urinous/sweaty	45–50
Isobuteraldehyde	Malty	36
1,8-cineole	Camphoraceous	33
ω-pentadecalactone	Musky	10
Trimethylamine	Fishy	6
Isovaleric acid	Sweaty	3

Data from Labows and Wysocki.[118] Modified from Mela DJ, Mattes RD.[128] ©Williams and Wilkins, 1988, with permission from the publisher.

Environmental and experiential factors may also contribute to individual variability in perceptions of many stimuli. For example, systematic training such as that undertaken by professional perfumers and wine tasters can lead to the ability to select out and identify subtle tastes and smells that might go unnoticed by untrained observers. Such training may expand people's capability to exploit the potential of their sensory systems, but does not alter their physical characteristics. In hedonic ratings, past experience and attitudes toward the stimulus can create a significant potential for cognitive bias. This phenomenon has been most clearly illustrated in the food labeling, marketing and branding arena,[122,123] but merits consideration in biomedical sensory evaluation research, particularly if clinical populations (eg, subjects who are obese or have eating disorders) are of interest.

APPLICATIONS OF SENSORY EVALUATION METHODS IN NUTRITION AND DIETETICS RESEARCH

Unsupported statements about nutrition and the role of sensory function in food selection pervade the sensory evaluation literature. Many sensory evaluation studies make assumptions or claims about the relevance of various measures to diet, without actually carrying out valid, detailed assessments of food intake or nutritional status. Similarly, unsupported statements about the role of sensory function in food selection are common in the nutrition literature. Nutrition studies rarely contain a sensory evaluation component, yet may commonly contain assumptions about the importance of sensory phenomena. This situation probably exists because of the multidisciplinary nature of both of these fields and the small number of research groups with expertise in both areas. Several recent reviews discuss the relationships between nutrition and sensory evaluation,[91, 124–129] and the reader is directed to these sources to gain a perspective on the present status of knowledge in this area. General factors affecting food acceptance, including sensory aspects, have also been the subject of a number of recent reviews.[130,131]

While it is clear that frank nutritional deficiencies can alter taste function,[124] most research in this area has focused on relationships between sensory function, preferences, and food intake or nutrient utilization in healthy subjects. The influence of the chemical senses on nutrient utilization and metabolism has been reviewed recently by Mattes,[125] and a number of issues for further research on that topic are identified.

It has proved difficult to document clear associations between sensory and dietary intake measures, despite strong indications from common experience that such relationships are important. At one extreme, recent studies of patients with chemosensory disorders indicate that, although they report pathology-related changes in eating habits and substantial loss of eating enjoyment, they are not at great nutritional risk.[132] The recent review by Shepherd and Farleigh[91] presents a clear and comprehensive overview of the use of sensory methods in relation to food selection and consumption in the normal population. Mattes[41] has also described some of the methodologic considerations important in characterizing diet-taste relationships. It is unclear how individual measures of "food acceptability"—however that construct may be measured—translate into the selection and consumption of foods and nutrients. The literature on this topic clearly points to hedonic measures as having the closest relationships with dietary intake; yet that relationship generally holds poor predictive and explanatory power. The incorporation of additional attitudinal and psychosocial information into these studies could help resolve differences between the sensory and dietary data.

CONCLUSIONS

The selection of sensory methods is clearly dependent on the research hypotheses under consideration. Although it is likely that hedonics will be the focus of interest for many types of nutrition studies, it may be of some value to investigate other measures of sensory function, particularly in clinical populations. There is a large literature on sensory evaluation, and because the techniques often lack the external validity of, for example, biochemical tests, investigators may be easily distracted by the many different and often conflicting methodologic approaches. Unfortunately, while there is generally no "right" way to conduct sensory analyses, there can be many wrong ways.

Researchers new to the area of sensory evaluation are strongly advised to consult the substantial existing literature. Numerous different types of measures have been applied to the assessment of human perceptions and acceptance of foods and food components. It is inadvisable to try to attempt to develop experimental protocols or devise new sensory tests without a clear understanding of the theoretical and practical problems encountered in both the conduct and interpretation of studies of human perception.

The capacity for humans to detect, recognize, enjoy, and desire the great variation in sensory qualities of foods may serve to ensure consumption from a wide diversity of safe nutrient sources. With proper use and consideration of underlying psychological and nutrition principles, substantial progress can be made in understanding the factors affecting sensory perceptions and their relationships with human eating behavior.

Acknowledgments

The author is grateful to Dr Wendy Brown for preparing the section on texture perception, and to other colleagues in the Consumer Sciences Department for their helpful discussions on the general subject matter. Some portions of the text and Tables 13.1, 13.2, 13.4, and 13.5 are modified from Mela DJ, Mattes RD.[128] ©Williams and Wilkins, 1988, with permission from the publisher.

APPENDIX: TEXTS INCORPORATING SENSORY EVALUATION METHODS

American Society for Testing and Materials. *Basic Principles of Sensory Evaluation.* Philadelphia, Pa: ASTM; 1968. ASTM special technical publication 433.

American Society for Testing and Materials. *Manual on Sensory Testing Methods.* Philadelphia, Pa: ASTM; 1968. ASTM special technical publication 434.

Amerine MA, Pangborn RM, Reossler EB. *Principles of Sensory Evaluation of Food.* New York, NY: Academic Press; 1965.

Arthur D. Little, Inc. *Flavor Research and Food Acceptance.* New York, NY: Reinhold; 1958.

Bourne MC. *Food Texture and Viscosity: Concept and Measurement.* New York, NY: Academic Press; 1982.

Finger TE, Silver WL, eds. *Neurobiology of Taste and Smell.* New York, NY: John Wiley and Sons; 1987.

Kuznicki JT, Rutkiewic AF, Johnson RA, eds. *Selected Sensory Methods: Problems and Approaches to Measuring Hedonics.* Philadelphia, Pa: American Society for Testing and Materials; 1982. ASTM special technical publication 773.

McBride RL, MacFie HJH, eds. *Psychological Basis of Sensory Evaluation.* London, England: Elsevier; 1990.

McBurney DH, Collings VB. *Introduction to Sensation/Perception.* Englewood Cliffs, NJ: Prentice-Hall; 1977.

Meiselman HL, Rivlin RS, eds. *Clinical Measurement of Taste and Smell.* New York, NY: Macmillan Publishing Co; 1986.

Moskowitz HR. *Product Testing and Sensory Evaluation of Foods: Marketing and R&D Approaches.* Westport, Conn: Food and Nutrition Press; 1983.

Piggott JR. *Sensory Evaluation of Foods.* 2nd ed. London, England: Elsevier; 1988.

Thomson DMH. *Food Acceptability.* London, England: Elsevier; 1988.

Williams AA, Atkin RK, eds. *Sensory Quality in Foods and Beverages: Definition, Measurement and Control.* Chichester, UK: Ellis Howard; 1983.

References

1. Miller IJ Jr. Variation in human fungiform taste bud densities among regions and subjects. *Anat Record.* 1986;216:474.
2. Nilsson B. The occurrence of taste buds in the palate of human adults as evidenced by light microscopy. *Acta Odontol Scand.* 1979;37:253.
3. Henkin RI, Christiansen RL. Taste localization on the tongue, palate, and pharynx of normal man. *J Appl Physiol.* 1967;22:316.
4. Miller IJ Jr, Reedy FE. Variation in human taste bud density and taste intensity perception. *Physiol Behav.* 1990;47:1213.
5. McBurney DH, Gent JF. On the nature of taste qualities. *Psychol Bull.* 1979;86:151.
6. Avenet P, Lindemann B. Perspectives of taste perception. *J Membrane Biol.* 1989;112:1.

7. Bruch RC, Kalinoski DL, Kare MR. Biochemistry of vertebrate olfaction and taste. *Ann Rev Nutr.* 1988;8:21.
8. Kinnamon SC. Taste transduction: a diversity of mechanisms. *Trends Neurosci.* 1988;11:491.
9. Cardello AV. Chemical stimulation of single human fungiform taste papillae: sensitivity profiles and locus of stimulation. *Sensory Processes.* 1978;2:173.
10. Collings VB. Human taste response as a function of locus of stimulation on the tongue and soft palate. *Percep Psychophys.* 1974;16:169.
11. Sandick B, Cardello AV. Taste profiles from single circumvallate papillae: comparison with fungiform profiles. *Chem Senses.* 1981;6:197.
12. Hänig DP. Zur Psychophysik des Geschmackssinnes. *Phil Stud.* 1901;17:576.
13. Bartoshuk LM. The psychophysics of taste. *Am J Clin Nutr.* 1978;31:1068.
14. Moskowitz HR. *Product Testing and Sensory Evaluation of Foods: Marketing and R&D Approaches.* Westport, Conn: Food and Nutrition Press; 1983.
15. Anholt RRH. Primary events in olfactory reception. *Trends Biochem Sci.* 1987;12:58.
16. Ohloff G. Chemistry of odor stimuli. *Experientia.* 1986;42:271.
17. Snyder SH, Sklar PB, Pevsner J. Molecular mechanisms of olfaction. *J Biol Chem.* 1988;263:13971.
18. Hornung DE, Mozell MM. Smell: human physiology. In: Meiselman HL, Rivlin RS, eds. *Clinical Measurement of Taste and Smell.* New York, NY: Macmillan Publishing Co; 1986:117.
19. Mozell MM, Hornung DE, Leopold DA, Youngentob SL. Initial mechanisms basic to olfactory perception. *Am J Otolaryngol.* 1983;4:238.
20. Goodspeed RB, Catalanotto FA, Gent JF, et al. Clinical characteristics of patients with taste and smell disorders. In: Meiselman HL, Rivlin RS, eds. *Clinical Measurement of Taste and Smell.* New York, NY: Macmillan Publishing Co; 1986:451.
21. Murphy C, Cain WS. Taste and olfaction: independence vs interaction. *Physiol Behav.* 1980;24:601.
22. Murphy C, Cain WS, Bartoshuk LM. Mutual action of taste and olfaction. *Sensory Process.* 1977;1:204.
23. Frank RA, Byram J. Taste-smell interactions are tastant and odorant dependent. *Chem Senses.* 1988;13:445.
24. Silver WL. The common chemical sense. In: Finger TE, Silver WL, eds. *Neurobiology of Taste and Smell.* New York, NY: John Wiley and Sons; 1987.
25. Silver WL, Mason JR, Adams MA, Smeraski CA. Nasal trigeminal chemoreception: Responses to *n*-aliphatic alcohols. *Brain Res.* 1986;376:221.
26. Doty RL, Brugger WE, Jurs PC, Orndorff MM. Intranasal trigeminal stimulation from odorous volatiles: psychometric responses from anosmic and normal humans. *Physiol Behav.* 1978;20:175.
27. Johansson RS. Tactile afferent units with small and well demarcated receptive fields in the glabrous skin area of the human hand. In: Kenshalo DR, ed. *Sensory Functions of the Skin of Humans.* New York, NY; Plenum; 1979:129.
28. Verillo RT, Grescheider GA. Psychophysical measurements of enhancement, suppression, and surface gradient effects in vibrotaction. In: Kenshalo DR, ed. *Sensory Functions of the Skin of Humans.* New York, NY: Plenum; 1979:153.
29. Mela DJ. Sensory assessment of fat content in fluid dairy products. *Appetite.* 1988;10:37.
30. Mela DJ, Christensen CM. Sensory assessment of oiliness in a low moisture food. *J Sensory Stud.* 1988;2:273.
31. Pfaffmann C. Afferent impulses from the teeth from pressure and noxious stimulation. *J Physiol.* 1939;97:207.
32. Christensen CM, Vickers ZM. Relationships of chewing sounds to judgements of food crispness. *J Food Sci.* 1981;46:574.
33. Szczesniak AS. Instrumental methods of texture measurement. *Food Technol.* 1972;26:50.
34. McBurney DH, Collings VB. *Introduction to Sensation/Perception.* Englewood Cliffs, NJ: Prentice-Hall; 1977.
35. American Society for Testing and Materials. *Manual on Sensory Testing Methods.* Philadelphia, Pa: ASTM; 1968. ASTM special technical publication 434.
36. Amerine MA, Pangborn RM, Reossler, EB. *Principles of Sensory Evaluation of Food.* New York, NY: Academic Press; 1965.

37. American Society for Testing and Materials. *Compilation of Odor and Taste Threshold Values Data.* Philadelphia, Pa: ASTM; 1978. ASTM publication DS48A.

38. Stevens JC, Cain WS, Burke RJ. Variability of olfactory thresholds. *Chem Senses.* 1988;13:643.

39. Robinson JO. The misuse of taste names by untrained observers. *Br J Psychol.* 1970;61:375.

40. Cornsweet TN. The staircase-method in psychophysics. *Am J Psychol.* 1962;75:485.

41. Mattes RD. Gustation as a determinant of ingestion: methodological issues. *Am J Clin Nutr.* 1985;41:672.

42. Mattes RD. Reliability of psychophysical measures of gustatory function. *Percept Pyschophys.* 1988;41:107.

43. Mela DJ. Gustatory function and dietary habits in users and non-users of smokeless tobacco. *Am J Clin Nutr.* 1989;49:482.

44. Harris H, Kalmus H. The measurement of taste sensitivity to phenylthiourea (P.T.C.). *Ann Eugen.* 1949;15:24.

45. Kelly MF, Mayer J. Rapid determination of taste threshold: a group procedure. *Am J Clin Nutr.* 1971;24:177.

46. Cain WS, Gent J, Goodspeed RB, Leonard G. Evaluation of olfactory dysfunction in the Connecticut Chemosensory Clinical Research Center. *Laryngoscope* 1988;98:83.

47. Cain WS, Rabin MD. Comparability of two tests of olfactory functioning. *Chem Senses.* 1989;14:479.

48. Smith DV. Assessment of patients with taste and smell disorders. *Acta Otolaryngol* 1988;458(suppl):129.

49. Lawless H. Contextual effects in category ratings. *J Test Eval.* 1983;11:346.

50. McBride RL. Stimulus range influences intensity and hedonic ratings of flavour. *Appetite* 1985;6:125.

51. Riskey DR. Use and abuses of category scales in sensory measurement. *J Sensory Stud.* 1986;1:217.

52. Moskowitz HR. Univariate psychophysical functions. In: Powers JJ, Moskowitz HR, eds. *Correlating Sensory Objective Measurements—New Methods for Answering Old Problems.* Philadelphia, Pa: American Society for Testing and Materials; 1976. ASTM special technical publication 594.

53. Poulton EC. The new psychophysics: six models for magnitude estimation. *Psychol Bull.* 1968;69:1.

54. Stevens SS. On the theory of scales of measurement. *Science.* 1946;103:677.

55. Stevens SS. On the psychophysical law. *Psychol Rev.* 1957;64:153.

56. Stevens SS. To honor Fechner and repeal his law. *Science* 1961;133:80.

57. Stevens JC. Psychophysics. In: Sills DL, ed. *International Encyclopedia of the Social Sciences.* New York, NY: Crowell Collier and Macmillan Inc; 1968;13:120.

58. Moskowitz HR. Magnitude estimation: notes on what, how, when, and why to use it. *J Food Qual.* 1977;1:195–227.

59. Doehlert DH. Methods for measuring degree of subjective response. In: American Society for Testing and Materials. *Basic Principles of Sensory Evaluation.* Philadelphia, Pa: ASTM; 1968:58. ASTM special technical publication 433.

60. Stevens SS. The surprising simplicity of sensory metrics. *Am Psychol.* 1962;17:29.

61. Bartoshuk LM, Gent J, Catalanotto FA, Goodspeed RB. Clinical evaluation of taste. *Am J Otolaryngol.* 1983;4:257.

62. Bartoshuk LM, Marks LE. Ratio scaling. In: Meiselman HL, Rivlin RS, eds. *Clinical Measurement of Taste and Smell.* New York, NY: Macmillan Publishing Co; 1986:117.

63. Butler G, Poste LM, Wolynetz MS, Agar VE, Larmond E. Alternative analyses of magnitude estimation data. *J Sensory Stud.* 1987;2:243.

64. Stevens JC, Marks LE. Cross-modality matching functions generated by magnitude estimation. *Percept Psychophys.* 1980;27:379.

65. Stevens JC, Plantinga A, Cain WS. Reduction of odor and nasal pungency associated with aging. *Neurobiol Aging.* 1982;3:125.

66. Lawless HT. Logarithmic transformation of magnitude estimation data and comparison of scaling methods *J Sensory Stud.* 1989;4:75.

67. Moskowitz HR. Utilitarian benefits of magnitude estimation scaling for testing product acceptability. In: Kuznicki JT, Rutkiewic AF, Johnson RA, eds. *Selected*

Sensory Methods: Problems and Approaches to Measuring Hedonics. Philadelphia, Pa: American Society for Testing and Materials; 1982. ASTM special technical publication 773.

68. Birnbaum MH. Problems with so-called "direct" scaling. In: Kuznicki JT, Rutkiewic AF, Johnson RA, eds. *Selected Sensory Methods: Problems and Approaches to Measuring Hedonics.* Philadelphia, Pa: American Society for Testing and Materials; 1982. ASTM special technical publication 773.

69. Giovanni MA, Pangborn RM. Measurement of taste intensity and degree of liking of beverages by graphic scales and magnitude estimation. *J Food Sci.* 1983;48:1175.

70. Tuorila H. Suprathreshold odour intensity assessment: individual variation in scaling. In: Schrier P, ed. *Flavour '81.* New York, NY: Walter de Gruyter; 1981:53.

71. Lawless HT, Malone GJ. The discriminative efficiency of common rating scaling methods. *J Sensory Stud.* 1986a;1:85.

72. Lawless HT, Malone GJ. A comparison of rating scales: sensitivity, replicates and relative measurement. *J Sensory Stud.* 1986b;1:155.

73. Lee WE, Pangborn RM. Time-intensity: the temporal aspects of sensory perception. *Food Technol.* 1986;40:71.

74. Liu Y-H, MacFie HJH. Methods for averaging time-intensity curves. *Chem Senses.* 1990;15:471.

75. Cain WS, Gent JF. Use of odor identification in clinical testing of olfaction. In: Meiselman HL, Rivlin RS, eds. *Clinical Measurement of Taste and Smell.* New York, NY: Macmillan Publishing Co; 1986:170.

76. Doty RL, Shaman P, Dann M. Development of the University of Pennsylvania Smell Identification Test: a standardized microencapsulated test of olfactory function. *Physiol Behav.* 1984;32:489.

77. Wright HN. Characterization of olfactory dysfunction. *Arch Otolaryngol Head Neck Surg.* 1987;113:163.

78. Schiffman S. Food recognition by the elderly. *J Gerontol.* 1977;32:586.

79. Laing DG, Francis GW. The capacity of humans to identify odors in mixtures. *Physiol Behav.* 1989;46:809.

80. Laing DG, Livermore BA, Francis GW. The human sense of smell has a limited capacity for identifying odors in mixtures. In: *ECRO IX Programme Abstracts.* Ninth Congress of the European Chemoreception Research Organization. 1990:51.

81. McBurney DH. Taste, smell, and flavor terminology: taking the confusion out of fusion. In: Meiselman HL, Rivlin RS, eds. *Clinical Measurement of Taste and Smell.* New York, NY: Macmillan Publishing Co; 1986:117.

82. Gross-Isseroff R, Lancet D. Concentration-dependent changes of perceived odor quality. *Chem Senses.* 1988;13:191.

83. Peryam DR, Pilgrim FJ. Hedonic scale method of measuring food preferences. *Food Technol.* 1957;11:9.

84. Schutz HG. A food action rating scale for measuring food acceptance. *J Food Sci.* 1965;30:365.

85. Drewnowski A, Greenwood MRC. Cream and sugar: human preferences for high-fat foods. *Physiol Behav.* 1983;30:629.

86. Drewnowski A. New techniques: multidimensional analyses of taste responsiveness. *Int J Obesity.* 1984;8:599.

87. Drewnowski A, Moskowitz HR. Sensory characteristics of foods: new evaluation techniques. *Am J Clin Nutr.* 1985;42(suppl):924.

88. Shepherd R, Smith K, Farleigh CA. The relationship between intensity, hedonic, and relative-to-ideal ratings. *Food Qual Pref.* 1989;1:75.

89. Mattes RD, Lawless HT. An adjustment error in optimization of taste intensity. *Appetite.* 1985;6:103.

90. Mattes RD, Mela DJ. Relationships between and among selected measures of sweet taste preferences and dietary intake. *Chem Senses.* 1986;11:523.

91. Shepherd R, Farleigh CA. Sensory assessment of foods and the role of sensory attributes in determining food choice. In: Shepherd R, ed. *Handbook of the Psychophysiology of Human Eating.* Chichester, UK: John Wiley and Sons; 1989:25.

92. Lucas F, Bellisle F. The measurement of food preferences in humans: do taste-and-spit tests predict consumption? *Physiol Behav.* 1987;39:739.

93. Meiselman HL. Personal communication. 1990.

94. Schutz HG. Personal communication. 1990.
95. MacFie HJH. Assessment of the sensory properties of food. *Nutr Rev.* 1990;48:87.
96. Thomson D. Recent advances in sensory and affective methods. *Food Sci Technol Today.* 1989;3:83.
97. Lawless HT. Multidimensional scaling. In: Meiselman HL, Rivlin RS, eds. *Clinical Measurement of Taste and Smell.* New York, NY: Macmillan Publishing Co; 1986:86.
98. MacDougall DB. Effects of pigmentation, light scatter, and illumination on food appearance and acceptance. In: Solms J, Booth DA, Pangborn RM, Raunhardt O, eds. *Food Acceptance and Nutrition.* San Diego, Calif: Academic Press; 1987:29.
99. Hoffman JA: Principles of psychophysical test methods (judgmental methods—appearance). In: American Society for Testing and Materials. *Basic Principles of Sensory Evaluation.* Philadelphia, Pa: ASTM; 1968:98. ASTM special technical publication 33.
100. Mela DJ. Sensory preferences for fats: what, who, why? *Food Qual Pref.* 1990;2:95–101.
101. Mela DJ, Sachetti DS. Sensory preferences for fats in foods: relationships to diet and body composition. *Am J Clin Nutr.* 1991;53:908.
102. Drewnowski A, Shrager EE, Lipsky C, Stellar E, Greenwood MRC. Sugar and fat: sensory and hedonic evaluation of liquid and solid foods. *Physiol Behav.* 1989;45:177.
103. O'Mahony M. Sensory adaptation. *J Sensory Stud.* 1986;1:237.
104. Berglund B, Berglund U, Lindvall T. Theory and methods for odor evaluation. *Experientia.* 1986;42:280.
105. Wysocki CJ, Beauchamp GK. Ability to smell androstenone is genetically determined. *PNAS* 1984;81:4899.
106. Kelly FB, Heymann H. Contrasting the effects of ingestion and expectoration in sensory difference tests. *J Sensory Stud.* 1989;3:249.
107. Bartoshuk LM, Rennert K, Rodin J, Stevens JC. Effects of temperature on the perceived sweetness of sucrose. *Physiol Behav.* 1982;28:905.
108. Rolls BJ, Rowe EA, Rolls ET. How sensory properties of foods affect human feeding behavior. *Physiol Behav.* 1982;29:409.
109. Schiffman SS. Taste and smell in disease. *N Engl J Med.* 1983;308:1275,1337.
110. Willoughby JMT. Drug-induced abnormalities of taste sensation. *Adverse Drug React Bull.* 1983;100:368.
111. Frye RE, Schwartz BS, Doty RL. Dose-related effects of cigarette smoking on olfactory function. *JAMA.* 1990;263:1233.
112. Janowitz HD, Grossman MI. Gusto-olfactory thresholds in relation to appetite and satiety sensations. *J Appl Physiol.* 1949;2:217.
113. Pangborn RM. Influence of hunger on sweetness preferences and taste thresholds. *Am J Clin Nutr.* 1959;7:280.
114. Cabanac M. Physiological role of pleasure. *Science.* 1971;173:1103.
115. Moskowitz HR, Kumraiah VK, Sharma KN, Jacobs HL, Sharma SD. Effects of hunger, satiety and glucose load upon taste intensity and taste hedonics. *Physiol Behav.* 1976;16:471.
116. Pangborn R. Individuality in responses to sensory stimuli. In: Solms J, Hall RL, eds. *Criteria of Food Acceptance. How Man Chooses What He Eats.* Zurich, Switzerland: Foster Verlag AG; 1981:177.
117. Allison AC, Blumberg BS. Ability to taste phenylthiocarbamide among Alaskan eskimos and other populations. *Hum Biol.* 1959;31:352.
118. Labows JN, Wysocki CJ. Individual differences in odor perception. *Perfumer Flavorist.* 1984;9:21.
119. Sevenants MR, Sanders RA. Anatomy of an off-flavor investigation: the "medicinal" cake mix. *Anal Chem.* 1984;56:293A.
120. Dorries KM, Schmidt HJ, Beauchamp GK, Wysocki CJ. Changes in sensitivity to the odor of androstenone during adolescence. *Development Psychol.* 1989;22:423.
121. Wysocki CJ, Dorries KM, Beauchamp GK. Ability to perceive androstenone can be acquired by ostensibly anosmic people. *PNAS.* 1989;86:7976.
122. Allison RI, Uhl KP. Influence of beer brand identification on taste perception. *J Marketing Res.* 1964;1:36.
123. Martin D. The impact of branding and marketing on perceptions of sensory qualities. *Food Sci Technol Today.* 1990;4:44.

124. Mattes RD. Effects of health disorders and poor nutritional status on gustatory function. *J Sensory Stud.* 1986;1:275.
125. Mattes RD. Sensory influences on food intake and utilization in humans. *Hum Nutr Appl Nutr.* 1987;41A:77.
126. Szczesniak AS. Relationship of texture to food acceptance and nutrition. In: Solms J, Booth DA, Pangborn RM, Raunhardt O, eds. *Food Acceptance and Nutrition.* San Diego, Calif: Academic Press; 1987:157.
127. Mela DJ, Kare MR. Healthy eating: the benefits of flavor. In: Manley CH, Morse RE, eds. *Healthy Eating, A Scientific Perspective.* Wheaton Ill: Allured Publishing; 1988:165.
128. Mela DJ, Mattes RD. The chemical senses and nutrition: part I. *Nutr Today.* 1988;23(2):4.
129. Mattes RD, Mela DJ. The chemical senses and nutrition: part II. *Nutr Today.* 1988;23(3):19.
130. Booth DA. Objective measurement of determinants of food acceptance: sensory, physiological, psychosocial. In: Solms J, Booth DA, Pangborn RM, Raunhardt O, eds. *Food Acceptance and Nutrition.* San Diego, Calif: Academic Press; 1987:1.
131. Shepherd R. Factors affecting food preferences and choice. In: Shepherd R, ed. *Handbook of the Psychophysiology of Human Eating.* Chichester, UK: John Wiley and Sons; 1989:3.
132. Mattes RD, Cowart BJ, Schiavo MA, et al. Dietary evaluation of patients with smell and/or taste disorders. *Am J Clin Nutr.* 1990;51:233.

14. RESEARCH IN FOODSERVICE PRODUCTION MANAGEMENT AND INFORMATION SYSTEMS IN FOODSERVICES

Denise Ouellet, MBA, DtP, and M. Eileen Matthews, PhD, RD

To undertake research in foodservice production management and foodservice information systems, the investigator needs to get acquainted with the goals pursued by foodservice researchers and the tools and techniques they use.

The goals of foodservice research are related intimately with the goals of foodservice managers. The foodservice industry constantly adapts to new lifestyles and eating habits. Foodservices rapidly become obsolete if they do not reevaluate themselves continuously and update their operations. Additionally, foodservices face scarce resources. Research is essential to provide dietitians with effective and efficient management tools to keep them competitive as foodservice managers. Research in production management provides them with methods to analyze and rationalize their operations and the use of each resource. Information systems must support the operations by gathering relevant information and providing computing power. Furthermore, food science, business, and engineering provide not only methods to improve resource utilization in foodservices, but also the tools to evaluate the impact of the changes made.

All research must start with the identification of a problem. Involvement of practitioner dietitians is essential to identify the problems on which research should focus. Practitioners are also needed to implement and evaluate the methods proposed by researchers. Once a problem has been identified, the researcher must look for information about what has been done to solve similar problems in the past. Solving the problem may consist of new ideas, improving existing methods, or applying to foodservices the methods developed by related fields such as food science, business, or engineering.

To gain knowledge of foodservice production management and foodservice information systems, the first step is to get acquainted with the content of textbooks on foodservice management. Next, specialized foodservice textbooks addressing the topic under study may be consulted. Third, current literature should be reviewed. Articles on these topics may be found in the *Journal of The American Dietetic Association* and other nutrition journals, in hospital administration journals, in business journals, in food science journals, and in food management journals. Finally, to learn more about particular techniques used in research, textbooks in related fields, should be consulted. *Table 14.1* presents selected textbooks on foodservice management and related fields.

Table 14.1
Selected Textbooks for
Information on Foodservice
Management

Topic	References
Foodservice management	Spears[1]
	West, Woods, Harger, et al[2]
Production management	
Introduction	Chase and Aquilano[3]
	Stevenson[4]
Operations research	Buffa and Dyer[5]
	Hillier and Lieberman[6]
Productivity management in foodservices	Halling, Lafferty, and Feller[7]
Work analysis in foodservices	Kazarian[8]
Energy management in foodservices	Unklesbay and Unklesbay[9]
Information systems	
In business	Burch and Grudnitski[10]
	Hicks[11]
In foodservices	Kaud[12]
	Pellegrino[13]
	Kasavana[14]
Food science	
Microbiological analysis of food	AOAC[15]
	Speck[16]
Nutrition analysis of food	AOAC[15]
	Augustin, Klein, Becker, et al[17]
Sensory evaluation	Stone and Sidel[18]

FOODSERVICE PRODUCTION MANAGEMENT

Foodservice production management consists of the managerial activities required in selecting, designing, operating, controlling, and updating food production systems. The objective is to produce quality products at the desired rate and at minimum cost. This is achieved by continuously updating the concepts and techniques used in food production. Research is needed to supply new concepts and techniques. The research approach follows acceptable scientific problem-solving methodology to investigate a problem and to create new, generally applicable knowledge.

The field of foodservice production management is a broad area that incorporates all the resources used by foodservice managers. These resources are classified as human, material, facilities, and operational.[1] In research, studies have been done on the selection and design of systems for foodservice and food production, on the planning and scheduling of the operations, and on the control and evaluation of the products and processes.

How to Do Research on Foodservice Production Management

Identification of the research problem is the primary step in any research project. Ideas for research topics may be gathered through contact with practitioners or by a literature review. Practitioners could advise researchers of the new challenges and problems they are facing. For researchers interested in a particular area, reviewing the literature on a specific topic may generate ideas for further research; no topics have been entirely researched.

The tools used for research in foodservice production management are borrowed from related fields, mainly, food science, business, and statistics. To engage in research in foodservice production management, a dietitian needs a good background in those three areas. A basic knowledge is usually acquired through undergraduate dietetic coursework; course work and reading can update and extend that knowledge.

Summary of Completed Research

A variety of research methods is used in foodservice production management. Descriptive research is used to develop and implement concepts and methods and to survey foodservice operations. Experimental research evaluates and compares methods under controlled conditions in laboratories or in actual operating foodservices.

A glimpse into past foodservice production management research illustrates the variety of topics as well as the tools and techniques used to conduct research in this field. An overview of the topics is presented in *Table 14.2.*

The early literature on foodservice production management primarily presented guidelines on operations. Topics included job analysis,[19] standardization methods,[20,21] and menu planning techniques.[22,23] Descriptive research compared employee performance[24] and food and labor costs among hospital foodservices.[25]

In the 1940s, the increasing number of meals eaten away from home brought concerns about the quality of the food served in restaurants and cafeterias. Experimental research was undertaken to analyze the vitamin content of food held hot for periods of time. The main vitamins studied were ascorbic acid, thiamin, and riboflavin. A review of this research was done by Snyder and Matthews in 1984.[26] In the late 1940s and during the 1950s, the safety of institutional food also was investigated. Experimental research was conducted in either foodservices or in laboratories to analyze the effects of different cooling methods on microbial growth.[27-29] In the 1960s, different cooking processes were studied for their impact on the microbial content of food.[30-32]

After World War II, industrial engineering methods were introduced in foodservices. The first publications illustrated how to use operation charts, time and motion studies, and work simplification[33,34] to improve work organization. Researchers investigated the effectiveness of applying these techniques in foodservices.[35,36] Motion studies such as cross charts also were used to improve foodservice layout design.[37,38] Work sampling techniques were introduced in the 1960s to improve staffing and scheduling.[39-41] In work sampling, random observations of workers' activities provided a detailed description of how working time was spent.

In the late 1970s, Waldvogel and Ostenso worked on the development of master standard data (MSD) for food production scheduling.[42,43] This industrial engineering technique determines time standards for each activity. Once standards are established, a manager can better predict the time required to complete a task. The MSD technique was later expanded and evaluated by Zemel and co-workers.[44-46] In the 1980s, Stinson and Guley used computer simulations to improve food production scheduling.[47,48]

Table 14.2
Selected Articles on Foodservice
Production Management

Topic	Research Design		
	Descriptive	Analytical	
		Observational	Experimental
		References	
Foodservice systems	80		60
Conventional,			
Commissary,			
Ready-prepared,			
Assembly-serve			
Food production systems			
Compare systems:	74,75	83	84
Cook/chill	80		
Cook/freeze	81		85
Cook-hot hold			
Heat-serve			
Planning			
Queuing			49
Transport models	86	87	88
Assembly line balancing	51,52		
Productivity			
Labor	89,90		
Productivity management	7,91		
Job design			
Job analysis	92		96,97
Work sampling	93–95		
Food production scheduling			
Master Standard Data		42–44	45
Priority sequencing		48	47
Material requirement planning		98	
Inventory management			
Economic order quantity	99		
Inventory policies			53
Purchasing policies			54
Quality control			
HACCP	76		77
Time and temperature studies	100–103		
Food analysis			
Microbiological	104		107,108
Sensory			66,67,109
Nutritional			70
Energy	105,106		110

Simulations for experimental purposes were introduced in foodservice research in the 1960s. They consisted of mathematical models that imitated actual conditions. With simulations, solutions could be derived or tested without conducting an experiment on the phenomenon itself. Simulations have been used to study customer flow in cafeterias and dining rooms,[49,50] and work division on tray lines.[51,52] In the 1970s, simulations were also used to develop inventory management models. These models were used to study the impact of storage space and of menu variety on food cost.[53,54]

The energy crisis of the 1970s created concerns about energy management in foodservices. Research was undertaken to develop research models[55,56] and analyze the energy usage in the different types of foodservice systems.[57-59]

Alternate foodservice and food production systems were introduced in the late 1960s.[60] Instead of cooking, holding hot, and serving, some systems chilled or froze food after cooking and rethermalized it just before service. On-site production could be reduced to a minimum and centralized kitchens could provide food for numerous facilities. These new systems created needs for research on the safety, quality, and economics of the food they produced. Research first addressed the sensory, microbiological, and nutritional quality of the food. This research area, introduced in the 1970s, was pursued throughout the 1980s and is continuing into the 1990s.[61-73] The economical aspect of these systems was studied by Greathouse and Gregoire in the late 1980s.[74,75]

In 1978, a new concept, hazard analysis critical control points (HACCP) was proposed for microbiological quality control in foodservices.[76,77] HACCP is a quality control system by which potential microbiological dangers are identified so that preventive monitoring can be done. Implementation of that quality concept in the industry is still pursued in the 1990s.[78]

Illustration With Example

In 1986, Hsieh and Matthews conducted research to determine the energy consumption, cooking time, and product yield of turkey rolls under three convection oven loads at three oven temperatures.[79] They also investigated the energy impact of three different holding loads in a hot-holding cabinet after one and two hours of hot-holding. The data collected included the internal temperature of the turkey rolls during the cooking and the holding process, the internal temperature of the oven, the energy used by the oven and the holding cabinet, and the weight of the turkey rolls, before and after the cooking and the holding process. For the internal meat temperature and oven temperature, thermocouples were used and monitored with a recording potentiometer. The amount of energy used was recorded by an energy monitor at predetermined intervals.

Analysis of the data was done using extensive inferential statistics. A two-way analysis of variance was performed with the temperature and the number of turkey rolls per load as factors. Covariance analysis was done for the time it took to reach the target internal meat temperature. Finally, regression analysis was performed to determine the significance of the difference between the cooking time required for each load.

This research concluded that the least amount of energy was required when the largest oven load was used at the lowest temperature. The authors also concluded that product yield was greater with lower oven temperature. This research provided foodservice managers with production scheduling information. To reduce energy cost and increase product yield in convection ovens, managers should tend toward using larger oven loads at lower temperatures. These decision criteria need to be balanced with other criteria, such as the availability of employees and of equipment, and the amount of product needed.

INFORMATION SYSTEMS

Hussain and Hussain[111] define an "information system" as an organized set of components designed to produce information for decision making. Information is data that has been transformed into a meaningful and useful form for specific needs. Information processing has been done mainly with computers in the past few decades, making "information systems" a synonym of "computer systems" in the general usage.

An essential function of managers is decision making. Even though some decisions might be based on a certain amount of intuition, they always rely on what a manager knows about a situation or information; the basis of decision making is information. Better information allows managers to better evaluate consequences of decisions as well as to consider more alternatives. Research in foodservice information systems covers all the resources used by foodservice managers: human, material, facilities, and operational resources such as time, money, energy, and information.

How to Do Research on Information Systems

The main purpose of information systems research is to develop efficient ways to produce current, timely, accurate, and relevant information. Facing an information problem, a researcher has to identify which information is needed, how it could be gathered, and how it should be processed. Reviewing the literature provides a good sense on how previous researchers selected, collected, and processed information in foodservices.

Both descriptive and analytical research have been conducted on information systems in foodservices. Descriptive research has focused on computer usage in foodservices, the selection and evaluation of information systems, and concepts for systems design. Analytical research was completed on the evaluation of systems and the development of models to build the systems. An overview of selected articles on information systems in foodservices is presented in *Table 14.3.*

Table 14.3
Selected Articles on Information
Systems in Foodservices

Topic	Research Design		
	Descriptive	Analytical	
		Observational	Experimental
	References		
Computer usage in foodservices			
Applications	112–114, 128		
Status reports	129–133		
Case reports	134		
Selection and evaluation	135,136		
Systems design	125–127, 137,138	139	140–142
Quantitative models			
Customer flow simulations			49,50,97 120,143
Menu planning			119,144
Purchasing		123	124
Production scheduling		48,98	47

The design of a system consists of transposing foodservice management principles into a computable format. Dietitians provide and/or generate concepts, guide the development, and implement and evaluate systems.

To build an information system, quantitative and conceptual models are required. Quantitative models provide the logical and mathematical processes to transform data into information. These models are developed by operations and production management research. Computers and quantitative models are intimately related, because most of these models will be practically unusable without the computing power.

Conceptual models provide the overall structure of the system and indicate how data, information, and knowledge should be organized and manipulated. Conceptual models are also needed to define the reasoning strategies used by the systems. Conceptual models are developed by combining concepts and principles from computer science and from foodservice management.

The tools used to build systems are drawn from foodservice management, business, and computer science. The programming part frequently is done in collaboration with computer science specialists. If a computer specialist is not available, "fourth-generation languages" (eg, spreadsheets or database software packages) might be used. These languages were developed to simplify and automate the tedious task of programming. They are used primarily for simple systems and prototyping, and they may become inefficient to use with complex or large systems.

A researcher may decide to program with a common programming language (eg, Fortran, Basic, Cobol). Programming requires knowledge of computer programming techniques and language(s), and a considerable amount of time. Because of the abilities required, the time involvement, and the availability of fourth-generation languages, programming is not recommended. If programming is selected, structured coursework in programming is a must.

General information on foodservice information systems may be found in the literature mentioned at the beginning of this chapter. In the 1980s, two major bibliographies[112,113] and a historical overview[114] were published. Information on how to design computer systems may be found in business and in computer science literature. Useful information may be accessed by completing a course on information systems, consulting business information systems textbooks, or reviewing popular microcomputing trade journals. If more technical details are required, use of computer science textbooks addressing specific software is recommended. Computer science research articles are not recommended because their high technical content will confuse the novice.

Summary of Completed Research

The tools and techniques used in foodservice information system research are numerous. The best way to get acquainted with what is used is to go through a brief historical review of the research completed in this area.

Early work on information systems for dietetics focused on methods for record keeping and accurate data collection.[115,116] The first reported foodservice computer systems, in the 1960s, were designed to execute routine, time-consuming tasks such as tallies,[117] food costing, and inventory control.[118] At the same time, researchers such as Balintfy,[119] Knickrehm,[120] and their co-workers developed quantitative models for better planning with information systems. Linear programming was applied to menu planning by Balintfy and co-workers[119] and queuing theories were used by Knickrehm and co-workers to plan a cafeteria line layout and dining room capacity.[50,120]

During the 1970s and 1980s, foodservice information systems were expanded to include major management functions such as inventory control, purchasing, production control, recipe adjustment, menu planning, meal counts, and nutritional analysis. The development of these systems required new quantitative models. As examples, sequencing[47,97] and forecasting models[121,122] were developed for food production scheduling systems. Forecasting models were also used for purchasing systems.[123,124]

In the 1980s, information systems went from batch systems to on-line or interactive systems.[125] Decision support systems used the interactive user-computer communication mode to provide greater analysis power to managers. A decision support system for foodservices was designed and implemented by Matthews, Norback, and Hicks.[126,127]

In the late 1980s, microcomputers made computerized information systems accessible to small facilities that were unable to afford the cost of mainframe computers. That was followed with an explosion of software available to dietitians at very affordable costs.

Illustration With Example

This example illustrates the tools and techniques that were combined to develop and implement a new information system for planning and control activities in foodservices.

Matthews and Norback developed their approach by combining foodservice principles with methods developed by managerial economics, accounting, mathematics, and information systems.[126] To better estimate the real cost of menu items, the concept of input-output was taken from managerial economics. The costing model came from the full cost accounting system: the cost of a menu item should include food and labor cost and a fair share of inventory, marketing, general, and administration costs.

To build the system, the researchers used a mathematical technique called a matrix data structure. This algebraic technique is an efficient method to organize and manipulate huge amounts of numerical data. By combining matrices, retrieval and transformation of data into information become rapid and convenient. The matrix structure also enables the integration of various pieces of data about the resources used. For example, matrices could quickly consolidate the data on quantity, price, and nutritive values for all ingredients in a recipe, or for all items in a menu.

The system was built with concepts of decision support systems (DSS). The main concept in DSS is that computer systems should help managers utilize data and mathematical models to solve unstructured problems: problems with no predetermined procedure to solve them. The key characteristic in DSS is an interactive computer-user interface that enables the manager to access all information directly, generate new reports, perform different mathematical analysis adapted to any specific situation, and do "what-if" analysis.

As described by Hicks, Matthews, and Norback, the system was implemented in an extended care facility and tested.[127] Using programming techniques and a programming language (Fortran), the system was developed and installed on a mainframe computer. Data from a long-term care facility consisting of a six-week menu cycle that included 983 menu items and 660 ingredients were entered into the system.

To evaluate the system, three unstructured problems were developed, based on typical situations faced by a foodservice dietitian. The three problems were solved using the computer system and a hand calculator. The computer system solved each problem, ten times faster than the hand calculator method. The authors also concluded that the computer system was able to handle unstructured problems.

The development part of this research illustrated to dietitians how foodservice management principles are applied to the conceptualization of an information system. It depicted the type of data entered and the information generated by a system using a conversational interaction mode. An efficient method to organize and manipulate data was also proposed. The implementation part provided information for dietitians on the benefits of using this foodservice information system.

CONCLUSION

As illustrated in this chapter, research in food production management and in foodservice information systems covers a very broad area and requires numerous tools and techniques. One does not need to master all these tools and techniques to undertake research, only those that apply in their specific area of foodservice research.

Coping with constant changes in foodservice systems will continue to be a major challenge for dietitians. The unique characteristics of foodservices, coupled with the diverse information needed for decision making about resource utilization, justifies the need for on-going research of both foodservice production and information systems. Although researchers and practitioners have their own special role, both need to work in a complementary manner to bridge gaps between research and practice in dietetics.

References

1. Spears MC. *Foodservice Organizations: A Managerial and Systems Approach.* 2nd ed. New York, NY: Macmillan Publishing Co; 1991.
2. West BB, Wood L, Harger VF, et al. *Foodservice in Institutions.* 6th ed. New York, NY: Macmillan Publishing Co; 1988.
3. Chase RB, Aquilano NJ. *Production and Operations Management: A Life Cycle Approach.* 5th ed. Homewood, Ill: Richard D Irwin Inc; 1989.
4. Stevenson WJ. *Production And Operations Management.* 3rd ed. Homewood, Ill: Richard D Irwin Inc; 1990.
5. Buffa ES, Dyer JS. *Management Science/Operations Research: Model Formulation and Solution Methods.* 2nd ed. New York, NY: John Wiley and Sons; 1981.
6. Hillier FS, Lieberman GS. *Introduction to Operations Research.* 5th ed. New York, NY: McGraw-Hill; 1990.
7. Halling JF, Lafferty LJ, Feller KS, eds. *Productivity Management for Nutrition Care.* Chicago, Ill: The American Dietetic Association; 1986.
8. Kazarian EA. *Work Analysis and Design For Hotels, Restaurants and Institutions.* Wesport, Conn: Avi Publishing Co; 1979.
9. Unklesbay N, Unklesbay K. *Energy Management in Foodservice.* Westport, Conn: Avi Publishing Co; 1982.
10. Burch J, Grudnitski G. *Information Systems: Theory and Practice.* 5th ed. New York, NY: John Wiley and Sons; 1989.
11. Hicks JO Jr. *Information Systems in Business: An Introduction.* 2nd ed. St Paul, Minn: West Publishing Co; 1990.
12. Kaud FA, ed. *Effective Computer Management in Food and Nutrition Services.* Rockville, Md: Aspen Publishers; 1989.
13. Pellegrino TW. *Selecting a Computer-assisted System for Volume Food Service.* Chicago, Ill: American Hospital Publishing Inc; 1986.
14. Kasavana ML. *Computer Systems For Foodservice Operations.* New York, NY: Van Nostrand Reinhold Co; 1984.
15. Association of Official Analytical Chemists. *Official Methods of Analysis of the Association of Official Analytical Chemists.* 15th ed. Washington, DC: Association of Official Analytical Chemists; 1990.
16. Speck ML, ed. *Compendium of Methods for the Microbiological Examination of Foods.* 2nd ed. Washington, DC: American Public Health Association; 1984.
17. Augustin J, Klein BP, Becker D, et al, eds. *Methods of Vitamin Assay.* 4th ed. New York, NY: John Wiley and Sons; 1985.
18. Stone H, Sidel JC. *Sensory Evaluation Practices.* Orlando, Fla: Academic Press; 1985.
19. Rush G. Job analysis of lunchroom and cafeteria management. *J Am Diet Assoc.* 1925;1:130–137.
20. Wheeler R. Standardization of institutional feeding. *J Am Diet Assoc.* 1926;2:6–9.
21. Denman I. Standardization trends in food administration. *J Am Diet Assoc.* 1931;7:95–109.
22. Smith GE. Controlling food cost through menu planning. *J Am Diet Assoc.* 1943;19:104–106.
23. Bradshaw TF. Institutional food cost control under wartime conditions. *J Am Diet Assoc.* 1943;19:413–415.
24. Enochs M, Yoder D. A comparative labor study of full-time and part-time employees. *J Am Diet Assoc.* 1932;8:56–60.
25. Western Washington Dietetic Association: A comparative study of amounts and costs of food and labor: report of administration section. *J Am Diet Assoc,* 1934;9:382–388.
26. Snyder PO, Matthews ME. Microbiological quality of foodservice menu items produced and stored by cook/chill, cook/freeze, cook/hot-hold and heat/serve methods. *J Food Protection.* 1984;47:876–885.

27. Black LC, Lewis MN. Effect on bacterial growth of various methods of cooling cooked foods. *J Am Diet Assoc.* 1948;24:399–404.

28. Longrée K, White JC. Cooling rates and bacterial growth in food prepared and stored in quantity. I. Broth and white sauce. *J Am Diet Assoc.* 1955;31:124–132.

29. Miller WA, Smull ML. Efficiency of cooling practices in preventing growth of micrococci. *J Am Diet Assoc.* 1955;31:469–473.

30. Wilkenson RJ, Mallman WL, Dawson LE, et al. Effective heat processing for the destruction of pathogenic bacteria in turkey rolls. *Poultry Sci.* 1964;44:131–136.

31. Woodburn M, Kim CH. Survival of *Clostridium perfrigens* during baking and holding of turkey stuffing. *Appl Microbiol.* 1966;14:914–920.

32. Strong DH, Repp NM. Effect of cookery and holding on hams and turkey rolls contaminated with *Clostridium perfrigens. Appl Microbiol.* 1967;15:1172–1179.

33. Thomas OM. Job analysis in institutional kitchen. *J Am Diet Assoc.* 1947;23:505–508.

34. Spickler JC. Work simplification as a tool of management. *J Am Diet Assoc.* 1948;24:598–600.

35. Rosa E. Work simplification—a tool in reducing food costs. *J Am Diet Assoc.* 1951;27:952–956.

36. Mundel ME. Motion study in food service. *J Am Diet Assoc.* 1956;32:546–547.

37. Bloetjes MK, Gottlieb R. Determining layout efficiency in the kitchen. *J Am Diet Assoc.* 1958;34:829–835.

38. Gottlieb R, Couch MA. Using cross chart in planning kitchen layouts. *J Am Diet Assoc.* 1960;36:585–592.

39. Wise BI, Donaldson B. Work sampling in the dietary department. *J Am Diet Assoc.* 1961;39:327–332.

40. Schell ML. Work sampling—an approach to a problem. *J Am Diet Assoc.* 1962;41:456–459.

41. Marteney AL, Ohlson MA. Work sampling of a dietary staff. *J Am Diet Assoc.* 1964;45:212–217.

42. Waldvogel CF, Ostenso GL. Master Standard Data Code: quantity food production labor time. *J Am Diet Assoc.* 1977;70:172–177.

43. Waldvogel CF, Ostenso GL. Labor time per portion and volume in foodservice. *J Am Diet Assoc.* 1977;70:178–181.

44. Zemel PC, Matthews ME. Master Standard Data quantity food production code: application to production of roast entrées under actual operating conditions in a hospital food service. *J Am Diet Assoc.* 1982;81:702–708.

45. Zemel PC, Matthews ME. Determining labor production time for roast entrées in hospital food services. *J Am Diet Assoc.* 1982;81:709–714.

46. Matthews ME, Waldvogel CF, Mahaffey MJ, et al. Master Standard Data quantity food production code: macro elements for synthesizing production labor time. *J Am Diet Assoc.* 1978;72:612–617.

47. Guley HM, Stinson JP. Computer simulation for production scheduling in a ready foods system. *J Am Diet Assoc.* 1980;76:482–487.

48. Stinson JP, Guley HM. Use of branch and bound algorithm to schedule food production in a semi-conventional food service system. *J Am Diet Assoc.* 1982;81:562–567.

49. Ostenso GL, Moy WA, Donaldson B. Developing a generalized cafeteria simulator. *J Am Diet Assoc.* 1965;46:379–383.

50. Knickrehm ME. Digital computer simulation in determining dining room seating capacity. *J Am Diet Assoc.* 1966;48:199–203.

51. McGary VE, Donaldson B. A model of a centralized tray assembly conveyor system for a hospital. I. Four strategic components. *J Am Diet Assoc.* 1969;55:366–371.

52. McGary VE, Donaldson B. A model of a centralized tray assembly conveyor system for a hospital. II. Station work content. *J Am Diet Assoc.* 1969;55:480–485.

53. Blondeau L, David BD. Choosing from alternatives in expanding storage space for frozen foods. *J Am Diet Assoc.* 1971;59:362–367.

54. Matthews ME, David BD. Effect of varying the number of entrée selections in the hospital menu. *J Am Diet Assoc.* 1971;59:575–581.

55. Barclay MJ, Hitchcock MJ. Energy consumption assessment in a conventional foodservice system. *J Foodserv Syst.* 1984;3:33–47.

56. Unklesbay NF, Brown NE, Matthews ME. Bentonite models simulate turkey rolls during convective heating. *J Am Diet Assoc.* 1988;88:928–931.

Key Techniques

57. McProud LM, David BD. Energy use and management in production of entrées in hospital food service systems. *J Am Diet Assoc.* 1982;81:145–151.

58. Thomas CJ, Brown NE. Use and cost of electricity for selected process specific to a hospital cook-chill/freeze food-production system. *J Foodserv Syst.* 1987; 4:159–169.

59. Biedrzycki K, Unklesbay N. Energy consumption during microwave reheating of turkey roll slices. *J Foodserv Syst.* 1988;5:1–11.

60. Quam ME, Fitzsimmons C, Godfrey RL. Ready-prepared vs. conventionally prepared foods. *J Am Diet Assoc.* 1967;50:196–200.

61. Cremer ML, Chipley JR. Satellite food-service system assessment in terms of time and temperature conditions and microbiological and sensory quality of spaghetti and chili. *J Food Sci.* 1977;42:225–229.

62. Cremer ML, Chipley JR. Time and temperature, microbiological, and sensory quality of meat loaf in a commissary foodservice system transporting heated food. *J Food Sci.* 1979;44:317–321, 326.

63. Snyder PO, Matthews ME. Effect of hot-holding on the nutritional quality of menu items in food service systems: a review. *School Food Serv Res Rev.* 1984;8:6–16.

64. Nicholanco S, Matthews ME. Quality of beef stew in a hospital chill foodservice system. *J Am Diet Assoc.* 1978;72:31–37.

65. Rollin JL, Matthews ME. Cook/chill foodservice systems: temperature histories of a cooked ground beef product during the chilling process. *J Food Protection.* 1977;40:782–784.

66. Brown NE, Bernard AI. Sensory and instrumental assessments of spaghetti and meat sauce subjected to three holding treatments. *J Am Diet Assoc.* 1988;88:1587–1588.

67. Sawyer CA, Naidu YM. Sensory evaluation of cook/chilled products reheated by conduction, convection, and microwave radiation. *J Foodserv Syst.* 1984;3:89–106.

68. Brown NE, Chyuan JYA. Convective heat processing of turkey roll: effects on sensory quality and energy usage. *J Am Diet Assoc.* 1987;87:1521–1525.

69. Brown NE, Moniz JC, Mohd-Jan A, et al. Effects of hot holding on spaghetti and meat sauce. *School Foodserv Res Rev.* 1987;11:20–24.

70. Snyder PO, Matthews ME. Percent retention of vitamin C in whipped potatoes after pre-service holding. *J Am Diet Assoc.* 1983;83:454–458.

71. Unklesbay NF, Brown NE, Matthews ME. Monitoring food temperatures during convective heating: implications for research procedures. *J Food Sci.* 1987;52:1438–1439.

72. Dahl CA, Matthews ME. Cook/chill foodservice system with a microwave oven: thiamin content in portions of beef loaf after microwave-heating. *J Food Sci.* 1980;45:608–612.

73. Bryan FL, Lyon JB. Critical control points of hospital foodservice operations. *J Food Protection.* 1984;47:950–963.

74. Greathouse KR, Gregoire MB. Variables related to selection of conventional, cook-chill, and cook-freeze systems. *J Am Diet Assoc.* 1988;88:476–478.

75. Greathouse KR, Gregoire MB, Spears MC, et al. Comparison of conventional, cook-chill, and cook-freeze foodservice systems. *J Am Diet Assoc.* 1989;89:1606–1611.

76. Bobeng BJ, David BD. HACCP models for quality control of entrée production in hospital foodservice systems. I. Development of hazard analysis critical control point models. *J Am Diet Assoc.* 1978;73:524–529.

77. Bobeng BJ, David BD. HACCP models for quality control of entrée production in hospital foodservice systems. II. Quality assessment of beef loaves utilizing HACCP models. *J Am Diet Assoc.* 1978;73:530–535.

78. Snyder OP. HACCP in the retail food industry. *Dairy Food Environ San.* 1991;11:73–81.

79. Hsieh J, Matthews ME. Energy use, time and product yield of turkey rolls at three oven loads and cooking temperatures in a convection oven. *J Foodserv Syst.* 1986;4:97–106.

80. Unklesbay NF, Maxcy RB, Knickrehm ME, et al. *Foodservice Systems: Product Flow and Microbial Quality and Safety of Foods.* Columbia, Mo: University of Missouri–Columbia, Agriculture Experiment Station; 1977. Research bulletin 1018.

81. Ridley SJ, Matthews ME. Temperature histories of menu items during meal assembly, distribution, and service in a hospital foodservice. *J Food Protection.* 1983;46:100–104.

82. Frakes EM, Arjmandi BH, Halling JF. Plate waste in a hospital cook-freeze production system. *J Am Diet Assoc.* 1986;86:941–942.

83. Carroll GH, Montag GM. Labor time comparison of a cook-freeze and a cook-serve system of food production. *J Can Diet Assoc.* 1979;40:39–45, 48–49.

84. Dahl-Sawyer CA, Jen JJ, Huang PD. Cook/chill foodservice systems with conduction, convection, and microwave reheat subsystems. Nutrient retention on beef loaf, potatoes, and peas. *J Food Sci.* 1982;47:1089–1095.

85. Cardello AV, Maller O, Kluter R. Multi-user assessment of a hospital cook-freeze foodservice system. *J Foodserv Syst.* 1984;3:153–169.

86. Boziuk JS. *Efficient Use of Modularization in Transportation Systems.* Natick, Mass: Army Natick Development Center; 1974.

87. Norback JP. Routing school food service vehicles: formal analysis for assistance in decision making. *School Foodserv Res Rev.* 1980;4:96–100.

88. Mann SH. The problem of distribution and transportation in a centralized food production facility. *J Hosp Educ.* 1976;1:44–56.

89. Lieux EM, Manning CK. Productivity in nutrition programs for the elderly that utilize an assembly-serve production system. *J Am Diet Assoc.* 1991;91:184–188.

90. Mayo CR, Olsen MD, Frary RB. Variables that affect productivity in school foodservices. *J Am Diet Assoc.* 1984;84:187–193.

91. Brown DM, Hoover LW. Productivity measurement in foodservice: past accomplishments—a future alternative. *J Am Diet Assoc.* 1990;90:973–981.

92. Maloney S, Zolber K, Burke K, et al. Work function analysis of vegetarian entrée production. *J Am Diet Assoc.* 1986;86:237–241.

93. Choi VLF, Roach FR, Konz SA. Occurence sampling in a residence hall foodservice: entrée production times. *J Am Diet Assoc.* 1986;86:1698–1701.

94. Zolber KK, Donaldson B. Distribution of work functions in hospital food systems. *J Am Diet Assoc.* 1970;56:39–45.

95. Matthews ME, Zardain MV, Mahaffey MJ. Labor time spent in foodservice activities in one hospital: a 12-year profile. *J Am Diet Assoc.* 1986;86:636–643.

96. Heinemeyer JM, Ostenso GL. Food production materials handling. *J Am Diet Assoc.* 1968;52:490–497.

97. Beach BL, Ostenso GL. Entrée serving time: relationship of serving time to system capacity. *J Am Diet Assoc.* 1969;54:290–296.

98. Lambert CU, Beach BL. Computerized scheduling for cook/freeze food production plans. *J Am Diet Assoc.* 1980;77:174–178.

99. Montag GM, Hullander EL. Quantitative inventory management. *J Am Diet Assoc.* 1971;59:356–361.

100. Allington JK, Matthews ME, Johnson NE. Methods for evaluating quality of meals and implications for school food service. *School Foodserv Res Rev.* 1981;5:68–73.

101. Klein BP, Matthews ME, Setser CS. *Foodservice Systems: Time and Temperature Effects on Food Quality.* Urbana, Ill: University of Illinois–Urbana, Agricultural Experiment Station; June 1984. North Central Regional Research publication 293.

102. Garey JG, Simko MD. Adherence to time and temperature standards and food acceptability. *J Am Diet Assoc.* 1987;87:1513–1520.

103. Unklesbay N. Monitoring for quality control in alternate foodservice systems. *J Am Diet Assoc.* 1977;71:423–428.

104. Brown NE, McKinley MM, Aryan KL, et al. Conditions, procedures, and practices affecting safety of food in 10 school food service systems with satellites. *School Foodserv Res Rev.* 1982;6:36–41.

105. Unklesbay N. Integration of energy data into food industry decision making. *Food Technol.* 1983;37(12):55–59, 110.

106. Unklesbay N. Overview and foodservice energy research: heat processing. *J Food Protection.* 1982;45:984–992.

107. Tuomi S, Matthews ME, Marth EH. Temperature and microbial flora of refrigerated ground beef gravy subjected to holding and heating as might occur in a school foodservice operation. *J Milk Food Technol.* 1974;37:457–462.

108. Tuomi S, Matthews ME, Marth EH. Behavior of *Clostridium perfrigens* in precooked chilled ground beef gravy during cooling, holding, and regeating. *J Milk Food Technol.* 1974;37:494–498.

109. Cremer ML. Sensory quality of turkey rolls roasted and held in an institutional convection oven with and without chilled storage. *J Food Sci.* 1986;51:868–872.

110. Unklesbay N, Unklesbay K. Energy expended in alternate foodservice systems for chicken menu items. *J Am Diet Assoc.* 1978;73:20–26.

111. Hussain D, Hussain KM. *Information Processing Systems for Management.* Homewood, Ill: Richard D Irwin Inc; 1981.

112. Orta J. *Computer Applications in Nutrition and Dietetics: An Annotated Bibliography.* New York, NY: Garland Publishers; 1988.

113. Hoover LW. *Computers in Nutrition, Dietetics and Foodservice Management: A Bibliography.* 3rd ed. Columbia, Mo: Curators of the University of Missouri; 1981.

114. Youngwirth J. The evolution of computers in dietetics: a review. *J Am Diet Assoc.* 1983;82:62–67.

115. McAuley MF. Food control and the food ledger. *J Am Diet Assoc.* 1934;10:1–11.

116. Radell NH. Food control records. *J Am Diet Assoc.* 1936;11:528–535.

117. Lowder W, Medill C. Punch cards simplify selective menus. *Modern Hosp.* 1958;9(1):102, 104, 106.

118. Andrews JT, Tuthill BH. Computer-based management of dietary departments. *Hospitals.* 1968;42(July 16):117–123.

119. Balintfy JL, Nebel E. Experiments with computer assisted menu planning. *Hospitals.* 1966;40(June 16):88–96.

120. Knickrehm ME, Hoffmann TR, Donaldson B. Digital computer simulations of a cafeteria service line. *J Am Diet Assoc.* 1963;43:203–208.

121. Wood SD. A model for statistical forecasting of menu item demand. *J Am Diet Assoc.* 1977;70:254–259.

122. Messersmith AN, Moore AN, Hoover LW. A multi-echelon menu item forecasting system for hospitals. *J Am Diet Assoc.* 1978;72:509–515.

123. Webster DB, Drogan RA, Wingard RM, et al. A systems model for food purchasing. *J Am Diet Assoc.* 1981;78:255–260.

124. Wilcox MM, Moore AM, Hoover LW. Automated purchasing: forecasts to determine stock levels and print orders. *J Am Diet Assoc.* 1978;73:400–405.

125. Hoover LW, Waller AL, Rastkar A, et al. Development of on-line real-time menu management system. *J Am Diet Assoc.* 1982;80:46–52.

126. Matthews ME, Norback JP. A new approach to the design of information systems for foodservice management in health care facilities. *J Am Diet Assoc.* 1984;84:675–678.

127. Hicks ZR, Matthews ME, Norback JP. A computer-based decision support system aids distribution in planning and control of foodservices. *J Am Diet Assoc.* 1986;86:1182–1188.

128. Bender JR, Matthews ME. Computer systems in food services: a review of applications and potential benefits. *School Foodserv Res Rev.* 1989;13:150–156.

129. Sawyer CA. Computers in food service. *School Foodserv Res Rev.* 1986;10:128–135.

130. McCool AC, Garand MM. Computer technology in institutional foodservice. *J Am Diet Assoc.* 1986;86:48–56.

131. Kim SAL, Matthews ME. Needs for computer systems and software available for school food services. *School Foodserv Res Rev.* 1990;14:38–41.

132. Perkin JE, Kauwell GPA. A survey of computer education in coordinated undergraduate programs. *J Am Diet Assoc.* 1989;89:1500–1502.

133. Miller JL. Survey of computer technology in foodservice management education. *J Am Diet Assoc.* 1989;89:1279–1281.

134. Galloway ME, Kraus G. A computerized food management system for an extended care unit. *J Can Diet Assoc.* 1983;44:347–357.

135. Fowler KD. Evaluating foodservice software: a suggested approach. *J Am Diet Assoc.* 1986;86:1224–1227.

136. Bender JR, Matthews ME. Development of an evaluation model for computer foodservice management systems. *J Am Diet Assoc.* 1989;89:1465–1472.

137. Armstrong RD, Balintfy JL, Sinha P. The conceptual foundation of computerized food management information systems. *J Foodserv Syst.* 1982;2:47–58.

138. Snyder OP. A computerized flow chart system for food production. *J Foodserv Syst.* 1983;2:211–228.
139. Stinson JP, Guley HM. Use of microcomputer to determine direct costs of menu items. *J Am Diet Assoc.* 1988;88:586–590.
140. Gelpi MJ, Balintfy JL, Dennis LC, et al. Integrated nutrition and food cost control by computer. *J Am Diet Assoc.* 1972;61:637–646.
141. Anderson AL, Moore AN, Hoover LW. Development of an automated form generating system for menu item data. *J Am Diet Assoc.* 1977;71:124–128.
142. Chiang SF, Matthews ME, Norback JP. Methodology for incorporating nutritive values of prepared ingredients into matrices for foodservice decision-making. *J Foodserv Syst.* 1988;5:13–27.
143. Lopez-Soriano EM, Matthews ME, Norback JP. Improving the flow of customers in a hospital cafeteria. *J Am Diet Assoc.* 1981;79:683–688.
144. Balintfy JL, Jarret K, Paige F, et al. Comparison of type A-constrained and RDA-constrained school lunch planning computer models. *School Foodserv Res Rev.* 1980;4:54–62.

15. OPERATIONS AND HUMAN RESOURCE MANAGEMENT IN FOODSERVICE

Judy L. Miller, PhD, RD, and Mary B. Gregoire, PhD, RD

Spears[1] describes foodservice operations as open systems. Inputs into this system include human, material, operational, and facility resources. Foodservice managers are critical to ensuring that these resources are used effectively to produce outputs such as meals, clientele satisfaction, financial accountability, and personnel satisfaction. Research on mathematical techniques, investment and profit analysis, and human resource management can help foodservice managers achieve a more effective operation. The purpose of this chapter is to review foodservice management research literature and identify appropriate methods for research in management in dietetics.

IMPORTANCE OF MATHEMATICAL TECHNIQUES IN FOODSERVICE OPERATIONS AND RESEARCH

Mathematical techniques used in foodservice operations include many that have been used in business and industry. Terms often used to identify these concepts include *operations research*, *management science*, *quantitative approach*, *systems analysis*, and *operations analysis*. Techniques that have been used in operational applications in foodservice or in similar operations include linear programming, forecasting models, econometric models, and decision models. All of these terms and techniques represent quantitative approaches or tools to assist in management decision making.

The concept of mathematical techniques is important to foodservice operations because it enables the manager to make improved decisions and therefore manage scarce resources more effectively and efficiently. As resources become more limited and accountability increases, dietitians must have the tools to manage effectively and compete with others who may be interested in managing foodservice operations. Although the concepts are mathematical in nature, they are simple when approached in a step-by-step manner. The success of the management dietitian and survival in the management arena is dependent on utilization of the best tools available.

The opportunities for research applications in foodservice management are limitless. The ability to complete successful projects exists among practitioners and the outcomes represent tools for improved management. As dietitians develop research projects to accomplish desired outcomes, the projects often will result in improved management practice.

Discussion of these concepts in the *Journal of The American Dietetic Association* (JADA) has taken place since 1937.[2] Between 1945 and 1975, exploration of management science techniques were reported,[3] with food production and service applications as the main focus. Simulation models, queuing techniques, statistical forecasting, and linear programming appeared in this early literature.[4–7] Since 1976, the volume of literature appearing in JADA related to quantitative techniques has increased, reflecting growing interest among dietetics professionals. Computer technology has contributed to this increased utilization of quantitative applications.[8–15]

Practitioners can be involved in research that develops dietetic applications in quantitative management because it is critical to progress at the operational level. Academic researchers and graduate students can work with practitioners in operations to develop projects. Practitioners have the requisite background to apply these techniques and to structure projects in a way that contributes to the body of literature. Where academic programs exist, undergraduate and graduate students can reach out to operations for projects that contribute to improved management practice.

Research Using Quantitative Techniques Applied to Management Practice

The practitioner should first peruse the literature related to the particular topic. Brown and Hoover[3] provide an excellent reference and discussion of quantitative management techniques. Further review of management literature[16,17] could include research reported in journals or techniques discussed in operations management research textbooks often used in business production management courses. Review of other related management literature will provide the practitioner with examples of applications that involve similar operational problems. Many of the techniques previously tested in foodservice have been borrowed from other business applications.

The practitioner needs to have a level of comfort with mathematical and statistical techniques. If this was not accomplished in either the undergraduate program or subsequent experience or course work, the dietitian may want to consider self-study or structured course work approaches to become familiar with the techniques and jargon. The concepts are not difficult; they simply require a frame of reference if projects are to be completed successfully. Some of the management literature referenced in many of the articles appearing in the *Journal* are very readable and will help the practitioner gain confidence in pursuing these research studies.[18,19] Survey, case study, and experimental research methods can be used in these areas of research. Many project designs would be analytical or case study. Surveys of tools being used by practitioners have been completed in some areas. Exploring techniques used and updating past surveys would provide needed information.

To assist the practitioner in initiating research using mathematical or quantitative techniques, the following example is presented. Miller and associates[20] completed a study that utilized mathematical techniques to forecast food production (menu item demand) in a residence hall foodservice. Data were retrieved from residence hall foodservice production sheets and organized according to date of service, meal periods, time periods served, amounts served and forecast. Then they were plotted and analyzed for consideration of appropriate methods. Statistical analysis of the data enabled the researchers to adjust the data to permit better forecasts. The data then were used to forecast future meal period demand using mathematical forecasting models. Simple models have been found to be as effective as more complex models and are easily understood and applied to foodservice operation problems. Therefore, simple mathematical models were used to forecast menu item demand. These forecasts then were compared with past and future forecasts to evaluate the effectiveness of the models. Statistical procedures and other observational techniques can be used to evaluate model effectiveness.

IMPORTANCE OF INVESTMENT DECISION AND PROFIT ANALYSIS IN FOODSERVICE OPERATIONS AND RESEARCH

Investment decision and profit analysis techniques have been used in foodservice operations and other similar business and industry applications. The level of sophistication may vary but the basic concepts have been included in undergraduate and graduate dietetic curricula for many years. Among the terms one finds when discussing these concepts are: *return on investment* (ROI), *pay-back period*, *net present value* (NPV), *break-even analysis*, and various *cost/benefit*, *cost control*, and *cost analysis strategies*. Some of these concepts relate to direct operational management on an ongoing basis, while others represent capital budgeting techniques used primarily when major purchase decisions are made. All of these methods, often discussed in finance and accounting textbooks, represent tools to assist the dietitian in management decision making.

As resources are increasingly limited in their availability, the dietitian must be equipped to manage effectively and produce positive bottom-line results. Administrators are increasingly conscious of bottom line as a performance indicator for dietetic departments or foodservice operations of any type. The management dietitian must be able to justify all decisions in all areas of practice, including clinical, to the administration based on fiscally responsible practice. This means that these concepts are increasingly important tools for the dietitian to comprehend and utilize. These tools are straightforward, requiring only basic math skills, and a knowledge of the available tools.

The opportunities for applications are limitless as the management dietitian confronts daily and strategic decisions that impact cost accountability and fiscal management. Practitioners, having had basic coursework in food cost accounting, can use knowledge earlier acquired coupled with newly acquired knowledge gained from readily available finance and accounting resources. As dietitians develop projects, both operations and the body of literature resulting from the research will be enhanced.

Articles exploring cost issues appeared in JADA as early as 1926.[21] Numerous other studies have been reported since that time.[22-27] Examples also proliferate in the accounting and finance literature. Hospital administration literature is another source of related information. Textbooks discuss the concepts and provide examples that can become the basis for research projects.

Practitioners can become involved with research in the areas related to cost accountability, assuming that it impacts the survival of the department or foodservice operation. Having control of the numbers means that the dietitian can be more creative in solving problems related to revenue generation, cost accountability, and a positive bottom line. Virtually every cost-related problem encountered by the practitioner could become a research project if properly structured. By using this approach, the practitioner improves the performance of the operation while contributing to the body of literature from which others may profit. To compete with external forces that threaten departmental management, sound fiscal policies, based on quality information, are the best tools available to the practitioner. Perceiving cost-related problems as opportunities to excel in managing the foodservice will result in a stronger profession. Practitioners have the requisite background to succeed in this area. However, if assistance is needed, self-study guides, published examples, and graduate course work will help build confidence to pursue these strategies.

Research Using Cost Techniques

Research in the area of investment decision, profit analysis, or any cost-related functional area, as in any other research, should be preceded by perusal of the literature related to the particular topic of interest. Brown and Hoover[3] provide an excellent review of management-related articles that have appeared in JADA throughout the history of the publication. Articles range from basic discussion to research application. Further review of finance and accounting or hospital administration literature will provide a sound base for initiating the research effort. The review of other related management literature will provide the practitioner with examples of applications that involve similar operational problems. Many of the techniques previously tested have been borrowed from other business applications.

A level of comfort with mathematical and statistical techniques is required for research in this area. If this was not accomplished in either the undergraduate program or in subsequent experience or course work, the dietitian may want to consider self-study or structured course work to become familiar with the techniques and jargon. The concepts are not difficult, but simply require a frame of reference if projects are to be completed successfully. Many of the articles appearing in JADA and other accounting and finance literature and textbooks are very readable and will enable the practitioner to gain confidence in pursuing these research studies.

Documentary, survey, and experimental designs can be used. Operations projects probably would be classified as descriptive or analytical. Surveys have been conducted to assess current practice. Replications and newer applications could provide important information.

To assist the practitioner in initiating research using cost analysis tools, the following example is presented. Greathouse and associates[28] completed a study that compared financial data in three types of foodservices. A questionnaire was developed for collecting operational data, and financial information was obtained from the Health Care Financing Administration (HCFA). Four financial variables were created from these data for foodservice types, and costs in the different foodservice types were compared. Regression analysis was used to develop models for predicting financial variables using operational information such as full-time equivalents. Results of the study potentially could enable foodservice directors to predict operating costs for their systems.

IMPORTANCE OF RESEARCH IN HUMAN RESOURCE MANAGEMENT

One of the primary inputs into the foodservice system is human resources. Foodservice managers are responsible for achieving an organization's goals through its human resources, and understanding human behavior in the work environment is critical to effective foodservice operation. Increasing labor costs and a dwindling labor pool make human resource management an even greater challenge for foodservice managers.

Productivity, satisfaction, and *effectiveness* are terms commonly linked with human resource management. Productivity can be defined as the output achieved by an individual or group; satisfaction is the feeling an individual has about his or her work; and effectiveness is the degree to which an organization's goals are met. Foodservice managers are challenged to improve employee satisfaction and productivity and perform as effective managers. Research results can suggest effective ways for foodservice managers to improve productivity, satisfaction, and effectiveness.

Productivity Research

Foodservice managers interested in the output level of their staff often conduct research on productivity. Data for productivity studies is collected by stopwatch timing, occurrence sampling, or self-reports of time spent.

Heberlein[29] observed the time spent performing perpetual and physical inventory activities in a small hospital, using a stopwatch to time each activity. Data from her study provided information to the foodservice director for scheduling labor for the inventory functions. The cost of manually performing the inventory functions was calculated and used in the financial feasibility study of computerizing the inventory functions of the department. Although such timing of activities provides valuable data on the amount of time spent on various activities, it requires an observer to be watching and recording activity continuously.

A more commonly used technique for collecting productivity data is occurrence sampling, which involves observing behavior at predetermined intervals. The activity being performed at the time of the observation is recorded. These observations then are converted to a percentage of total activities, eg, 50 observations of cleaning activities of a total 1000 observations would suggest that 5% of an employee's time was spent performing cleaning activities. Estimates of time spent on activities then are made based on the percentage of time in each activity, ie, if an employee works an eight-hour shift, approximately 25 minutes of their time would be spent on cleaning. Block and associates[30] used this technique to determine cleaning times for selected vegetables. Choi et al[31] used occurrence sampling to determine time spent in direct work, indirect work, and delay time for entree production. Both of their studies were done in single operations and provided valuable information for managers who scheduled labor in those operations.

Lieux and Manning[32] observed workers in eight senior centers at five-minute intervals and recorded labor activities performed. By collecting information in several operations, their results on minutes spent per meal performing various activities such as service, processing, and cleaning provided useful information for managers scheduling labor in similar operations.

An example of a research project using self-reports of time spent is the work by Thies and Matthews.[33] In their study, consultant dietitians were asked in a questionnaire to estimate the time they spent performing selected functions. Results of their study could be used by current and prospective consultant dietitians to estimate the amount of time required for consulting activities.

Job Satisfaction Research

Research in the area of organizational behavior has explored the issue of job satisfaction in employees. Results of several research projects suggest that an employee's level of job satisfaction may affect his or her performance. Research in this area usually has involved administration of a standardized test such as the Job Diagnostic Survey (JDS) developed by Hackman and Oldham[34] or the Job Characteristics Inventory (JCI) developed by Sims et al.[35]

Several authors have explored the job satisfaction of foodservice employees. Hopkins and colleagues[36] focused their work on the satisfaction and work values of school foodservice personnel. Calbeck and associates[37] examined the work-related values and satisfaction of professional and nonprofessional hospital dietetic department personnel. Agriesti-Johnson and Broski[38] reported on-the-job satisfaction of dietitians. Dude and Sneed[39] studied the relationship between job characteristics and job satisfaction of university foodservice managers and employees. Kuntz et al[40] explored the relationship of educational background and job satisfaction of university foodservice managers. Each of these studies had participants complete a instrument, such at the JDS, to provide information on job satisfaction. Results of these studies provide foodservice managers with useful information on how to improve the satisfaction of employees.

Effectiveness Research

Effectiveness of management practice research has focused on several issues. The skills and abilities of the manager have been explored to determine what a manager does. The effectiveness of a foodservice operation has been examined using criteria such as accuracy of trays and satisfaction of patients. Data for effectiveness research usually is collected by having participants complete a questionnaire, or by observation of employee performance.

Management practice. The role of managers has been examined in various types of foodservice operations. Palacio and associates[41,42] explored whether the managerial roles identified by Mintzberg,[43] were characteristic of hospital clinical and administrative dietitians. In the Palacio study,[41] a questionnaire was developed and sent to dietitians in three organizational levels (lower, middle, and upper) and two practice areas (administrative and clinical) in hospitals with 300 or more beds. Dietitians were asked to indicate the importance and time demand of 81 activities.[42] Sultemeier and colleagues[44] used the instrument developed by Palacio and co-workers[41] to examine the managerial characteristics of college and university foodservice managers. Both studies provide information for educators and practitioners on the importance of managerial roles in dietetic practice and the amount of time being spent on such activities.

Yakes et al[45] surveyed hospital administrators to determine the competencies required of health care foodservice managers. They then requested information from dietetic educators on the degree of training provided on these same competencies. Dowling and associates[46] obtained information from hospital foodservice directors, hospital administrators, and foodservice management educators on the credentials and skills needed for a hospital food and nutrition department director. Results of research such as these provide dietetic educators with information to prepare students for practice and provide practitioners who are interested in foodservice management positions with information about the requirements and expectations of such positions.

Foodservice operations. Another major area of foodservice management research has been the evaluation of foodservice operations. Such work has focused on assessing the acceptability, quality, and accuracy of the food provided to patients and clients.

Glover and Keane[47] observed food items placed on patient trays and documented critical and general errors as a way to determine accuracy of hospital food service. Dowling and Cotner[48] developed a tray error monitoring system that quantified evidence of patient tray error and indicated the seriousness of these errors. Both studies are examples of quality control techniques that could be implemented by hospital management dietitians.

Patient or client acceptance of meals has been the focus of several projects. Cash and Khan[49] asked patients to complete a questionnaire to determine factors that affected their consumption of entree items. Harris and associates[50] had congregate program participants and managers complete a questionnaire to help determine perceptions of meal quality, meal acceptance, and program administration. Oldford[51] developed a questionnaire for measuring several components of hospital patients' satisfaction with foodservice. Having clients evaluate the food and service they received provides foodservice managers with information on how to continually improve their operation.

FUTURE RESEARCH IN MANY AREAS OF HUMAN RESOURCE MANAGEMENT

Future research is especially critical in quantitative areas of foodservice management practice. Due to the imperative for informed decision making, operations management techniques must be applied to foodservice problems if dietitians are to keep pace with management in other business and industry sectors.

Academicians, graduate students, and practitioners must work together to develop models and applications to serve management dietitians. With increasing accountability, the need for productivity and sound resource management are paramount. Fiscal responsibility, utilizing state-of-the-art financial management and accounting techniques is imperative.

As the labor pool of younger workers declines, more research is needed on effectiveness of various retention techniques. New labor markets, such as older workers and the handicapped, should be explained. Additional research is needed to determine factors that influence workers to choose their jobs, what benefits they expect, what type of training they need, and how managers should be prepared to work with them.

Service quality has become a major issue in commercial foodservice. Research is needed to clarify what service means in institutional foodservice management, how the trait of service orientation is developed in employees, and the relationship between having service-oriented employees and the quality of service provided.

SUMMARY

Foodservice management research can provide valuable information for practice, yet such research is limited. The objective of this chapter is to suggest techniques that can be used to conduct research in the area of human resource management. An increase in the publication of such research is a desired result. Operations, investment decision, and profit analysis research are primarily quantitative. Survey methods may be used to assess the status, while quantitative methods often will be required to conduct research. Research provides a systematic, objective way to establish, defend, or change beliefs about human resource management. Data for human resource management research usually is collected through observation of practice or completion of questionnaires by managers or employees. Foodservice management practitioners can use methods developed by others to examine concerns in their own operation.

References

1. Spears MC. *Foodservice Organizations: A Managerial and Systems Approach.* 2nd ed. New York, NY: Macmillan Publishing Co; 1991.
2. Dodge QO. Where administrators come from. *J Am Diet Assoc.* 1937;13:130–138.

3. Brown DM, Hoover LW. Quantitative management techniques in dietetics: improving practice through technology transfer. *J Am Diet Assoc.* 1988; 88:1567–1575.

4. Knickrehm ME, Hoffman TR, Donaldson, B. Digital computer simulations of a cafeteria service line. *J Am Diet Assoc.* 1963;43:203–208.

5. Blaker G, Donaldson B. Systems analysis—a tool for management. *J Am Diet Assoc.* 1969;55:121–126.

6. Mitchell ML. Production management in today's kitchen. *J Am Diet Assoc.* 1947;23:25–30.

7. Hoover LW, Moore AN. An educational model simulating computer-assisted dietetics: "Dietetic COM-PAK." *J Am Diet Assoc.* 1974;64:500–504.

8. Tienor CA, Donaldson B. A dietary department applies procedure for developing a demand forecasting system. *J Am Diet Assoc.* 1976;68:460–462.

9. Mackle M, David BD. Developing a demand forecasting system. *J Am Diet Assoc.* 1976;68:457–460.

10. Wood SD. A model for statistical forecasting of menu item demand. *J Am Diet Assoc.* 1977;70:254–259.

11. Messersmith AM, Moore AN, Hoover LW. A multi-echelon menu item forecasting system for hospitals. *J Am Diet Assoc.* 1978;72:509–515.

12. Matthews ME, Waldvogel CF, Mahaffey MJ, Zemel PC. Food production relationships between entrée combinations and forecasted demand. *J Am Diet Assoc.* 1978;72:618–621.

13. Stinson JP and Guley HM. Use of a branch and bound algorithm to schedule food production in a semi-conventional foodservice system. *J Am Diet Assoc.* 1982;81:562–567.

14. Miller JL, Shanklin CW. Forecasting menu-item demand in foodservice operations, *J Am Diet Assoc.* 1988;88:443–449.

15. Finley DH, Kim IY. Use of selected management science techniques in health care foodservice systems. *J Foodserv Syst.* 1986;4:1–16.

16. Armstrong JS. Research on forecasting: a quarter-century review, 1960–1984. *Interfaces.* 1986;16:77–89.

17. Gardner ES, Dannenbring DJ. Forecasting with exponential smoothing: some guidelines for model statistics. *Decision Sci.* 1980;11:370–383.

18. Wheelwright SC, Makridakis S. *Forecasting Methods for Management.* 3rd ed. New York, NY: John Wiley and Sons; 1980.

19. Simon JL. *Basic Research Methods in Social Science.* 2nd ed. New York, NY: Random House; 1978.

20. Miller JL, Thompson PA, Mahler M. Forecasting in foodservice: model development, testing and evaluation. *J Am Diet Assoc.* 1991;91:569–574.

21. Wheeler R, Moe V. An economic analysis of hospital food bills. *J Am Diet Assoc.* 1926;2:28–34.

22. Gillam SM. Labor organization, labor turnover, and food costs in the hospital dietary department for the year 1927–1928. *J Am Diet Assoc.* 1928;4:133–141.

23. Report of administrative section, Western Washington Dietetic Association: a comparative study of amounts and costs of food and labor. *J Am Diet Assoc.* 1934;9:382–388.

24. Brodner J. Institution food accounting and control problems. *J Am Diet Assoc.* 1941;17:771–777.

25. Sigmond R. Problems of fiscal control in hospital foodservices. *J Am Diet Assoc.* 1953;29:779.

26. Olsen MD. Obtaining meaningful cost information in dietary departments. II. Labor cost information. *J Am Diet Assoc.* 1975;67:55–59.

27. Tuthill BH. Dietitians use computer assistance to contain costs. *J Am Diet Assoc.* 1980;76:479–482.

28. Greathouse KR, Gregoire MB, Spears MC, Richards V, Nassar RF: Comparison of conventional, cook-chill, and cook-freeze foodservice systems. *J Am Diet Assoc.* 1989;89:1606–1611.

29. Heberlein E. *Determination of Time Spent Manually Performing Foodservice Inventory Activities in a Small Community Hospital.* Manhattan, Kan: Kansas State University, 1989. Thesis.

30. Block AA, Roach FR, Konz SA. Occurrence sampling in a residence hall foodservice: cleaning times for selected vegetables. *J Am Diet Assoc.* 1985;85:206–209.

Key Techniques

31. Choi VL, Roach FR, and Konz S.A.: Occurrence sampling in a residence hall food-service: entree production times. *J Am Diet Assoc.* 1986;86:1698–1701.
32. Lieux EM, Manning CK. Productivity in nutrition programs for the elderly that utilize an assembly-serve production system. *J Am Diet Assoc.* 1991;91:184–188.
33. Thies M, Matthews ME. Time spent in state-recommended functions by consultant dietitians in Wisconsin skilled nursing facilities. *J Am Diet Assoc.* 1991;91:52–56.
34. Hackman JR, Oldham GR. Development of the job diagnostic survey. *J Appl Psychol.* 1975;60:159–169.
35. Sims HP, Szilagiy AD, Keller RT. The measurement of job characteristics. *Acad Manage J.* 1976;19:195–203.
36. Hopkins DE, Vaden AG, Vaden RE. Some determinants of work performance in foodservice systems: job satisfaction and work values of school foodservice personnel. *J Am Diet Assoc.* 1979;75:640–647.
37. Calbeck DC, Vaden AG, Vaden RE. Work-related values and satisfactions. A cross-occupational analysis of professionals vs. nonprofessionals in hospital dietetic services. *J Am Diet Assoc.* 1978;75:434–440.
38. Agriesti-Johnson C, Broski D. Job satisfaction of dietitians in the United States. *J Am Diet Assoc.* 1982;81:555–559.
39. Dude KM, Sneed J. Research model for relating job characteristics to job satisfaction of university foodservice employees. *J Am Diet Assoc.* 1989;89:1087–1091.
40. Kuntz KA, Borja ME, Loftus MK. The effect of education on foodservice manager job satisfaction. *J Am Diet Assoc.* 1990;90:1398–1401.
41. Palacio JP, Spears MC, Vaden AG, Dayton AD. The effect of organizational level and practice area on managerial work in hospital dietetic services. *J Am Diet Assoc.* 1985;85:799–805.
42. Palacio JP, Spears MC, Vaden AG, Downey RG. Dimensions of managerial work in hospital dietetic services. *J Am Diet Assoc.* 1985;85:809–815.
43. Mintzberg H. *The Nature of Managerial Work.* New York, NY: Harper and Row Publishers Inc; 1973.
44. Sultemeier PM, Gregoire MB, Spears MC, and Downey R. Managerial functions of college and university foodservice managers. *J Am Diet Assoc.* 1989;89:924–928.
45. Yakes SC, Shanklin CW, Gorman MA. Competence of foodservice director/managers required in health care operations. *J Am Diet Assoc.* 1987; 87:1636–1639.
46. Dowling RA, Lafferty LJ, McCurley M. Credentials and skills required for hospital food and nutrition department directors. *J Am Diet Assoc.* 1990;90:1535–1540.
47. Glover NS, Keane TM. Examining the accuracy of foodservice in a hospital setting. *J Am Diet Assoc.* 1984;84:1018–1029.
48. Dowling RA, Cotner CG. Monitor of tray rates for quality control. *J Am Diet Assoc.* 1988;88:450–453.
49. Cash E, Kahn MA. An assessment of factors affecting consumption of entree items by hospitals. *J Am Diet Assoc.* 1985;85:350–352.
50. Harris LJ, Hodges PA, Johnson JM, Shifflet PA. Comparing participants' and managers' perception of services in a congregate meal program. *J Am Diet Assoc.* 1987;87:190–195.
51. Oldford C. Patients' Satisfaction With Foodservice: Development of a Validated Taxonomy and Measurement Tool. New York, NY: New York University; 1989. Dissertation.

16. COST-EFFECTIVENESS AND COST-BENEFIT ANALYSES: RESEARCH TO SUPPORT PRACTICE

Doris D. Disbrow, DrPH, RD, and Rebecca A. Dowling, PhD, RD

Cost-effectiveness and cost-benefit analyses continue to be important tools for nutrition practitioners as dietetic services are used to improve the health of Americans. These services are both effective and much less costly than many currently used methods of treatment and rehabilitation, but research is needed to substantiate this observation.[1]

The purpose of this paper is to provide the theoretical background on cost-effectiveness and cost-benefit analyses. The Ross Roundtable Report[2] is used to organize the research steps necessary to apply these analyses to dietetic services in a variety of practice settings. Two case studies are presented as examples that may be used as models. However, dietitians must keep in mind that each study has unique features and that there is no perfect model that can be copied directly.

ECONOMIC ANALYSES

There are never enough resources to provide all of the health services known to be beneficial, and difficult choices have to be made. The purpose of cost-effectiveness and cost-benefit analyses is to assist in these resource allocation decisions. These two forms of economic analysis can be used to compare the contributions made by dietetic services with the resources required to produce them. In other words, economic analysis, or cost-effectiveness analysis (CEA) and cost-benefit analysis (CBA) measure the pros (the effects and benefits) and cons (the costs) of a particular type of service. They may be applied to a national program, using the societal perspective; to a selected group of people, using a payer's analysis; or to a specific setting using the organizational perspective.

CEA and CBA were developed for application to public investments made by governments.[3,4] The proliferation of these studies in health care is a reflection of the concern of government officials over the cost of health care in the United States. Thirty years ago, federal, state, and local governments paid about 25% of these costs; today they pay more than 40%.[3,5] The concerns for access and quality care as a means to improve the health of the population are addressed through the analysis of effectiveness, whereas concerns about government expenditures are reflected in analysis of cost.

Cost-Effectiveness Analysis

CEA compares two or more alternatives to achieve the same objective[3,6]; therefore, CEA is useful when the outcomes of the care are the same. A nutrition alternative may be compared with another treatment method when both are expected to have the same result. For example, with the objective to reduce serum cholesterol, dietetic services might be compared with medications. Or one process of nutrition care delivery could be compared with another, such as personal counseling versus using videotapes to educate clients. The CEA case study compares two approaches intended to reduce the high cholesterol risk factor: screening and referral to customary medical care and screening and a worksite intervention.

The measurement of effect in cost-effectiveness studies is expressed in units of outcome, because the outcomes are the same in the different approaches being studied. Therefore, the effect of each approach is measured with appropriate clinical indicators, such as weight changes and laboratory values. An example of cost-effectiveness was provided by Splett and associates[7] when they presented their results in "costs per successful outcome." The outcome used was the weight gain of pregnant women and the alternative methods studied were nutrition care provided in two different settings. At a city health department, the cost-effectiveness was $231 for each woman's achieving her recommended weight gain, compared with $170 per woman at a county hospital. The researchers discussed the cost differences in light of the process of care at both sites.

Cost-Benefit Analysis

CBA is an extension of CEA because it not only measures the effects, but also places a dollar value on these outcomes.[6] The cost of the service is measured in the same way; the difference is in the expression of the outcomes. CBA may be used when the outcomes being compared are different. A hypothetical example is a comparison of dietetic services with physical therapy for Medicare beneficiaries. All would agree that both are important services for the elderly, but the intended effects are different and a direct comparison of cost and outcome is inappropriate. CBA compares the cost and the dollar value of the outcome for one service with those for the other. The results of this type of research often are used to negotiate the amount to invest in both services to achieve the greatest value for the consumer group.

The CBA case study cited at the end of the chapter would have been a CEA if the cost had been compared with the indicators of hematopoietic recovery or survival. However, it is a CBA because dollar values are assigned to the effectiveness measures. (Because the CEA and CBA case studies given in appendix 1 and 2 are referred to throughout this chapter, the reader might wish to scan them before proceeding.)

USING COST-BENEFIT AND COST-EFFECTIVENESS IN DIETETICS

Dietitians can use the information provided by CBA and CEA with department managers and organization administrators, with insurance company representatives and benefit managers of corporations, with government planners and evaluators, with legislators and other elected officials, as well as in making decisions about their own practices. The efforts to collect and analyze the information usually pay off in many more ways than were anticipated.

The results of CEA can assist dietitians when making decisions about the best way to deliver nutrition services. It can identify the method of delivery that gives the desired or best outcome for the least cost. The data needed for cost-effectiveness analysis may be available through quality assurance activities and productivity information acquired for different purposes. Quality assurance criteria spell out the desired outcomes of service,[8] which, when measured, produce the effectiveness information. On the other side of the equation, productivity studies contribute a major portion of the information needed for the cost side.

Figure 16.1 is a conceptual model that shows the relationship of dietetic practice and economic benefits.[9] The model begins with the delivery of dietetic service, which is anticipated to lead to measurable changes in health behaviors. The recipients of the service would be expected to have improved clinical indicators as signs of reduced risk factors. The anticipation of better health status is expected to slow the progression of the disease, and ultimately produce economic benefits for the individual, the health care industry, and society at large. This model provides a good framework for dietitians to use when developing research on the effectiveness and benefits of nutrition care.

Figure 16.1
Expanded model for measuring the benefits of nutritional care. Adapted from Olendsky MC, Tolpin, HG, Buckley, EL.[9]

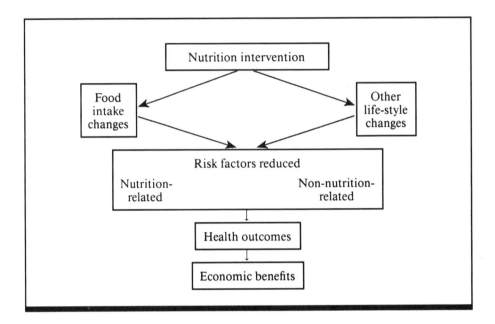

Research Questions

Research begins with questions for which answers are sought. Answers may be found in the literature, and questions may evolve from these previous works.[10-12] Questions to be answered as part of cost-benefit and cost-effectiveness research are:

1. Do dietetic services prevent the onset of illness? How much and in which illnesses?
2. Do dietetic services decrease the severity of illness? How much and in what illnesses?
3. Do dietetic services decrease the duration of illness? How much and in what illnesses?
4. Do dietetic services improve rehabilitation from treatment and illness?
5. Do dietetic services result in improved quality of life?
6. What is the value of the improvement?
7. What are the components of effective care?
8. How much do dietetic services cost?
9. Which method of nutrition care is most cost-effective?
10. Given several effective programs designed to achieve the same health outcome, do dietetic services deliver the outcome at less cost?
11. Does the dietetic service deliver a greater level of outcome than other services at the equivalent cost?
12. Are dietetic services an efficient use of resources when compared to its alternatives?

Key Techniques

Effectiveness is addressed by questions 1 through 5, while 6 attaches a dollar value to any health improvements measured. Question 7 describes the process used to deliver nutrition care. Question 8 provides the cost of the service, and 9 through 12 answer the efficiency concerns.

The term *dietetic services* is intentionally used in these questions to reflect the role of the dietitian as the provider. Nutrition services are provided by an array of businesses and health professionals, but the research needed is the cost and the effect of nutrition care provided by dietitians. Dietitians can best define, deliver, evaluate, and interpret the contributions made by dietetic services.[13]

Research Design

CEA and CBA research may be conducted prospectively or retrospectively. Prospective research is carried out from the present into the future. The advantages are the ability to control for confounding factors and potential bias, and as a result, a prospective study is a more powerful design. The disadvantage is the high amount of the dietitian's time required to complete client care and fulfill the research protocols as well. For example, completion of research forms may be necessary at the same time documentation is placed in the client's record. This doubles the paperwork and slows the dietitian in accomplishing the work of the day. Both case studies described at the end of the chapter used a prospective design.

Retrospective research is conducted in the present and looks into the past. This is a less powerful design because many confounding variables cannot be controlled. When this approach is used in patient care, the medical record is often the source of information. Interruption in the dietitian's practice is minimal because another person usually carries out the research protocol. This person could be a student, a nutrition assistant, or a volunteer who is trained to review the records and complete the data collection forms. The retrospective approach requires complete and consistent documentation, which may be a barrier for this research design.[14,15]

The Decision-Makers

The first consideration when planning an economic analysis is to anticipate which decision-makers will use the results.[16] In the CEA case study cited at the end of the chapter, the employer was interested because the disability costs from heart disease had been rising. Health promotion program directors and benefits managers also could use the results to justify work site programs. The CBA example was designed for hospital administrators and department managers. Clinical dietitians and physicians may also find the results useful as they strive to provide quality care in the cost-containment environment. Information about the nutrition implications of the problem and the dietitian's role are relevant to the decision-makers with whom the results will be used.[3,6,17]

People who make decisions about the use of resources are most interested in those areas where the greatest expenditures are made. Health problems with a high incidence and relatively small treatment cost, such as the common cold, are important because the total cost to society is great. Likewise, a medical problem with low incidence and a high treatment cost, such as the various types of cancer, will get attention.[18] In either case, the savings achieved through the reduction of medical care costs will be of interest to decision-makers.

There are three groups of decision-makers: people who use information to plan national and state policies for society, managers within organizations, and individual consumers. All use economic information, but need different data.[2,3] For example, when giving attention to nutrition services for hospitalized elders, the planner considering the inclusion of nutrition services in the Medicare payment system uses different pieces of information than the hospital administrator.

The Medicare analyst wants assurance that dietetic services are safe, effective, accepted by the medical community, appropriate, available, and cost-effective.[19] This planner is interested in dietitians' care if they save Medicare expenses by reducing the number of other procedures required for treatment for a large segment of the elderly.

The hospital administrator, as the recipient of Medicare moneys, is interested in the effect nutrition services will have on the length of stay, especially for those conditions for which the number of days extend beyond the amount of the pre-established payment. This person's concern is the effect of nutrition services on the hospital's finances.

Consumers want the best quality care as well as the smallest out-of-pocket payments. If dietitians can demonstrate the value of nutrition services to the public, the request for dietetic services will increase and influence the planners and administrators. The differences in the economic perspectives of the various decision-makers are outlined in the Ross Roundtable Report.[2]

PROCEDURES TO CONDUCT CBA AND CEA RESEARCH IN NUTRITION PRACTICE

Identify the Target Audience

The client group to be studied depends on the questions asked. Economic studies may focus on a specific medical problem; the health status of a particular group of people, or the efficient use of technology.[17] Specific medical problems may be defined as individual diseases or symptoms with a nutrition treatment, such as diabetes or high blood pressure. Pregnant women have been studied to show how dietetic services bring about improvement in their health status and pregnancy outcome.[7,20] A study, on the other hand, may focus on the improvement in the efficiency with which dietetic services are provided.

Calculate the Benefits

Before benefits can be measured, the objectives of the dietetic service must be elucidated and the anticipated health improvements specified. Assurance that the nutrition care is delivered consistently and based on standardized protocols is important to enable a description of the process by which benefits are achieved.[14]

Objectives must be reliable, understandable, specific, measurable, and achievable.[21] They may be the same as the outcome criteria established for quality assurance activities.[8] Objectives of a dietetic service need to be related to the health outcomes anticipated (reduced illness), or the intermediate outcomes,[17] such as weight changes and blood indices, that are associated with reduced illness and improved health status. Intermediate outcomes must be chosen carefully to ensure a relationship with the desired ultimate health outcome, such as improved health status, disease prevented, or deaths averted.[6]

When the efficiency of new protocols is to be studied, time needs to be allowed for staff development before a study begins. Baseline data may be collected under one process of delivering a service, then staff members must have time to become proficient in the new method of delivery before the study data are collected.

Type of analysis. Once the objectives of the service and the study have been determined, the next decision is the type of economic analysis to apply. It could be a CEA or a CBA; in addition, the best use of the research might come from presenting the results in both ways. The needs of the decision-makers who are expected to use the research must be considered when making this determination.

Expressions of benefits. For CEA, the benefits are the degree of effect the intervention has on the desired outcomes. The amount of weight loss from a weight management program, the percentage reduction in cholesterol, and the number of people with diabetes who improve their blood glucose levels are examples. Dollar values are not placed on these effects as they are in CBA.

Direct benefits. Economists classify benefits as direct, indirect, and intangible[3,22] when a CBA is conducted. Direct benefits are the expenditures that would otherwise have been spent on health care had dietetic services not been effective. It is expected that people who improve their health status through better nutrition practices after receiving care from a dietitian will use less of other medical services, and therefore, save resources. For example, Orstead and associates[20] calculated the number of low-birthweight babies that would have been born if nutrition services had not been expanded. The direct dollar benefit was the money saved from the reduction in neonatal intensive care days due to fewer low-birthweight babies. In the fire fighter case study described later, the fire district expected direct benefits from reduced heart disease treatment expenditures.

Direct benefits represent all types of health resources that are not spent; put in other terms, they represent resources that are saved because of the nutrition intervention. As in the Orstead study,[20] the resources may be saved in hospital care. But savings also may be measured in other areas, such as personnel, outpatient care, diagnostic tests, laboratory tests, medications, and other treatments. When Davidson and co-workers[23] demonstrated improved blood sugar control by changing the way dietetic services were provided for people with diabetes, one benefit was the reduction in insulin usage. Direct benefits also accrue to individuals; people with better nutritional status may, for example, save out-of-pocket expenses by reducing medication.

Indirect benefits. Indirect benefits of nutrition care are improvements in the quality of life. These benefits may be measures of well-being as well as an increased ability to carry out the daily tasks of living. Improvements in work attendance and performance are frequently used as proxies for improved health status. They are the savings of the indirect costs that have been estimated as part of the burden of illness.[17,18,24] These are measured in the National Health Interview Survey and are useful when assessing the indirect benefits of health care to consumers and to society.

Intangible benefits. Improvements in the quality of life also represent important benefits that cannot be expressed in dollar terms. These intangible benefits are very real to the people who experience them and contribute to the decision-making process. Intangible benefits express subjective well-being, improved mobility, and the avoidance of pain and suffering.[3,17] The reduced number of insulin shots reported by Davidson and colleagues[23] were intangible benefits for their clients. All decision-makers can understand improvement in the quality of life when people need fewer injections.

All payers are interested in direct benefits because they want to reduce their expenditures. Insurance companies began to pay for diabetes education in Maine when the savings in hospital costs were demonstrated.[25] However, payers and organization administrators are less concerned about indirect benefits and intangibles because they do not produce specific dollar savings for the sponsor. All three categories of benefits may occur in the same situation, but indirect and intangible benefits are not measured as frequently as direct benefits.

Anticipated benefits. Once the objectives of the service are defined and the type of analysis has been decided upon, the effect or benefit anticipated from the dietetic services can be identified. Then the research method to measure the benefits can be determined.

To determine the benefit of a new service or new protocol for delivering dietetic services, comparison information is needed. The strongest research design is the controlled experiment, which randomizes the clients into at least two groups: one that receives the dietetic service under study and one that does not (see chapters 8 and 9). In situations where clinical trials are not feasible, a carefully constructed quasi-experimental design may be used successfully.[13,26] It is important for a comparison group to be identified through standard research methodology. This will strengthen the results and therefore the usefulness of the economic analysis.

When conducting research in hospitals, seasonal variations of illness and deaths must be considered.[27] It may be necessary to collect baseline data one year prior to the experimental data, or to study two groups with the same diagnosis during the same study period, to control for this confounding factor.

Data need to be collected on all of the potential variables that could confound the results of the effectiveness of dietary change. For example, age, ethnicity, socioeconomic status, smoking, and alcohol habits may have an effect on the outcome of medical care, so this information has to be included to demonstrate that the health improvement was indeed related to the nutrition care. If the groups are selected randomly or matched on the key variables, there should be no statistical difference between the comparison and experimental groups in these descriptive variables. This allows the findings to be correlated to the service and diminish the problems of confounding and statistical interaction, which can lead to spurious results.

Expression of benefits. Benefits, or effects, in CEA are expressed in units of the desired outcome. Two methods for achieving the same objective are compared and the units are the same, so it is not necessary to value them in dollar terms.[6] In the CEA case study, the effectiveness measure was the total serum cholesterol level. In this example, the effectiveness was measured by the degree to which this biochemical value changed in each alternative under study. For this reason, CEA is easier to carry out.

For economic analyses, data that are measured, as well as data that are estimated may be used. The effect of dietetic services may be measured, but the value of that effect to society, third-party payers, or an organization may be estimated by using data from other sources. For a societal perspective in CBA, information collected by the federal government through national studies is often used. The National Center for Health Statistics conducts the National

Health Survey and publishes the results on a regular basis through the Vital and Health Statistics series. It might be useful to compare the length of stay of a group of patients receiving special dietetic services with that reported for the same diagnosis in the national study, and estimate the benefit from the potential cost savings if a shorter length of stay is found in the group receiving the special services. The benefits are expressed in dollar terms in CBA so they can be directly compared with the costs. The CBA case study provides an example of using measured data.

As mentioned earlier, intangible benefits may be identified, but not measured. These benefits are important to the consumers and, depending on the perspective, may be of interest to the decision-maker. A legislator considering a Medicare or Medicaid reimbursement policy, for instance, would be interested to know that the constituents' quality of life has improved through a reduction in pain or an increased ability to move and care for themselves. The Medicare administrator, however, would not find this information as useful because it has no impact on the direct costs of the Medicare program.

Calculate the Costs

Identify the costs. The costs of providing the service are, like benefits, categorized into: direct, indirect, and intangible.[3,22] They can be considered the "flip side of the coin" from the benefits. The researcher decides which costs to measure, based on the information needed by the decision-maker who will use the results.

Direct costs. Direct costs are the expenditures attributed to wages for all personnel (including administrative), fringe benefits, materials, space, travel, training, lab tests, equipment and computers, accounting and legal services, advertising, and all other operational costs of the service.[2,3,17,22,28,29] Direct costs may be increased by side effects and complications; for example, parenteral nutrition therapy has been associated with increased rates of infection and complications.[30–34] The cost of treating the problems associated with any treatment modality needs to be included in the cost calculations for both CEA and CBA.

Time studies may be necessary to assess the appropriate costs for personnel.[28] Data from productivity studies carried out in the organization may be appropriate as measures of the time allotted to specific activities. Other costs are measured by the amount used for the nutrition care. The time various pieces of equipment are in use for the service being studied is noted. The number of lab tests required and educational pieces used would be recorded as costs.

In economics, everything has a value; nothing is free. Opportunity costs are associated with everything. An opportunity cost is the value that would have been gained if resources had been used for the next best alternative. For example, public funds applied to drug treatments are not available for nutrition services. The opportunity cost for drug treatments is the value that could have been gained from the dietetic services had the money been applied to nutrition. Time is a cost, for example, when a dietitian volunteers to conduct a healthy-heart class and is not paid. During that period, other services, such as counseling for clients with diabetes, cannot be offered. The opportunity cost for the healthy-heart class is equivalent to the value of the time lost to the diabetes program.

Direct costs may be required of recipients of nutrition care as well as providers. Consumers have direct costs when they pay for special dietary products or supplements as a part of carrying out the directions to achieve the health benefit. In following recommendations from a cholesterol education program, the client may purchase oat bran and substitute canola oil for a less-expensive product. The cost of the oat bran is a direct cost, as is the increased expenditure for the oil used in food preparation.

Indirect costs. The value of consumers' time and expenditures associated with receiving the service are additional important costs. Time costs, including time waiting for a service to begin, travel costs, and child-care costs all are potential indirect costs to clients and are very important to the people receiving the service.[3,6] These costs are very influential in decisions to keep appointments and to adhere to the treatment prescription. The perspective of the study determines whether or not these indirect costs are included in the analysis.

Intangible costs. The fear, grief, worry or pain of the treatment experienced by consumers and their family members are intangible costs. These costs are difficult to measure and even more difficult to value in dollar terms, but they are very real to the client and his or her family. The intangible cost of breast cancer treatment is evident. Maintaining nutritional status during the treatment phase may reduce the intangible costs to the patient and her family. The loss of a loved one is a major intangible cost of fatal heart attacks. All illnesses and treatments have intangible costs, but they are rarely addressed.[29,35] They may be very influential pieces of information for decision-makers, however.

Once costs are identified and the units of cost are measured, the appropriate dollar values can then be assigned. Wages are frequently used to value indirect costs, and in spite of the potential inequities for women, minorities, and youth, are considered by economists to be the best measure of value. Wages must be used with caution and acknowledgment that indirect costs may be underestimated for some groups and overestimated for others.[3,6]

Evaluate the Results

The expression of results varies with the type of analysis and the information to be presented. The usefulness of the results may increase if both CEA and CBA are used.

Presenting cost-effectiveness results. CEA provides the cost for each desired outcome. Therefore, it is important to present first the expected health improvement from the service. Health improvements from dietetic services may best be expressed as intermediate outcomes, those that are indicators of health status such as weight for height, laboratory values, complication rates, and levels of function. The results are then presented as the cost per unit of outcome achieved. For example, in the CEA case study presented later, the chosen outcome variable was lowered blood cholesterol as an intermediary for preventing coronary artery disease. The cost-effectiveness results: for alternative I, screening and the intervention, $6.75 for each percent decrease in the mean cholesterol. For alternative II, screening and referral to customary medical care, it was $25.56 for no reduction in serum cholesterol.

Presenting cost-benefit results. A ratio is traditionally used to express the results of CBA research. It may be a cost-benefit ratio in which the cost is presented first, or a benefit-cost ratio in which the first expression is the benefit value.

$$\text{Cost-benefit ratio} = \frac{\text{Cost in dollars}}{\text{Benefit in dollars}} = 1:3$$

$$\text{Benefit-cost ratio} = \frac{\text{Benefit in dollars}}{\text{Cost in dollars}} = 3:1$$

In the CBA case study cited at the end of the chapter, the cost-benefit ratio is 1:3.5, and is expressed as "For every dollar spent, there were $3.50 of benefit." These same results may be given as a benefit-cost ratio, 3.5:1. This would be stated as "$3.50 of benefit were achieved for each dollar spent." One way of expressing the results is not better than the other. However, it is important that the numbers be consistent with the terms. To reverse them would be embarrassing and damaging to the dietitian's credibility.

Net benefits. It is important when presenting the results of CBA to include the net benefits or net costs. These dollar differences between the cost and the benefits allow the magnitude of the results to be considered, whereas presenting only the ratio conceals the size of the dollar value. For example, benefits of $3 million dollars gained from an expenditure of $1 million results in a 1:3 cost-benefit ratio. This same ratio can reflect benefits of $3000 and a cost of $1000. Although the ratio is the same, the first project would be far more important because of its greater size.

When the results are complete, nutrition practitioners need to interpret the findings and make recommendations for action. Dietitians are in the best position to explain the meaning of the analysis and the conclusions.

Other Concepts

Discounting, the changing value of money over time, sensitivity analysis, and ethical issues are important concepts that need to be considered as a part of carrying out an analysis. They also are not to be overlooked when reviewing cost-effective and cost-benefit studies others have prepared, as the ultimate results may be affected.

Discounting. Discounting adjusts for the preference people have for immediate consumption over future consumption.[3] People prefer to have $10 000 now than wait for ten years to receive it. The saying "a bird in the hand is worth two in the bush" reflects the essence of this preference.[6] If money is invested in a service now, people prefer to have the benefits immediately rather than in five years. People want immediate results and to have the money saved now rather than in the future. The discounting procedure needs to be applied whenever the period for the expenditure differs from the time when benefits occur. The purpose of discounting is to adjust the time periods of both to the present for comparison with other ways in which the money currently may be used.

Discounting is important when the costs and the benefits are expressed in different periods. If a healthy-heart program is begun this year for 10-year-old schoolchildren with the expectation of reducing the morbidity and mortality from heart disease when they are 50-year-old adults, the money spent now is of higher preference to society than the savings in 40 years. Because people place greater importance on money they have for spending or investing now than what will be available in the future, the social value of $10 000 now is greater than $10 000 in the future, and the two are not comparable. An adjustment must be made to make them comparable for the purpose of analysis. The rule of thumb says an analyst should apply discounting to any study when the time difference between investment and benefit is greater than one year. Both case studies described later measured effects or benefits within one year of the expenditures for the service; therefore, discounting was not carried out in either. This is an important concept for nutrition programs intended to prevent future health problems.

The formula for discounting[3,22,29] is:

$$PVC/B = C/B_0 + \frac{C/B_1}{(1+r)} + \frac{C/B_2}{(1+r)^2} + \ldots + \frac{C/B_n}{(1+r)^n}$$

where PVC/B = present value of costs or benefits
C/B_0 = dollar value of costs or benefits during the immediate period
C/B_1 = dollar value of costs or benefits during the first year
C/B_2 = dollar value of costs or benefits during the second year
C/B_n = dollar value of costs or benefits during each subsequent year until the end of the expenditures or the last year benefits are expected to accrue
r = the discount rate

"Present value tables" in microeconomic text books and on computer spreadsheet software programs simplify the process of discounting. The analyst, however, must choose the discount rate with care to avoid introducing bias into the results.

When presenting the results of a study to decision-makers, it is better to provide information using several different discount rates. These rates may vary between 2% and 10%.[6] If a low rate is used, the value of long-term costs and benefits is increased, whereas a higher discount rate increases the value of short-term costs and benefits. The rate is chosen by the analyst; hence, it is possible to manipulate the results to favor the long term, or the short term. Therefore, at a minimum, the middle of the range, or a 5% rate, is suggested.[6] It would be best, however, to carry out discounting at a low, middle, and high rate and present the results from all three calculations to decision-makers.[3,6]

Adjusting for the changing value of money. Discounting adjusts for the human preference for dollars spent and saved now rather than for those spent and saved in the future. A second type of adjustment, that of accounting for inflation, is often confused with discounting. This provides for the difference in the value of the dollar during different periods.[3,4,6] The appropriate consumer price index for the years included in the study allows the correction to be made.

The Consumer Price Index reflects the average change in prices of defined goods and services over specified periods. The US Department of Labor collects prices of selected items each month at multiple sites across the country. These are reported monthly by the Bureau of Labor Statistics in the "Consumer Price Index Detailed Report," and summarized annually in "Statistical Abstracts of the United States." The indices for food and beverages and medical care are especially useful for evaluating dietetic services.

The Consumer Price Index is important when the research is conducted over a period of years and inflation is known to have been a factor in the value of the dollar. Baseline data may have been collected during one year and compared with results attained years later.[20,23] When this occurs, the study is strengthened by expressing the costs and the dollar values of the benefits in constant dollars, such as those of current prices by using the Consumer Price Index to adjust for the inflation factors. According to Warner and Luce,[3] it is best to recalculate these dollar values before discounting is applied. This adjustment was not necessary in the case studies presented in this chapter because the period of both studies was short with little, if any, inflation.

Sensitivity analysis. Once the analysis has been done, it is important to analyze the sensitivity of the conclusions. Sensitivity analysis is the reanalysis of the data using different estimates for any assumptions that may be questioned. It informs the analyst and decision-makers of the degree to which specific assumptions affect the results. If the first results of the study change, the degree to which any factor influences the outcome is known. On the other hand, greater confidence can be placed in the results if the findings are supported by the repeated analyses.[3,6]

Questions will arise about the assumptions and aspects of the methodology in every CEA and CBA; therefore, dietitians need to identify the potential areas for questioning and attempt to recalculate the results using other estimates. For example, if personnel costs are based on the time needed to provide nutrition care, and the times are estimated, rather than measured, it may be appropriate to reanalyze the data using other time factors. If, for example, the maximum time needed to provide the service is used in the calculation, the sensitivity analysis would require reanalyzing the data using the midpoint and the minimum of the time range. The information from all of the analyses would be presented to the decision-maker. In this case, a manager could use this information as time boundaries when making judgments about the personnel to be included in nutrition care.

All major assumptions that might have an impact on the results need to be considered for reanalysis. The rates chosen for discounting and the wages used to value the indirect benefits of improved health are examples of important assumptions to be included in the sensitivity analysis. Reanalysis is not difficult; with a spreadsheet software program, the numbers for the second analysis can be substituted for those used in the first, and the computer quickly recalculates the results.

Sensitivity analysis could be applied to the cost-benefit case study at the end of the chapter. Perhaps the hospital has two different units where bone marrow transplant patients may receive care, and the cost per hospital day is $700 in one unit and $1000 in the other. The calculations would be repeated using $1000 in place of $700, and both results reported for consideration by the decision-makers.

Ethical issues. Ethical issues also need to be considered, and if any are identified, they need to be interpreted for the decision-maker. Keep in mind that many people who may use the report are planners or policy analysts who have no nutrition training. The ethical issues related to dietetic services must be brought to the forefront for inclusion in the review of the results. Two ethical issues in nutrition services have been discussed in the literature. One is the decision to use or withhold special products that have not been demonstrated to be effective in specific types of cases, such as total parenteral nutrition.[34-36] Equal access to dietetic services for all clientele is the second. Is it ethical that those who need repeated nutrition appointments for adequate treatment, such as clients with diabetes, cannot have the services because they lack the money to pay?

When an ethical issue, such as equal access to care for low-income people, is incorporated into the objectives of the CEA or CBA, an attempt should be made to measure and value the issue. When appropriate to the analysis, the ethical issues should be identified and discussed, even if it is not possible to measure or place a dollar value on them.[17] An example would be a study of the use of nutrition support; some people who need it do not receive it because of reimbursement questions or the policies of the care setting.[34,37]

Recommendations Based on Results

Once the results are known, and the sensitivity to the various assumptions have been tested, recommendations should be made to the decision-makers who will be using the information. Dietitians are the nutrition care experts; therefore, they know how to interpret the results and apply the conclusions to practice. It is appropriate and crucial for dietetic practitioners to make recommendations about nutrition care based on the results. It cannot be assumed that decision-makers understand the significance of the results on dietetic practice. It means taking a risk,[38] the investigator's sticking his or her neck out, giving the study a much greater chance to influence the decision-maker.

The results can also be used to review the delivery of dietetic services and to improve the efficiency of quality care. Clinical nutrition managers benefit from the identification of areas in which quality assurance standards are not being reached or the patients' health outcomes could be achieved with fewer inputs. The results will support the changes in practice necessary to make dietetic services more effective and efficient.

Every study has limitations that must be acknowledged. For example, the CBA case study described later found a three-day difference in the length of stay, but this finding was not statistically significant. As indicated in the case study, this can make an important difference financially, but it could have occurred by chance and could not be generalized to other groups of patients. Dietitians can use this information carefully to promote dietetic care if the results are used with integrity and the recognition that more research in the area will be needed.

CONCLUSION

Dietetic practitioners in all practice settings can work to contribute to the knowledge about the effectiveness and efficiency of nutrition care. CEA is recommended because it has fewer methodologic difficulties than CBA. Using data collected for quality assurance purposes can ease the burden of conducting CEA. Dietitians with management responsibilities can facilitate these activities by allocating time for staff to spend on planning, conducting, and reporting these projects.

Studies may be small and carried out in one facility, or they can be carried out with collaboration from several locations; all will add to the information needed to refine, improve, and market nutrition care. The results need to be shared through professional meetings and publications. It is up to dietitians to conduct the research and make the results available to the administrators, planners, regulators, legislators, and third-party payers who need this information to justify decisions to allocate resources to nutrition care. By working with these policy-makers, dietitians will learn about their different perspectives and, therefore, their data needs.

Evaluating the effectiveness of dietetic services is difficult and challenging. It is easier to evaluate the effectiveness of a medication because it involves measuring the differences between an experimental group that takes the drug and a control group that does not. There are many confounding factors in nutrition care research. The study must be designed carefully and the appropriate methodologies used. The better the study, the more valuable the results will be to the profession and to individual decision-makers. However, no study is perfect; there are always caveats. Dietitians need to go forward with cost-benefit and cost-effectiveness research, in spite of these limitations.

CEA and CBA are not the panacea for the dietetics profession. They are tools to provide more information about nutrition care. If used wisely, these tools will enable dietitians to continue to improve their service, increase their visibility with payers, and make progress in providing nutrition services that will have greater impact on the health of the public.

APPENDIX 1: CEA CASE STUDY

A prospective study was conducted to evaluate the effectiveness of a worksite nutrition intervention program designed to lower total serum cholesterol levels.* The target population was a group of 450 professional firefighters, all of whom participated in the worksite program. Of the 450, 52 men with elevated cholesterol volunteered to be in an experimental group for the study. The comparison group was 44 male volunteers from adjacent fire department districts.

Protocol

A three-phase intervention program was delivered to 450 firefighters. Phase I included a lipid screening and height and weight measurements. A questionnaire was also administered to collect information on diagnoses, medication use, family history of coronary heart disease (CHD), dietary practices, and so forth. In phase II, the treatment phase, dietitians interpreted lab results for each participant and provided an individualized behavior change plan based on those results. Phase II also included a variety of educational sessions, cooking demonstrations, and exercise prescriptions. Classes were 2.5 hours, each with 20 to 25 participants.

Phase III was the evaluation phase. A six-month follow-up lipid panel was completed. The lab results were reviewed and individual progress toward meeting specific goals was discussed. Motivational materials were provided to encourage continued compliance after completion of the program. The comparison group had the lipid panel analysis at the beginning and end of the project. They did not participate in the intervention program.

Results

Experimental group. At the six-month follow-up, the mean percentage change in total serum cholesterol for the 52 men in the experimental group was

*The authors appreciate the contribution made by Karen Bertram, MPH, RD

The CEA research was supported by funds from the Zellmer Trust Fund, California Dietetic Association.

a 10.4% decrease. Forty-five of the 52 men in this group (86.5%) had decreased their total serum cholesterol. The mean decrease for the 45 men was 32 mg/dL, with a range of 3 to 79 mg/dL.

Comparison group. Six of the 44 volunteers in the comparison group were lost to follow-up; repeat lipid panel analyses were completed on 38 men. Although serum cholesterol had decreased for 14 men, the mean percentage change in total serum cholesterol for the comparison group during the follow-up period was a 4.9% increase.

Benefit Analysis	Subtotal	Total

Identify the target audience.
The target audience was professional firefighters from one district. A random sample showed 60% to be at increased risk for CHD, based on blood lipid evaluation.

Calculate the benefits.
A. Specific benefits of the program: 10.4% decrease in total serum cholesterol.
B. Total dollar value of benefit: Not assigned a dollar value for cost-effectiveness.

Calculate the costs per participant.
A. *Alternative I*: Screening plus intervention (n = 52)
  1. Personnel time
     - RD—program development, administrative activities: 0.07 hours
     - RD—teaching, development of classes and individualized treatment plans: 0.74 hours
     - Nutrition assistant—teaching, counseling, blood draws: 0.74 hours
     - Clerical—typing, filing: 0.32 hours
  2. Hourly cost for each type of personnel
     - RD—$21.60/hour ($18.00/hour + 20% fringe benefits)
     - Nutrition Assistant—$13.20/hour ($11.00/hour + 20% fringe benefits)
     - Clerical—$6.60/hour ($5.50/hour + 20% fringe benefits)
  3. Personnel cost per participant per type of personnel
     - RD (program development, administrative activities)—$21.60/hour × 0.07 hours = $1.51
     - RD (teaching, treatment plans)—$21.60/hour × 0.74 hours = $15.98
     - Nutrition assistant—$13.20/hour × 0.74 hours = $9.77
     - Clerical—$6.60/hour × 0.32 hours = $2.11
  4. **Total personnel costs per participant** $29.37
  5. Costs of materials and supplies per participant
     - 2 blood analyses/participant × $11.00 = $22.00
     - Assessment forms = $0.27
     - Education materials = $1.67
     - Supplies = $0.27
     - Computer time and software = $3.44

	Subtotal	Total

Administrative costs per participant
- Travel= $0.33
- Advertising = $0.24
- Office space and equipment = $12.64

6. **Total material, supply and administrative costs per participant** — $40.86

7. **Total direct costs per participant** (personnel + materials/supplies and administrative costs) — $70.23
8. Calculate indirect costs per participant — 0.00
   Data on indirect costs were not collected for this study.
9. **Total costs per articipant** — **$70.23**

B. *Alternative II:* Screening with referral to standard medical care (n = 38). Since this group did not receive any intervention, the only costs are for the lipid analyses completed at the beginning and end of the project.
   1. Personnel time *per participant*
      - Nutrition assistant (blood draws)—0.27 hours
   2. Hourly cost for each type of personnel
      - Nutrition assistant—$13.20/hour ($11.00/hour + 20% fringe benefits)
   3. **Total personnel cost per participant**
      - Nutrition assistant—$13.20/hour × 0.27 — $ 3.56
   4. **Total cost of materials and supplies per participant**
      - 2 blood analyses/participant × $11.00 — $22.00
   5. **Total costs per comparison group participant** — **$25.56**

Evaluate the results	Results

A. *Alternative I:* Screening plus intervention (n = 52)
   1. Identify benefit
      10.4% mean decrease in total cholesterol
   2. Identify cost
      $70.23 per participant
   3. Express as ratio of cost per effect
      It cost $70.23 per participant to achieve 10.4% mean decrease in total cholesterol. This could also be expressed as $6.75 per each 1% decrease. — $70.23 per 10.4% decrease

B. *Alternative II:* Screening with referral to standard medical care (n = 38)
   1. Identify benefit
      There was no benefit. Participants had mean *increase* in total serum cholesterol of 4.9%.
   2. Identify cost
      $25.56 per participant.
   3. Express as ratio of cost per effect
      It cost $25.56 per participant yet no reduction in serum cholesterol was achieved. — $25.56 per no decrease

The worksite intervention program was effective in achieving the goal of reduction in serum cholesterol and, theoretically, reducing the risk of the participants for CHD. The results support the use of screening plus cholesterol education interventions by an RD when compared with cholesterol screening with no education.

Discussion of the Case Study

The experimental group (n = 52), all with elevated cholesterol, was self-selected, not assigned randomly to the group. Therefore, they were not necessarily representative of the total group of firefighters.

The results of the screening plus intervention study can be used to promote the continuation and expansion of this worksite program. Other fire districts as well as other public employee groups such as police and bus drivers would be obvious prospective clients. The trend toward self-insurance by large corporations also creates a growing opportunity for the marketing of this program and the value of the RD. The data would also be of interest to HMOs, which are structured to control health care costs by prevention of disease. With additional information, the study results could provide a basis for a cost-benefit study. Documenting the CHD-related health care costs for experimental and comparison group participants over time may reveal differences between the groups that would further support the value of the RD, as well as this type of intervention.

APPENDIX 2: CBA CASE STUDY

A prospective, randomized clinical trial was conducted by Szeluga and associates to compare the effectiveness of two methods of nutrition support for bone marrow transplant (BMT) recipients: total parenteral nutrition (TPN) and an individualized enteral feeding program (EFP), which included specially prepared high-protein snacks and/or tube feeding.[39] At the time of the study, parenteral nutrition was the common feeding modality for BMT recipients. The two feeding methods were compared for their effectiveness in preserving body composition and for clinical outcomes, including frequency of catheter-related complications, medication use, abnormalities in serum chemistries, rate of bone marrow recovery, length of hospitalization, survival, and costs. (See reference 39 for full protocol and outcome data.)

The goal of the study was to provide clinical decision-makers with data required to select a primary treatment protocol for BMT recipients in this specific institution. A secondary goal was to provide the hospital administrator with data regarding resources required to provide nutrition care for BMT recipients. The results also would be of interest to third-party payers.

Results

The study did not demonstrate clearly superior results for either method of nutrition support (TPN or EFP) when considering any of the clinical outcome measures identified for the study. Hematopoietic recovery rate, length of hospitalization, and survival were similar for both treatments.

Certain medications were used for a longer period, and catheter-related complications were more frequent in the TPN patients. The enteral feeding program was less effective in maintaining weight, but this did not seem to influence other clinical outcomes.

Although the clinical effectiveness (outcome) of the two treatments were similar, the costs required to achieve those results for each group were different.

Benefit Analysis	Subtotal	Total

Identify the target audience.

The target audience for the protocols was 57 BMT recipients. The two treatment groups were comparable with respect to demographic characteristics and baseline nutritional status.

Calculate the benefits.

A. List the specific benefits

The length of stay (LOS) for EFP recipients was three days shorter than that of TPN recipients. Although this difference is not statistically significant, the difference is financially significant. The mean LOS for TPN recipients was 36 days; the mean LOS for EFP recipients was 33 days.

- Three-day reduction in LOS per patient.
- Other benefits realized in the EFP but not measured in a manner to allow costing are the reduction in the catheter-related complications and the reduction in days of medication.

B. Determine the dollar value of each benefit measured

- Hospital day variable cost $700.00/day (includes room cost and overhead)

C. Multiply the dollar value of the benefit by the number of benefits

- 3-day reduction in LOS
  @ $700.00/day = $2100.00

D. **Total financial benefit per patient**   **$2100.00**

Calculate the costs per patient*

A. EFP recipients (costs for 33-day LOS).

1. Personnel time per patient
- RD assessment—2.25 hours (3 assessments at 45 minutes each)
- RD monitoring—8.25 hours (daily visits at 15 minutes each)
- Registered pharmacist (RPh)—0.35 hours (for mixing TPN solution for patients who failed EFP)
- Food preparation personnel—6.60 hours (to purchase and prepare special-request food products not available from hospital kitchen)

*Note: All costs as originally reported by the researchers were updated to reflect current costs of supplies and personnel.

2. Hourly cost for each type of personnel
   - RD—$16.20/hour ($13.50/hour + 20% fringe benefits)
   - RPh—$21.60/hour ($18.00/hour + 20% fringe benefits)
   - Food preparation—$12.00/hour ($10.00/hour + 20% fringe benefits)
3. Personnel cost per type of personnel
   - RD—$16.20 × 10.5 hours = $170.10
   - RPh—$21.60 × 0.35 hours = $7.56
   - Food preparation personnel—$12.00 × 6.60 hours = $79.20

4. **Total personnel costs per EFP patient** $ 256.86

5. Direct per-patient costs of materials and supplies
   - Enteral products = $3.65
   - Magnesium riders = $41.27
   - Oral vitamins = $1.65
   - Feeding tubes = $4.00
   - Feeding pump cassettes = $6.13
   - Special food products = $17.50

   Cost of required conversion to TPN for patients who failed EFP protocol
   - Placement of catheter line (or time and materials) = $73.84
   - IV tubing sets = $24.41
   - TPN solution including amino acids = $103.07
   - Pump cassette = $42.44
   - Catheters = $12.10
   - Dressing change kits = $11.04

6. **Total material and supply costs per patient** $ 341.10

7. **Total direct costs** (personnel + material/supplies) $ 597.96

8. **Indirect cost per patient** For this study, indirect costs were not calculated.   0.00

9. **Total costs per EFP patient** $ 597.96

B. TPN recipients (costs for 36-day LOS).
   1. Personnel time per patient
      - RD assessment—1.0 hours (3 assessments at 20 minutes each)
      - RD monitoring—9.0 hours (daily visits at 15 minutes each)
      - Registered pharmacist (RPh)—36.0 hours (1 hour/patient/day for mixing TPN solution)
   2. Hourly cost for each type of personnel
      - RD—$16.20/hour ($13.50/hour + 20% fringe benefits)
      - RPh—$21.60/hour ($18.00/hour + 20% fringe benefits)

	Subtotal	Total

3. Personnel cost per type of personnel
   - RD—$16.20 × 20 hours = $162.00
   - RPh—$21.60 × 36 hours = $777.60
4. **Total personnel cost per TPN patient** $ 939.60
5. Direct per patient costs of materials and supplies
   - Placement of catheter lines (for time and materials) = $840.64
   - IV tubing sets = $82.75
   - TPN solution, including amino acids = $609.09
   - Lipids emulsions
     10% = $22.90
     20% = $13.62
   - Pump cassettes = $142.92
   - Catheters = $83.78
   - Dressing change kits = $112.26
   - Enteral products = $0.96
6. **Total material and supply costs per TPN patient** $1909.92
7. **Total direct costs per TPN patient** (personnel + materials/supplies) $2849.52
8. **Indirect cost per patient**
   Not determined 0.00
9. **Total costs per TPN patient**   **$2849.52**

Evaluate the results	Results

A. Calculate net savings of EFP
   1. Record the number of patients involved in the protocol
      - 30 patients were in the EFP
   2. Subtract the total cost from the total benefits
      - $2100.00 (reduction in LOS)
        − 597.96 (cost per EFP patient)
        $1502.04 Net value, or
                   benefit of EFP
   3. Multiply net value of benefit times the number of patients involved.
      Net savings = $1502.04 × 30 = $45 061.20 $45 061.20
      Note: The $45 061.20 saving was for EFP recipients only.
B. Calculate benefit-cost ratio
   - Benefit : Cost Ratio for EFP
   - $2100.00 : $597.96 = 3.5:1 3.5:1
   For every $1.00 invested in EFP, a benefit of $3.50 is realized when compared to the TPN program.

EFP was less costly in terms of personnel and materials/supply costs per patient than the TPN program ($597.96 and $2849.52, respectively). Fewer infections and other catheter-related complications occurred in the EFP group, which also underwent fewer days of medication. Although the costs of these differences were not captured, increased infections, complications, and medications would have increased the cost of TPN treatment and certainly negatively affected the quality of life for those patients.

Discussion of the Case Study

This study was primarily designed to compare clinical outcomes, and cost data were not fully captured (eg, use of all medications, nursing time, physician time). The true costs associated with each feeding regimen were therefore underestimated, and the cost difference between the TPN and EFP groups probably would be even greater.

It also must be recognized that the three-day difference in LOS between the TPN and EFP treatment groups was not statistically significant and may or may not hold true in other studies based on these protocols. The lack of a statistically significant difference may be related to the relatively small sample size. Because of the potentially large financial benefit accrued from the reduction in LOS for this study, additional research would be warranted. Designs and techniques such as those used in this study could be applied to other patient groups as well to evaluate the relative benefit of alternative nutrition therapy regimens.

Several ethical issues must be mentioned as potential weaknesses. Weight loss from the body cell mass and body fat compartments did occur in the EFP group, although this certainly was not a goal of the nutrition therapy. These patients were closely followed, however, and they received vitamin, mineral, and amino acid supplements, when appropriate. Clearly, important clinical outcomes (survival, length of hospitalization, time until bone marrow recovery, and so forth) were not affected adversely. Additionally, it must be emphasized that the enteral program was designed to provide promptly any requested food item. Most hospital settings are not staffed to provide this type of service to BMT or any type of patient.

Another ethical issue is that several of the EFP patients whose voluntary oral intake was inadequate refused nasoenteric feeding. Although patients have the right to refuse any treatment, it is difficult to justify using central venous nutrition in a patient with a functional gastrointestinal tract. Many patients and some health care professionals believe that nasoenteric feeding is more "traumatic" than central venous feeding because the feeding tube extends visibly from the nose.

This trauma is psychological in nature, different from the physical trauma of central line placement, constant line and exit site care, and the risk of infection. However, the central IV line is generally not seen by visitors or others and therefore is more socially acceptable than the feeding tube. Nevertheless, using the intestinal tract, when it is functional, is less expensive and safer and may be more healthful physiologically than using the parenteral route.

References

1. Disbrow DD. Costs and benefits of nutrition services. A literature review. *J Am Diet Assoc.* 1989;89(suppl):S-6–S-64.

2. Dowling RA, Smith AE, eds. *Benefits of Nutrition Services: A Costing and Marketing Approach, Report of the Seventh Ross Roundtable on Medical Issues.* Columbus, Ohio: Ross Laboratories; 1987.

3. Warner KE, Luce BR. *Cost-Benefit and Cost-Effectiveness Analysis in Health Care. Principles, Practice and Potential.* Ann Arbor, Mich: Health Administration Press; 1982.

4. Gramlich EM. *Benefit-cost Analysis of Government Programs.* Englewood Cliffs, NJ: Prentice-Hall Inc; 1981.

5. Renn SC. The structure and financing of the health care delivery system of the 1980s. In: Schramm CJ, ed. *Health Care and Its Costs.* New York, NY: WW Norton and Co; 1987.

6. Drummond MF, Stoddart GL, Torrance GW. *Methods for the Economic Evaluation of Health Care Programmes.* Oxford, England: Oxford University Press; 1987.

7. Splett PL, Caldwell HM, Holey ES, Alton IT. Prenatal nutrition services: a cost analysis. *J Am Diet Assoc.* 1987;87:204.

8. Kaufman M, ed. *Guide to Quality Assurance in Ambulatory Nutrition Care.* Chicago, Ill: The American Dietetic Association; 1983.

9. Olendsky MC, Tolpin HG, Buckley EL. Evaluating nutrition intervention in atherosclerosis: some theoretical and practical considerations. *J Am Diet Assoc.* 1981;79:9.

10. Adamow CL, Clipper AJ. Is prospective payment inhibiting the use of nutrition support services? Discussion and research implications. *J Am Diet Assoc.* 1985;85:1616.

11. Dahl T. *Cost Benefits of Nutrition Education.* St Paul, Minn: United Hospitals; 1984.

12. Robbins S. Documenting the cost effectiveness of nutrition services. *Dietitians in Pediatric Practice.* 1984;7(2):2–3.

13. Green LW, Lewis FM. *Measurement and Evaluation in Health Education and Health Promotion.* Palo Alto, Calif: Mayfield Publishing Co; 1986.

14. Mason M, Hallahan IA, Monsen E, Mutch PB, Palombo R, White HG. Requisites of advocacy: philosophy, research, documentation. Phase II of the costs and benefits of nutrition care. *J Am Diet Assoc.* 1982;80:213.

15. Wills BB. Documentation: the missing link in evaluation. *J Am Diet Assoc.* 1985;85:225.

16. Smith PE. A benefit-driven approach to marketing nutrition services in a cost-conscious health care economy. In: Dowling RA, Smith AE, eds. *Benefits of Nutrition Services: A Costing and Marketing Approach, Report of the Seventh Ross Roundtable on Medical Issues.* Columbus, Ohio: Ross Laboratories; 1987.

17. Office of Technology Assessment. *The Implications of Cost-effectiveness Analysis of Medical Technology. Background Paper 1: Methodological Issues and Literature Review.* Washington, DC: Office of Technology Assessment; 1980.

18. Scheffler RM, Andrews NC, Phillips KA, eds. *Cancer Cure and Cost: DRGs and Beyond.* Ann Arbor, Mich: Health Administration Press Perspectives; 1989.

19. Medicare program; criteria and procedures for making medical services coverage decisions that relate to health care technology. *Federal Register.* 1989;54(18):4302.

20. Orstead C, Arrington D, Kamath SK, Olson R, Kohrs MB. Efficacy of prenatal nutrition counseling: weight gain, infant birth weight, and cost-effectiveness. *J Am Diet Assoc.* 1985;85:40.

21. Vermeersch JA. How will we know we got there? Evaluation of quality assurance standards for ambulatory nutritional care. In: Kaufman M, ed. *Quality Assurance in Ambulatory Nutritional Care. Proceedings of a National Conference.* Durham, NC, June 17–20, 1979.

22. Drummond MF. *Principles of Economic Appraisal in Health Care.* New York, NY: Oxford University Press; 1980.

23. Davidson JK, Delcher HK, Englund A. Spin-off cost/benefits of expanded nutritional care. *J Am Diet Assoc.* 1979;75:250.

24. Rice DP. *Estimating the Cost of Illness.* Washington, DC: US Dept of Health Education and Welfare; 1966. Health Economic Series 6, Public Health Service.

25. Impact of diabetes outpatient education program—Maine. *MMWR.* 1982; 31:307.

26. Campbell DT, Stanley JC. *Experimental and Quasi-Experimental Designs for Research.* Chicago, Ill: Rand McNally; 1963.

Research to Support Practice

27. Veney JE, Kaluzny AD. *Evaluation and Decision Making for Health Services Programs.* Englewood Cliffs, NJ: Prentice-Hall Inc; 1984.
28. Splett P, Caldwell M. *Costing Nutrition Services: A Workbook.* Chicago, Ill: Dept of Health and Human Services, Region V; November 1985.
29. Disbrow D, Bertram K. *Cost Benefit and Cost Effectiveness Analysis: A Practical, Step-by-Step Guide for Nutrition Professionals.* Concord, Calif: Center for Health Education; 1984.
30. Bower RH, Talamini MA, Sax HC, Hamilton F, Fischer JE. Postoperative enteral vs parenteral nutrition. *Arch Surg.* 1986;121:1040.
31. Nehme AE. Nutritional support of the hospitalized patient. The team concept. *JAMA.* 1980;243:1906.
32. Faubion WC, Wesley JR, Khalidi N, Silva J. Total parenteral nutrition catheter sepsis: impact of the team approach. *JPEN J Parenter Enteral Nutr.* 1986;10:642.
33. Copeland EM, Daly JM, Dudrick SJ. Nutrition as an adjunct to cancer treatment in the adult. *Cancer Res.* 1977;37: 2451.
34. Pillar B, Perry S. *Evaluating Total Parenteral Nutrition: Final Report and Core Statement of the Technology Assessment and Practice Guidelines Forum.* Washington, DC: Georgetown University School of Medicine; 1990.
35. Klarman HE. The road to cost-effectiveness analysis. *Milbank Mem Fund Quart. Health Soc.* 1982;60:585.
36. Schiller MR. Ethical issues in nutrition care. *J Am Diet Assoc.* 1988;88:13.
37. Nutrition support and hydration. In: US Congress, Office of Technology Assessment. *Life-Sustaining Technologies and the Elderly.* Washington, DC: US Government Printing Office; 1987. OTA-BA-306.
38. Helm KK. Risk taking isn't risky like it used to be. *J Am Diet Assoc.* 1989;89:488.
39. Szeluga DJ, Stuart RK, Brookmeyer R, Utermohlen V, Santos GW. Nutritional support of bone marrow transplant recipients: a prospective, randomized clinical trial comparing total parenteral nutrition to an enteral feeding program. *Cancer Res.* 1987;47:3309.

Key Techniques

17. RESEARCH TECHNIQUES USED TO SUPPORT MARKETING MANAGEMENT DECISIONS

Sara C. Parks, MBA, RD

Dietetics professionals face marketing research problems every day, as illustrated in the following typical examples:

- To combat declining occupancy rates and increasing competition, hospital administrators hire a marketing research firm "to study population demographics, life-styles, and buyer behavior patterns" in their service delivery areas. The head of the nutrition department is asked to prepare a listing of important factors. What population characteristics in each of the three categories should she request? How should she approach the task? What should she do with the information once it is provided?

- A dietitian has been offering a supermarket tour for the past several years. Sales were great at first, but recently consumer interest appears to be only limited. The dietitian had expected the project to have a more enduring life cycle. How can he determine if supermarket tours still have market potential? What kind of information should he collect? How can he find out what customers really think about the tours? The pricing? The competition? What information should go to potential customers to attract them?

- A dietetic consultant wants to begin to advertise professional services. Where should she advertise? Yellow Pages, newspaper, radio, church bulletins? What should the ads say? How can she measure the effectiveness of her advertising? How much does she know about present or potential customers? What do they read or listen to? How much are they willing to spend on nutrition services?

These are a few of the typical marketing research problems that dietetics professionals must address. Answers to these and similar questions are available to any manager or practitioner who understands simple market research techniques. Even those with a limited knowledge of modern research methods can develop better solutions to the questions just raised if they understand the critical role that marketing research plays in marketing decision making.

If it is true that the central focus of marketing (and therefore of any organization) is consumer satisfaction, then it is also true that every organization is constantly conducting "market research." Most of the time, people within organizations face a constant stream of consumer-related questions that they must address: A chef wonders whether a new menu item will be received by cafeteria customers. A dietetic consultant who is successful at one location contemplates opening a second office on the other side of town. A hospital with a new "senior wellness" program must decide whether to stick with physicians or to look for a new sales distribution channel. These people ponder the answers to important marketing management decisions. Often they ask friends, family, or co-workers, an approach that is not true research and could lead to future trouble.

Successful organizations cannot afford to make costly errors. Modern marketing research methods result in more effective solutions to problems and fewer mistakes in judgment than the less sophisticated techniques many dietetics professionals use to make marketing strategy decisions.

The purpose of this chapter is to help dietetics professionals improve their marketing decision making ability through the effective use of primary and secondary research. To that end, a definition of marketing research will be presented, along with a discussion of the important role it plays in understanding consumer behavior. The primary focus of this chapter is to discuss the steps in the marketing research process, secondary sources of marketing research data, and the more prevalent primary research methods used to support marketing management decisions. Finally, this chapter will look at how the various research pieces fit together to support marketing management decisions.

MARKETING RESEARCH DEFINED

There are many ways to approach the study of marketing research and to define the term. First, marketing research can be defined as a process to collect data and information about a specific market situation. Second, marketing research can be defined in terms of how it is used. There are two widely accepted uses of marketing research: to build the theoretical framework for the discipline and to provide data to support marketing-related decisions. Finally, marketing research can be defined relative to the techniques used to collect primary and secondary data. Both qualitative and quantitative techniques will be discussed in this chapter.

Among the attempts to describe marketing research briefly and accurately, the definitions presented by the American Marketing Association[1] and by Philip Kotler[2] are the more widely accepted. In 1987, the American Marketing Association approved the following definition[1]:

Marketing research is the function which links consumers, customers, and the public to the marketer through information—information used to identify and define marketing opportunities and problems; generate, refine, and evaluate marketing actions; monitor marketing performance and improve understanding of marketing as a process.

Marketing research specifies the information required to address these issues; designs the method for collecting information; manages and implements the data collection process; analyzes the results; and communicates the findings and their implications.

This definition enlarges the role of marketing research to include marketing management decision-support as well as the development of theory. This definition has three important parts. First, it deals with all phases of marketing; second, it emphasizes the systematic gathering and processing of data; and third, it links consumers to environmental opportunities and challenges. Earlier definitions of marketing research were limited to the first two parts of this definition.

An additional definition of marketing research that has been widely accepted is one proposed by Kotler. He describes marketing research as "the systematic design, collection, analysis, and reporting of data and findings relevant to a specific marketing situation."[2] The specific marketing situation usually involves a marketing decision such as introducing a new product, changing a promotional appeal, or monitoring market conditions and competitive pressures. Another important dimension of the definition of marketing research was presented by Eugene Kelley, the former president of the American Marketing Association. Kelley describes marketing researchers as the "investigators, the eyes, and ears of our profession,"[3] and predicts that marketing research will become the "strategic lifeline" for business decision makers.

THE FOUR *P*s OF MARKETING

A brief look at some of the typical applications of marketing research activities will show its scope and value.

Most marketing research evolves from a need to understand market potential and characteristics, and the four *P*s of marketing—*price, product, place*, and *promotion*. Kress[4] identifies the most prevalent uses of marketing research to include measuring market potential, analyzing market share, and determining market characteristics. More specifically, market research on target audiences will forecast demand for existing and new products and services, provide information on general trends, and provide data needed to segment markets. Looking at research on products and services, the author cites new product (services) testing, packaging evaluation, and comparison studies on competitive product (services) as a major use of marketing research. Pricing research examines identifying price elasticities, cost analysis, and testing alternative pricing strategies with various market segments. Research on place involves site analysis and distribution methods, while research on promotion comprises testing different advertising messages, establishing sales territories, and selecting and evaluating advertising effectiveness.

According to Kress,[4] marketing research relating to corporate marketing functions and responsibilities is least important. Instead, the key outcomes to marketing research should be to help firms understand and satisfy consumers' needs, to provide input for marketing decisions, and to serve as key ingredients of marketing information systems.

A FRAMEWORK FOR STUDYING CONSUMER BEHAVIOR

If marketers completely understood consumer behavior, poor decisions about the four *P*s would be rare. Unfortunately, product failures are commonplace, advertising campaigns are less than effective, and pricing strategies do not always reflect consumers' willingness to pay. Does this mean that marketers know little about buyer behavior? Although marketers probably will never have a complete grasp of consumer behavior, they know a great deal about why people buy products or services. Research related to how knowledge of consumer behavior assists marketers in making better decisions regarding the four *P*s is based in the social and behavioral science literature; in particular, that of sociology, psychology, and anthropology.

Patti and Frazer[5] define buyer behavior as "a process that includes the actions, internal and external, involved in identifying needs, and in locating products and services." These authors go on to say that the process consists of five steps: recognizing the marketing problem or consumer need, searching for solutions, evaluating alternative solutions, making a purchase decision, and evaluating (post-purchase) the decision. The length of time it takes a person to work through these five steps varies with need and with the overall market situation. A product or service such as health care may be more important if a health crisis exists than it would be in a health promotion program. On the other hand, each step might be influenced through the manipulation of one or more of the four *P*s. For example, advertisers might attempt to shorten the search for appropriate solutions by letting consumers know how certain products or services will satisfy their needs. This assumes that advertisers know what factors most strongly affect purchase behavior.

Peter and Olsen[6] present a general framework that many researchers use to study consumer behavior. It consists of four major elements: cognition, behavior, environment, and relationship to developing marketing strategies. In this framework, cognition is referred to as "everything that goes on inside consumer minds, including rational, emotional, and subconscious processes."[6] Examples of cognitive behaviors studied by marketing researchers include memory, knowledge, belief, attitude, and intention.

The second component is behavior. A review of the literature reveals that little attention has been given to what consumers actually do. The focus of most consumer behavior research is on what consumers say they think and feel or what they report that they do; actual purchase behavior is rarely measured, in spite of its relevance to understanding consumers and developing appropriate marketing strategies. Because purchase behaviors are rarely the result of a one-step process, and because they are sometimes impulse decisions, designing and controlling a study aimed at measuring such behavior is difficult. This is one of the reasons why measuring purchase-related attitudes has become so important in the marketing research literature. When actual behavior is studied, it is generally done through personal observations of each of the steps in the buyer behavior process and how various marketing strategies influence the process.

The study of environmental influences is the third component of the Peter and Olsen consumer behavior model. Broadly defined, the "social environment includes all human activities and interactions" that the consumer interacts with.[6] The social environment is important because much of a consumer's knowledge about products, stores, prices, and advertising is influenced by the opinions of other people who are known as key influentials. This is why, for example, many consumers purchase the same products as parents or friends. Culture and reference groups—groups that serve as guides to shaping individual behavior—not only influence marketing strategies, but also play an important role in creating a consumer's social and physical environments.

The uniqueness of the Peter and Olsen model is that it takes consumer behavior research beyond the one-way, cause-and-effect relationship between knowledge and behavior often discussed in the marketing research literature. Earlier models suggested that knowledge change would automatically lead to attitude change, which would then cause behavior change.[8] While these one-way causal approaches do have value, they often ignore the relationships among cognition, behavior, and environments.

The fourth component of the Peter and Olsen[6] marketing framework is marketing strategy. According to the authors, marketing strategy provides the physical and social stimuli (ie, products, promotional materials, price, and information) needed to attract consumer purchases. Marketing strategies are aimed at influencing future consumer cognitions and behaviors to purchase the products in question. Typically, marketing strategies are based on past cognitions and behaviors as defined or documented through marketing research, with the assumption that future cognitions and behaviors will be similar to those of the past. As a consumer's environment becomes increasingly saturated with promotional messages, the task of reaching a consumer with a single product, service, or message becomes considerably more complex and burdensome. The task becomes one of collecting appropriate research data to increase the probability that the best strategy will be selected.

MARKETING RESEARCH

Categories

Most marketing research carried out in business can be placed in one of three categories: basic research, applied research, and simple fact gathering.[4] Basic research includes those studies whose sole purpose is discovery of new knowledge or theory; applied research is used to support operational decision-making; and simple fact gathering is the gathering of some predetermined data. The nature of the marketing decision determines the type of research to be done. For instance, if a dietetics professional planning a weight management program wants to know how many competitors are in a given geographical area, the task is merely one of collecting data. Thus, simple fact gathering is the appropriate strategy. On the other hand, if the same practitioner wants to measure the effectiveness of a promotional strategy in reaching a weight management audience, applied research is probably the more appropriate research technique.

A more useful categorization is provided by Weiers,[7] who uses the functional objective of the research investigation as the basis of categorizing four major research designs: exploratory, descriptive, causal, and predictive.

Exploratory studies are designed to help one become familiar with a problem situation, to identify important variables, and to help establish which avenues of future research can be studied within budgetary constraints. The literature survey, focus group analysis, and interviews of experts are all examples of exploratory techniques. Descriptive studies are the most frequently used in marketing research. They describe or provide information about such issues as the characteristics of users of a given product, percentage of the market that recognizes the name and image of a given product, and usage rates of various media sources by specific market profile. Causal and predictive studies are less often used in marketing research. The goal of causal studies is to determine cause-and-effect relationships between such variables as advertising and package design on sales. Predictive studies are used to forecast sales based on the relationship of variables to sales. For example, the Ajzen-Fishbein model predicts consumer behavior by looking at the relationship of beliefs, attitudes, and subjective norms to a consumer's intention to make a purchase.[8,9]

Sequence of Steps

Although each research problem imposes its own special requirements, a marketing research project can be viewed as a sequence of six steps.

The first step of the research process, formulating the marketing problem and research question, requires that the researcher translate the decision problem into a research question.[10] If sales for a given product are not at a desirable level, the manager must make decisions about what to do to improve those sales records. If the manager attributes the poor sales to inappropriate advertising, the research question should address a hypothesis regarding advertising. In this example, the researcher might set up a comparative study and measure the percentage of a television audience that recalls features of two ads from two competing organizations. Defining the problem situation and important variables often requires exploratory research. At a minimum, the research problem must be defined clearly enough to state hypotheses and objectives or research questions for the project.

Determining information requirements and information sources, the second and third steps in the research process, involve making a list of information needed to satisfy the research objectives. Some information will not be available, making it necessary to make appropriate assumptions about the project. Additionally, caution must be exercised not to collect information that is interesting but not directly related to the project. In developing the list of information, the researcher becomes increasingly aware of the primary and secondary sources of data that are available.

The fourth step in the process is the examination of decision implications of potential findings. Whereas most market researchers agree that this is the most difficult step in the process, it is nevertheless important to the final success of the project. Weiers[7] views this issue particularly strongly: "If the answer to a particular research question has no influence on the ultimate decision reached, then resources should not be expended on attempting to answer the question."

Estimating time and cost requirements and preparing the research proposal are the last two steps in the marketing research model. Both time and cost are critical to the decision context; the research proposal outlines the steps needed to execute the study and to report its findings. It should be noted that the market research is extremely costly, as the number of study participants usually must be relatively large if the results are to be generalizable. Larger sample sizes are needed with research related to decision support because those response rates are typically lower than for other types of research. It is not unusual for managers to use the results of studies that have 30% to 40% response rates; however, in basic research this response would be unacceptable. Nevertheless, the timing of data collection and the cost of continuing inappropriate marketing strategies often does not allow for the follow-up procedures usually conducted in other types of research.

Common Errors

Weiers,[7] Churchill,[10] and Kress[4] discuss common research errors that reduce the accuracy and usefulness of marketing research studies. Weiers[7] identifies four categories of error: problem definition error, informational error, experimental error, and analysis error. The most difficult step in the research process is trying to define the "right" question to ask: If the problem is not well-defined, the research results will be not useful. If the researcher studies consumers' reactions to the quality of hospital food, but it is actually the time when food is served that makes a difference to consumers, then the wrong question is being addressed. This is an example of a problem definition error.

There are two types of informational errors, sampling and nonsampling. Sampling errors arise because a sample is used instead of the entire population; nonsampling errors occur when sample values are distorted by a variety of conditions that result in errors that are not reflected in the actual population. Response and nonresponse biases are additional examples of nonsampling errors. Response bias occurs because of a subject's tendency to exaggerate (eg, amount of income, amount of product used) or underestimate usage (eg, cigarette or alcohol consumption). Nonresponse bias occurs when the researcher does not attempt to document the differences (characteristics, actions, and attitudes) between segments of the sample respondents and nonrespondents.

Experimental errors are closely tied to validity, reliability, and objectivity.[4] Validity refers to how well the research measures what it claims to measure; reliability identifies the stability of the results over time or different population groups; and objectivity addresses the researcher's ability to avoid preconceived notions as to the study outcome. These errors can be minimized if a researcher does not work with his or her own population, but rather has a more neutral person conduct such research.

Finally, analysis errors may result from applying incorrect analytical techniques to a set of data. Powerful statistical tools often are applied to descriptive or ordinal data when, in fact, the only statistics that can be legitimately applied to the data are simple measures of central tendency. Analysis error results when inappropriate statistical measures are used to analyze research findings.

RESEARCH USING SECONDARY DATA SOURCES

To collect information about major competitors is not an easy task and usually requires primary research techniques. Thus, one must rely on secondary sources, such as state and local government information, annual company or hospital financial reports, media reports, advertisements, and other formal and informal observations. The following example illustrates the internal and external secondary data sources that might be readily available:

Suppose your facility has just initiated a new policy requiring marketing research proposals for all new food and nutrition projects under development. No one on staff is experienced with marketing research. Since you need information before completing a plan, you ask your facility's marketing department to provide data from internal records, and you ask your assistant to visit the city library to collect external data available on the general characteristics of the proposed market area. The alternative to doing the secondary data research yourself is to hire a marketing research consultant; but your budget does not provide for that luxury.

Internal Data

Internal secondary data that exist within an organization generally are collected for reasons other than the project at hand. In a hospital, for example, both the medical records and the admissions departments have excellent demographic data on the facility's current and past clients. Most hospitals also collect information on some health behaviors, disease status, and geographical location of its target audiences. This information is invaluable when segmenting markets for any new product line. The accounting department often collects revenue and expense data and usually does so by the various product or service lines offered by the facility. To the extent that the organization maintains a formal marketing department, the data are more likely to be in the format that is readily usable for the project at hand.

Other internal sources of secondary information include previous marketing studies, periodic reports on facility sales, customer correspondence and surveys, and reports from pertinent departments; for example, long-range plans and admissions data.[7] Being able to access secondary data substantially reduces the cost and time needed to conduct the study.

External Data

One of the biggest problems in collecting secondary research is finding the key words needed to access the articles or periodicals to be used. The listing in *Table 17.1* should make the task of external data collection easier.

Table 17.1
Secondary External Data
Sources

Periodical indexes

Information on trends can be located in a large variety of periodicals, so several periodical indexes need to be consulted for an overall view of the field.

Bibliography of Agriculture. Phoenix, Ariz: Oryx Press.

Bibliography of Hotel and Restaurant Administration. Ithaca, NY: Cornell University.

A subject bibliography to retrospective books, pamphlets, periodcals, and articles relating to food service and nutrition; extensive cross references are a useful feature. Publication ceased with the 1985 index.

Biological and Agricultural Index. New York, NY: Wilson; 1964– .

Subject index that includes nutrition, the food industry, and related topics.

Business Index. Menlo Park, Calif: Information Access Corp.

Cumulative index (1979–present) to business journals and newspapers.

Business Periodicals Index. New York, NY: Wilson; 1958– .

Covers fields of accounting, advertising, marketing, personnel, and specific industries; a very important index for most health fields.

Consumer Health and Nutrition Index. Phoenix, Ariz: Oryx Press.

Cumulative Index to Nursing and Allied Health Literature.

Indexes all major English language nursing journals, plus some major medical journals. Useful for information on foodservices in nursing homes and hospitals.

F & S Index of Corporations and Industries. Cleveland, Ohio: Predicasts Inc; 1960– .

Indexes mostly journal articles and covers business trends, new products, technological developments, consumer spending, and company profiles. Access by company name and by Standard Industrial Classification (SIC) number.

Hospital Literature Index. Chicago, Ill: American Hospital Association 1959– .

Primarily journal articles on hospital and instructional subjects, but does include some relevant articles under "food service" and "dietary department." This is one of the few indexes that cover foodservice in institutional settings.

The Hospitality Index: An Index for the Hotel, Foodservice and Travel Industries. Washington, DC: The Consortium; 1988– .

A comprehensive index produced by a consortium of academic and industry specialists.

Public Affairs Information Service Bulletin. New York, NY: PAIS, 1915– .

An important subject index to books, pamphlets, reports, journal articles, and selected government publications, with good coverage of economic and social conditions. Includes indexing of the Cornell HRA Quarterly.

Readers' Guide to Periodical Literature. New York, NY: Wilson, 1905– .

Indexes articles from popular, general-interest magazines on a wide variety of topics. Good for general overview of a subject, and for current, if "trendy" articles.

World Agricultural Economics and Rural Sociology Abstracts. Farnham Royal, England: Commonwealth Agricultural Bureau; 1959– .

Forecasting and trends

The following books are useful for information on trends:

Casale AM. *USA Today: Tracking Tomorrow's Trends: What We Think About Our Lives and Our Future.* Kansas City, Mo: Andrews McMeel and Parker; 1986.

Naisbitt J, Aburdene P. *Megatrends 2000: Ten New Directions for the 1990s.* New York, NY: Morrow; 1990.

Newspaper indexes

New York Times Index. New York, NY: The New York Times; 1851–   .
Subject index with exact reference to data, page, and column. Contains summaries and extensive cross references to related topics.

Wall Street Journal Index. New York, NY: Dow Jones; 1959–
Two-part index with sections for corporate and general news.

Newspaper Abstracts Ondisc. Louisville, Ky: UMI/Data Courier; 1984–1988.
A compact disc index to the *New York Times, Wall Street Journal, Los Angeles Times, Chicago Tribune, Christian Science Monitor, Atlanta Constitution,* and *Boston Globe.* Indexes only most recent years.

Reference sources

These sources gather together statistics on trends and projections in the health care industry and on the economy as a whole.

American Statistics Index. Washington, DC: Congressional Information Service; 1973–   .
A master guide and subject index to statistics in US government publications. The subject heading "Projections" is of particular interest.

Predicasts. Cleveland, Ohio: Predicasts Inc; 1960–   .
A useful quarterly source for short- and long-range forecasts. Accompanying each forecast is a date and page reference to the current journal, government report, or special study from which the statistics were taken.

Standard and Poor's Statistical Service. New York, NY: Standard and Poor's Corp; 1977–   .
Provides current and basic statistics in many areas, including agriculture, energy, and building.

Statistical Reference Index. Washington, DC: Congressional Information Service.

Demographic, economic, and market information

Advertising Age. Chicago, Ill: Crain Communications Inc; weekly.

American Households and Their Money. Ithaca, NY: American Demographics; 1986.
An analysis of household trends based on the Census Bureau's March 1986 Current Population Survey.

American Households and Their Spending: Focus on Food. Ithaca, NY: American Demographics; 1988.

The Gallup Poll: Public Opinion. Wilmington, Del: Scholarly Resources; 1972–   , annual.
Compilation of all polls conducted each year by the American Institute of Public Opinion.

Handbook of Labor Statistics. Washington, DC: US Bureau of Labor Statistics; 1927–   .
A compendium of statistical data relating to the labor force.

Hispanic Shoppers. Washington, DC: Food Marketing Institute, 1984.
A research study of Hispanic Americans as consumers.

Sales and Marketing Management. "Survey of Buying Power"
(Part 1 is special July issue of journal; part 2 is special October issue). Population, effective buying income, and retail sales estimates for state, county, and metropolitan areas; includes special reports on most affluent markets and population shifts.

Simmons Market Research Bureau, Inc. *Study of Media and Markets.*
Multi-volume set of data compiled by a private market research company in order to give information on various consumer products and services.

(Continued.)

Table 17.1 (continued)
Secondary External Data
Sources

The Sourcebook of Demographics and Buying Power for Every Zipcode in the U.S.A. Arlington, Va: CACI; 1984–1989.
Includes "Purchasing Potential Index" for dining out.
Mediamark Research, Inc. (MRI)
Provides a comprehensive source of media and product information.
Burrelle's Special Groups Media Directory, Update. Livingston, NJ: Burrelle's Media Directories; updated regularly.
Cable TV Publicity Outlets—Nationwide. Depot, Conn: Cable TV Publicity Outlets; updated regularly.
Media Market Guide. New York, NY: Gannett Newspapers; updated regularly.
Statistical Abstract of the United States. Washington, DC: US Bureau of Census; 1879– .
A compilation of American social, economic, and political statistics.

Restaurant/Foodservice industry
Consumer Behavior and Attitudes Toward Fast Food and Moderately Priced Family Restaurants. Washington, DC: National Restaurant Association; 1987.
Consumer Expectations with Regard to Dining at Atmosphere Restaurants. Washington, DC: National Restaurant Association; 1983.
Consumer Expectations with Regard to Dining at Fast Food Restaurants. Washington, DC: National Restaurant Association; 1983.
Consumer Nutrition Concerns and Restaurant Choices. Washington, DC: National Restaurant Association; 1986.
A market study of the impact of nutrition on restaurants. The market is divided into four groups: traditional consumers, weight conscious consumers, health conscious consumers, and the uncommitted.
Consumer Preferences for Ethnic Foods in Restaurants. Washington, DC: National Association; 1984.
Consumer Preferences for New Restaurant Concepts. Washington, DC: National Restaurant Association; 1985.
Consumer Reactions to and Use of Restaurant Promotions. Washington, DC: National Restaurant Association; 1982.
Consumer Restaurant Behavior: A View Based on Occasion Segmentation. Washington, DC: National Restaurant Association; 1984.
Dinner Decision Making: A Consumer Attitude Survey. Washington, DC: National Restaurant Association; 1989.
Food Marketing Facts. Washington, DC: Food Marketing Institute.
Foodservice and Energy to the Year 2000. Washington, DC: National Restaurant Association; 1988.
Foodservice in Convenience Stores. Chicago, Ill: IFMA, 1989.
Foodservice Industry, Forecast. Washington, DC: National Restaurant Association; 1989.
The Gallup Annual Report on Eating Out. Princeton, NJ: The Gallup Organization; 1984– . A detailed study of the consumers, foods and trends of the eating away from home market.
How Consumers Make the Decision to Eat Out. Washington, DC: National Restaurant Association; 1982.
Market Research for the Restaurateur: A Do-It-Yourself Handbook for Market Research. Washington, DC: National Restaurant Association; 1981.
Shopping A La Cart; the Changing Environment of the Takeout Food Market. Washington, DC; Food Marketing Institute; 1987.
The Take Out Market. Washington, DC: National Restaurant Association; 1986.
The Technomic 100. Chicago, Ill: Technomic; 1987.
Trends: Consumer Attitudes and the Supermarket. Washington, DC: Food Marketing Institute; annual.

Table 17.1 (continued)
Secondary External Data
Sources

Hospitals, health care, and institutional feeding

American Hospital Association Guide to the Health Care Field. Chicago, Ill: American Hospital Association; 1972–
A state by state directory of hospitals in the United States. Accompanying statistical data includes number of beds and occupancy rates.

Hospital Statistics. Chicago, Ill: American Hospital Association; 1974–
Detailed data on hospital utilization, personnel and finances. Introductory section analyses trends in American hospitals.

Directory of Multihospital Systems, Multistate Alliances, and Networks. 6th ed. Chicago, Ill: American Hospital Publishing; 1985.
Provides directory and statistical information for multihospital systems and their hospitals.

Directory of Investor-Owned Hospitals, Hospital Management Companies and Health Systems. Little Rock, Ark: Federation of American Health Systems; 1987–
A geographical listing of investor-owned hospitals providing information on size, type of ownership. The "Statistical section" provides an EL profile of the growth of the investor-owned hospital industry.

The Med Tech Directory. South Orange, NJ: Med Tech Services; 1982–   . Data given includes latest available four fiscal year net sales or revenues, net profits, earnings per share, and stock price range.

Directory of Nursing Homes. 2nd ed. Phoenix, Ariz: Oryx Press; 1984.
A state-by-state listing of facilities and services. Description indicates whether dining facilities are provided, number of beds, and level of care provided.

National Directory of Retirement Facilities. Phoenix, Ariz: Oryx Press; 1986.
A state-by-state directory to more than 12 000 housing facilities for the elderly. Each entry indicates facility type and capacity.

Nursing Home Industry. Philadelphia, Pa: Laventhol and Horwath; annual.

Prevention Index. Emmaus, Pa: Rodale Press; 1984–

Statistical Handbook on Aging Americans. Phoenix, Ariz: Oryx Press; 1986.
Demographic, social, economic, financial, and medical data about the aging population in the United States.

The Condition of Education. Washington, DC: National Center for Education Statistics; 1975–
Focuses upon different issues from year to year but the first section always provides an overview of trends in education at all levels.

Data should not be overcollected; in most cases, more data will exist than needed. Furthermore, bias may be present in secondary data, and it must be controlled if the data are used to support a research design. Sponsoring organizations, interviewees, researchers, and editors all bring a bias to data that they present; thus, the user of secondary data has an obligation to identify in the study the bias that specific authors place on the data. Additionally, when selecting the data, care must be exercised to make certain that the research methodology is sound. Questions such as the following must be considered: Is the sample size reliable for the level of accuracy desired? Is the statistical analysis consistent with the data set? Can the results be generalized? The answers to these and other questions, will help to avoid some of the pitfalls of using secondary data sources.

Steps in Collecting Secondary Data

Table 17.2 summarizes Breen and Blankenship's[11] tips for collecting general marketing information from secondary sources, adapted to make them applicable to dietetics.

Table 17.2
Tips for Collecting Secondary
Marketing Research Data

1. Start by consulting the most promising guides, ie, *Reader's Guide to Periodical Literature, The New York Times Index,* the *Business Periodicals Index,* and the *Index to Health Care Literature.* These indexes will provide access to current business literature.

2. Refer to the Standard Industrial Classification (SIC) Manual to obtain SIC codes. These will allow you to access specific statistics regarding specific industries in both printed and on-line databases.

3. Use free government information sources, eg, Department of Commerce, Bureau of the Census, Department of Aging, and National Institutes of Health. The federal government prepares three census reports—population, housing, and business. State, county, and local governments have similar statistics.

4. Learn about other government sources. *American Statistics Index, Statistical Abstract of the United States,* and *Survey of Current Business* are excellent sources of business and general economic statistics.

5. Check state and local (city or county) government sources. Start by writing to the state departments of commerce, development, or libraries. At the local level, try city or county planning offices and the economic development commission; they generally have data regarding present and future growth plans.

6. Use business and professional associations. When the new professional member database is available, The American Dietetic Association should be one of the first places to check. The National Center for Nutrition and Dietetics and the National Agricultural Library also are excellent food and nutrition sources.

7. Check directories, such as *Dun and Bradstreet, Moody's Manuals,* and *Thomas Register.* These sources will provide data on various organizations and businesses in a given market area.

8. Check other sources of commercial printed information. The *Sales Management Annual Survey of Buying Power* provides local information on population, income, retail (including eating and drinking establishments), and an index of market potential. *Restaurants and Institutions* magazine publishes market surveys, generally in the July and October issues. *Gallup Poll* publishes studies about food, eating habits, and health trends on an annual basis.

9. Learn about existing databases and data banks that can provide useful demographic, buyer behavior and psychographic data. There are more than 5000 on-line data banks that have both general and specific information. To access them, check *Directory of On-Line Information Resources* (CSG Press, Rockville, Maryland) and *Database Catalog* (Dialog, Palo Alto, California).

10. Select the right specialist to work with. Information brokers provide such services on a fee basis. Many public and university libraries offer database searches for a minimal fee. Your local library should, at a minimum, be able to tell you where to go to access the information.

An Illustration

There is little question that the marketing environment for dietetics professionals has changed dramatically over the past decade: the profession has shifted from a product orientation ("you must follow this diet prescription") to a customer-driven emphasis ("these are your options"). Marketing and other factors have forced the profession to shift from identifying unique nutrition programs (products) and searching for potential users to focusing on target audiences, individual customer preferences, consumer demographics, and lifestyles prior to product development. Moreover, with greater competition for food and nutrition services, the need to promote them to motivate customers to purchase what dietetics professionals have to offer increases. More important is the profession's recognizition of the need to improve market performance by "targeting" products and services to specific audiences. The world is no longer a feasible market.

These changes require vast amounts of data from a variety of sources: internal information about customers' purchase behavior and external segmentation data such as geo-demographic, psychographic, life-style, and financial data. All of these data are critical elements of the new marketing behaviors just described and serve as the basis for the following example.

Any City Hospital wants to develop a segmentation plan for a new weight management program recently developed by its dietetic staff. Its goal is to make the program a revenue-generating project. With limited advertising dollars, the hospital's marketing and nutrition departments have agreed that they should collect information about potential clients for the program. They are under time constraints, so they decide to rely primarily on secondary data sources.

The first step in searching out information about potential markets is to decide on the project's research objectives. A typical research question might be "to determine what percentage of women older than 25 years has purchased weight management programs during the immediate past calendar year."

There are several ways to segment the weight management market. A geographic sales analysis of other weight management programs might be conducted. Demographic data (income, marital status, education, and so forth) could be studied. Product consumption (Weight Watchers, diet books, television programs, and so forth) could be evaluated. Additionally, hospital records could be explored to determine specific clients who are overweight or who have had weight-management programs prescribed during the period in question.

The following illustrates some of the most common segmentation characteristics in action. A study of geographic data shows that most women purchase weight management programs close to their work or homes. Approximately 75% buy programs within a 3-mile radius of these two locations. Of prime importance is demographics. The external reports evaluated indicate that the majority of women interested in weight-management, as opposed to weight-loss, are college graduates, unmarried, and employed in professional positions. Benefits sought by this market segment are time, convenience, and the ability to have reasonable weight-management options that can be adapted to busy life-styles. Psychographic research shows that this market segment has a positive attitude toward a healthy life-style and a negative perception about returning to the local hospital to make the purchase. All data that must be incorporated into the decision-making process when the four P strategies are developed.

The aforementioned segmentation dimensions are some common data studied, but by no means all of the alternatives, and the reader is cautioned against some common misconceptions that oversimplify the market segmentation process. First, market segmentation is not a partitioning process. Rather, it is a gathering of information about potential customers and an assembling of this information around commonalities. Second, segmentation is not merely a marketing process; its real impact is what it brings to an organization's market plans and strategies. Finally, it is a myth to say that everyone is a part of a segment in a given market. It is likely that a small percentage of a population is unclassifiable, based on specified segmentation criteria.

This section reviewed the common sources of internal and external secondary market research data available to decision makers and provided an illustration of how a secondary data search might work. The benefits of secondary data sources—including timely and cost-effective data collection methods—probably override the negative aspects of this research tool.

METHODS FOR OBTAINING PRIMARY DATA

Most primary data used to support marketing decisions can be produced in one of two ways: by questioning people or by observing selected activities. A number of researchers also include experimental research designs. With surveys, "data are collected by asking questions of individuals thought to have the desired information."[4] A number of survey techniques generally are used to collect market research data: mail and telephone surveys, interviews, consumer panels, and focus groups. Observational research involves a researcher who "observes the objects or actions of interest—and [the observation process] can be performed by a human or mechanically."[4] In developing experiments, the researcher "controls or manipulates one or more independent variables and determines the effect of such manipulation(s) on the dependent variable."[7]

There is general agreement among marketing researchers that the purpose(s) of the research should determine the method used to collect primary data. Because it is often difficult to identify the appropriate research method, there are generally accepted criteria for making that determination: validity of findings, cost and timeliness, versatility, and accuracy.[4] For example, if advertising expenditures and sales revenues are key variables to a given decision context, the method used to study these variables must provide sufficient data to test the relationship between advertising and sales. Researchers often rely on mail or telephone surveys to collect market research data because they usually meet the cost and timeliness criteria. Marketing research is costly, so these factors often take precedence over validity, versatility, and accuracy. Because marketing research projects generally seek information about more than a single variable, versatility becomes a third factor to consider in method choice. For that reason, the observation method is rarely used alone; it is often combined with the survey method. Finally, accuracy and representativeness are Kress's[4] final criteria for selecting a research method. These factors assess the quality of the results and the extent results can be generalized from a small sample to a total population.

Methods Used to Collect Primary Data

There are numerous ways of collecting survey data. Five of these methods will be discussed in this chapter: mail surveys, telephone surveys, personal interviews, consumer panels, and focus groups.

Mail surveys. The mail survey method is the most frequently used technique in collecting market research data, but it is also the most frequently misused method. Various authors provide tips to increase the method's validity and reliability. Vichas[12] presents ten criteria to consider for successful mail surveys:
1. Choose a sample that is homogeneous or has a common problem large enough to be representative
2. Compose questions that are reflective of the objectives of the project
3. Keep the questionnaire at a reasonable length: six to eight pages maximum
4. Code questions to ensure quick data entry
5. Lay out the questionnaire with an interesting format
6. Develop a professional, yet motivational cover letter

7. Test internally with co-workers and externally with a small number of sample respondents and rewrite
8. Produce in a quality, upscale printed format
9. Know how to increase participation rates
10. Review examples of other mail questionnaires

Other techniques used to increase the reliability and validity of surveys include an expert review for content validity; applying statistical methods to determine the instrument's reliability prior to use; and determining face validity by pretesting the instrument with sample respondents. The reader is referred to Vichas[12] and to Dillman[13] for more specific details on each of the ten steps just listed.

Telephone surveys. Another way to collect qualitative and quantitative market research data is through telephone surveys. As are written surveys, this method is fraught with both sampling and nonsampling errors that are of concern to marketers. (Sampling errors have to do with getting the right numbers and kinds of people to respond; nonsampling errors occur when the true intent of the variables under question are distorted by the interviewer or interviewee.) With the increased use of household telephone answering services and devices, reaching the appropriate sample can be hampered. The following questions may help the researcher determine the existence of response errors: Is the true meaning of the question being reflected by the interviewer? Does the respondent know the right answer? Is the respondent willing to provide true answers? Is the wording of the question likely to elicit a biased response?[7]

Computer-assisted telephone interviewing (CATI) and mechanical computer surveys are two additional methods used successfully to obtain marketing data. CATI involves programming a questionnaire into a computer; the interviewer reads the questions from the computer screen and records answers on the keyboard. Random-digit dialing helps overcome the problems caused by unlisted numbers or outdated directories. This method generates lists of possible numbers, either randomly or through some other systematic process, and reduces the number of nonworking or unlisted telephone numbers.

Personal interviews. Personal interviews are a third survey method for obtaining marketing information. While written and telephone surveys are a good way to collect data, most marketing researchers say they should be supplemented by personal interviews. There are four basic types of interviews: structured and direct; unstructured and direct; structured and indirect; and unstructured and indirect.[12] An unstructured interview appears to have no fixed pattern or order of questioning, but it does have a clear objective or purpose. The direct interview starts by telling respondents the purpose, while the indirect technique does not have a specific objective. Interviews are particularly valuable in helping researchers observe subtle feedback that otherwise would be unavailable.

Consumer panels. This method is often used to test new products using the same persons in several tests. Marketing researchers assemble a group of study participants for a variety of projects. There are several problems with consumer panel designs: panel members do not always represent the buying population; seldom are all population segments represented on the panel; people who state their opinions for pay do not always give honest answers; and some panel members prevent others from expressing their true feelings.[12]

Focus groups. Focus groups continue to be one of the most used and abused marketing research techniques in today's society. This method is based upon the assumption that people feel more comfortable and provide more useful information in small groups. Focus groups have four primary purposes: to provide input on new products, new markets, and new packaging; to aid in identifying key variables used in more quantitative studies; to provide input into the development of new products and services; and to obtain research data quickly and inexpensively.[14] To ensure some credibility of focus group results, the leaders must be well-trained, the group composition should be homogeneous, and the procedures for running the group must be clearly defined. More specific details on setting up focus groups is given by Greenbaum[14] and Vichas.[12]

In summary, primary market data can be obtained by either questioning people or observing their activities. Questioning can be completed through surveys, interviews, consumer panels, and focus groups. Each method has advantages and disadvantages, and the selection should be based on the research question.

ATTITUDE MEASUREMENT

This chapter has focused on research techniques used to collect data about the who, what, when, where, and how of making marketing decisions. Attitude research in marketing is particularly important because it answers the question of why consumers buy a given product; what their preferences are; what factors motivate them toward repeat purchases; and why some consumers are brand loyal and others are not.

Attitudes are so important to the marketing process that millions of dollars per year are spent in advertising aimed at maintaining or changing consumer attitudes toward products and services of all types. Most attitude research is done either to measure consumer attitudes or, once those attitudes are known, to help devise strategies for shaping them. The California Raisin Advisory Board's "I Heard it through the Grapevine" and Wendy's "Where's the Beef?" campaigns are often cited in the advertising literature as two promotional activities that had tremendous effects on attitude change. The raisin commercials took a product with a negative image and created a positive, upbeat feeling about it. Wendy's commercials, on the other hand, were aimed at changing attitudes regarding competitive products.

Earlier in this chapter, attitudes are identified as cognitions, and they are often considered either strengths or weaknesses in marketing efforts. Attitudes generally can be defined as "a person's point of view toward an object or an idea."[4] Kress goes on to say that determining attitudes in marketing is the process of identifying people's feelings about product attributes and how important those attributes are to them. Fishbein and Ajzen[8] are considered two of the leading researchers in the application of attitude theory to various marketing contexts.

Several types of scales are used to collect information on attitudes: semantic differential, projective and expressive psychological techniques, ranking, and Likert Summated and Thurstone Differential Scales.[12] Of these techniques, Vichas and others identify the semantic differential scale as the most frequently used data collection method in marketing research.

Semantic Differential

Vichas defines semantic differential as the "repetitious measurement of a concept compared against a series of descriptive polar-adjective scales."[12] It is a technique designed to look at how much customers like or dislike a company, product, sales force, or competitor. Vichas[12] lists five steps to success in semantic differential measurement: defining study objectives, developing questions and responses, pretesting the questionnaire, administering the instrument, and analyzing the data. Consumers' responses to advertisements are often measured with a semantic differential scale. In the Cobb-Walgren and Sleszynski[15] study of consumer reactions to physicians' Yellow Pages ads, a semantic differential scale was used to determine receptivity to a number of different advertisements. Consumers were asked to rate, on a scale, their perceptions of the ad and specific attributes of the ad.

In step 1 of the process, the definition of objectives, the researcher asks the question relative to the purpose of the study. To arrive at the study purpose(s), Vichas[12] suggests that ads be reviewed, comparative ad studies be constructed, or consumer buying profiles be considered. Step 2 in the semantic differential methodology involves developing the questions and response scales. *Table 17.3* provides an example of a modified semantic differential questionnaire on which the scale ranges in four steps from excellent to unsatisfactory. The pairs of terms (eg, high quality–low quality) were identified in focus groups, employee panels, and foodservice publications.

Table 17.3
Example of a Semantic
Differential Questionnaire

Question: What do you think of foodservice in this hospital?

	Excellent	Satisfactory	Okay	Unsatisfactory	
High quality	4	3	2	1	Low quality
Large selection	4	3	2	1	Small selection
Friendly	4	3	2	1	Unfriendly
Low prices	4	3	2	1	High prices
Helpful employees	4	3	2	1	Unhelpful employees
Many specials	4	3	2	1	Few specials
Flexible	4	3	2	1	Inflexible

Table 17.4 provides an example of a semantic differential scale used to define certain consumer characteristics relative to two weight management programs. The seven steps on the scale are, for example, extremely slow weight loss, very slow weight loss, slightly slow weight loss, neither slow nor fast, fast weight loss, very fast weight loss, or extremely fast weight loss. The terms *expensive, professionalism of consultants, convenience,* and *friendly atmosphere* are substituted for *weight loss* using the same modifiers. Four to seven levels of intensity are generally considered adequate for a semantic differential scale.[4,7] There is considerable debate over whether the semantic scale should have even or odd numbers of responses; even numbers are considered by Vichas[12] as forcing respondents away from the middle or "safe" response categories.

The final steps in the semantic differential process are similar to those of almost any other research technique: pretesting to improve the questionnaire, administering the instrument, and analyzing data. The advantages of the semantic differential method are cost, time, and improved validity and reliability. This latter is particularly true if the adjectives are generated by consumer focus groups or panels.

Table 17.4
Profile of Two Weight Management Programs from Semantic Differential Scores of 150 Consumers

Slow weight loss	1	2	3	4	5	6	7	Fast weight loss
Inexpensive	1	2	3	4	5	6	7	Expensive
Nonprofessional nutrition consultants	1	2	3	4	5	6	7	Professional nutrition consultants
Inconvenient	1	2	3	4	5	6	7	Convenient
Unfriendly	1	2	3	4	5	6	7	Friendly

Likert Summated and Thurstone Differential Scales

In the Likert Summated Scale, respondents are given a series of statements and are asked to rate each statement on the strength of their personal feelings toward it. The statements used in the survey usually are selected from a larger list that had been generated by exploratory research with consumers. *Table 17.5* provides an example of a questionnaire using a Likert Scale for measuring the effectiveness of a nutrition consultation. A four-point scale is used as an example; however, the scale could have as many as seven descriptors. A particularly good feature of Likert scales is the ability to separate respondents into three groups based on their total scores: favorable, somewhat neutral, and unfavorable. This separation allows for comparisons among respondent groups.

Table 17.5
Example of a Likert Scale Used to Measure Effectiveness of a Nutrition Consultation

How useful was the information provided?

	Very Useful	Somewhat Useful	Not Useful	Do Not Use
a. Consultation	1	2	3	4
b. Handout	1	2	3	4
c. Verbal instruction	1	2	3	4
d. Video	1	2	3	4

The Thurstone Differential Scale is a method in which respondents are asked to select from a list of 100 or more statements the 20 or 25 with which they most agree[4]. Once again, the original list is generated by a panel of experts and confirmed by consumer focus groups. Respondents are asked to identify and rank those 20 or 25 statements that they most favor. The statements deal with the same subject, eg, either the organization's products or its advertising, but not both. Most statisticians believe that this process only develops a set of ordinal data and thus cannot be used to predict other people's behaviors. Measures of central tendency can be applied to the data collected using this method.

Projective and Expressive Psychological Techniques

Vichas[12] identifies four projective and expressive techniques currently used in marketing research: association, completion, expression, and construction. The purpose of each of these techniques is to induce study respondents to write, or to respond to verbally, their initial thoughts about a term, phrase, or comparison. Another variation of the projective technique is to ask subjects to respond to a series of terms, phrases, or comparisons just with words that come to mind, or to complete a sentence.

The real question about projective and expressive psychological techniques is whether they are of value to developing marketing strategies. The answer to that question is very little by themselves. When accompanied by other research techniques, psychological techniques may be useful with new product testing. These methods continue to provide excellent results when used in basic research and have made substantial contributions to the generation of knowledge. Additionally, these methods are generally valid only when prepared by trained psychologists, making the method much more costly than others.

SUMMARY

This chapter had three primary purposes:
1. To help dietetics professionals make marketing decisions based on research findings, rather than hunches
2. To help readers understand that the basis for virtually all marketing decisions is consumer behavior
3. To provide definitions of marketing research and the techniques peculiar to each of these definitions

This chapter does not present all market research techniques, but it does introduce readers to many reference sources that can be used to help guide applied and fact-finding research. Of particular value should be the listing of secondary data sources that are found internal and external to most organizations. Throughout the chapter, an attempt was made to provide specific examples of how to apply each of the techniques.

Marketing research is a complex arena that brings logic and meaning to management decision making.

References

1. New marketing research definition approved. *Marketing News.* January 2, 1987.
2. Kotler P. *Principles of Marketing.* 3rd ed. Englewood Cliffs, NJ: Prentice-Hall Inc; 1986.
3. Kelley E. Marketing researchers will become "strategic lifelines" of corporations. *Marketing News.* January 21, 1983.
4. Kress G. *Marketing Research.* 3rd ed. Englewood Cliffs, NJ: Prentice-Hall Inc; 1988.
5. Patti CH, Frazer CF. *Advertising: A Decision-Making Approach.* Chicago, Ill: Dryden Press; 1988.
6. Peter JP, Olsen JC. *Consumer Behavior: Marketing Strategy Perspectives.* Homewood, Ill: Richard D Irwin Inc; 1987.
7. Weiers RM. *Marketing Research.* 2nd ed. Englewood Cliffs, NJ: Prentice-Hall Inc; 1988.
8. Fishbein M, Ajzen I. *Belief, Attitude, Intention, and Behavior: An Introduction to Theory and Research.* Reading, Mass: Addison-Wesley Publishers; 1975.
9. Ajzen I, Fishbein M. *Understanding Attitudes and Predicting Social Behavior.* Englewood Cliffs, NJ: Prentice-Hall Inc; 1980.

10. Churchill GA Jr. *Marketing Research: Methodological Foundations.* Chicago, Ill: Dryden Press; 1989.
11. Breen G, Blankenship AB. *Do-It-Yourself Marketing Research.* 3rd ed. New York, NY: McGraw-Hill Publishing Co; 1989.
12. Vichas RP. *Complete Handbook of Profitable Marketing Research Techniques.* Englewood Cliffs, NJ: Prentice-Hall Inc; 1982.
13. Dillman DA. *Mail and Telephone Surveys: The Total Design Method.* New York, NY: John Wiley and Sons, Inc; 1978.
14. Greenbaum TL. *The Practical Handbook and Guide to Focus Group Research.* Lexington books series, Lexington, Mass: DC Heath and Co; 1988.
15. Cobb-Walgren CJ, Sleszynski H. Responses to physician advertising in the Yellow Pages. In: Leigh JM, Martin CR, eds. *Current Issues and Research in Advertising.* Ann Arbor, Mich: University of Michigan Press; 1987.

18. DIETETIC EDUCATION RESEARCH

Mary B. Gregoire, PhD, RD

Dietetic education is defined in The American Dietetic Association's Standards of Education as a dynamic and complex process that translates the theoretical and ideal into actual application and practice. The Standards stress that dietetic education should reflect the needs of its participants as well as the current and future needs of society.[1]

Discussion of dietetic education programs dates back to the early 1900s, when formal dietetic training began. A three-month course for "pupil dietitians," which required work experience and classroom instruction, was established by Corbett in 1903.[2]

Dietetic education research began in the 1920s as a way to find reliable answers to education questions, discover the best ways of educating future dietitians, and establish principles for dietetic education. The first issue of the *Journal of The American Dietetic Association,* published in 1925, contained a questionnaire from the education section of the Association designed to solicit information on the courses given to student dietitians in hospitals.[3]

Dietetic education research published since that time has focused on a variety of topics, most commonly assessment and evaluation. Assessment, a fact-finding activity, describes conditions existing at a particular time. No hypotheses are proposed or tested, no variable relationships are examined, and no recommendations for action are suggested. Evaluation is concerned with the application of findings and implies some judgment of the effectiveness, social utility, or desirability of a process or program in terms of carefully defined and agreed-upon objectives or values.

Borg and Gall[4] identify several factors that they suggest contribute to the complexity of education research. Subjects in an education research project often are exposed to complex stimuli; these people differ in how they process a given stimulus, and their individual reactions to a given stimulus typically are complex. Thus, dietetic education researchers often have many variables to address simultaneously in a single research project.

RESEARCH DESIGN

An Example of Analytical Research Design

Analytical research designs have been used in dietetic education, most often to assess the effectiveness of a particular teaching method. Cloninger and colleagues,[5] for example, used an analytical design to examine the effectiveness of a microcomputer instructional simulation for teaching food inventory concepts. Students, randomly assigned to treatment and control groups, completed a pretest and attended two lectures on inventory concepts. The treatment group completed a microcomputer simulation program of food item inventory systems, which permitted application of inventory management concepts to solve a case study problem. All students then completed a posttest. Data analysis focused on evaluating the difference between pretest and posttest scores to determine the impact of the independent variable, the use of the computer simulation.

An Example of Descriptive Research Design

The focus of descriptive designs, such as survey and case studies, is on exploring, describing, or explaining existing conditions. No attempts are made to modify variables; rather, data are collected and relationships examined retrospectively.

Survey design, the most common descriptive design used for dietetic education research, uses data collected from a sample to make generalizations about the population of interest. Dietetic education research using the survey design has been conducted for a variety of objectives, such as assessing need for programs, comparing content taught in programs, determining graduates' perceptions of program quality, and evaluating continuing education.

Research by Deskins and Spicher,[6] for example, used survey design to assess the current status of food science instruction in dietetic programs. The authors sent questionnaires to directors of Plan IV and Coordinated Programs in Dietetics to elicit information on faculty teaching food science courses, content of those courses, and perceived changes needed in course content. Results provided information to dietetic educators on how food science is being taught.

Tests

Tests are any series of questions or exercises developed for assessing human performance. Standardized tests have consistent and uniform procedures for administering, scoring, and interpreting behavior and have been demonstrated to have strong validity and reliability. Numerous standardized tests are available for measuring personality, reading, intelligence, achievement, and so forth. The most common references that list standardized measuring instruments are the *Mental Measurement Yearbooks*[8] and their companion volume, *Tests in Print.*[9]

Moore[7] suggests that tests that are not standardized usually do not have an established procedure for administration and have not been constructed using procedures to minimize error. Use of nonstandardized tests is commonly reported in dietetic education research. Researchers who have developed their own tests have documented steps taken to ensure the reliability and validity of such tests. A common use of researcher-developed tests is to measure knowledge or behavior before and after an educational program is initiated. Miller and Shanklin,[10] for example, developed a test to measure behavioral objectives related to forecasting. The test was given before and after completion of a self-instructional module on foodservice forecasting, and data analysis focused on the change in test scores.

Dietetic education researchers collecting data using either standardized or nonstandardized tests need to be concerned about the effect of retesting and test anxiety. Retesting effect is of primary concern in analytical designs that use a pretest and a posttest as part of the methodology. Retesting effect refers to the improvement in test scores that occurs on subsequent tests because a previous test had been taken on the same material. The amount of this effect varies depending on the type of test, the sophistication of the test taker, and the amount of time between the two testings. Anderson and associates[11] suggest that, although reduction of the retesting effect may be difficult, having a control group that takes both the pretest and posttest provides researchers with a way to statistically control for the effect of retesting.

Test anxiety is a concern because it may affect the meaning of test scores and thus influence inferences made based on those scores. Dietetic education researchers can try to reduce the likelihood of test anxiety before data are collected, or they can try to assess the level of test anxiety and then take its influence into account in analysis and interpretation.

Questionnaires

A questionnaire is a group of printed questions used to elicit information from respondents by means of self-report. The questions may be open-ended, requiring respondents to answer in their own words; closed-ended, requiring respondents to select one or more answers from among those provided; or a combination of the two. Questionnaires are the most common data collection technique reported in dietetic education research. Perkin discusses the design and use of questionnaires in chapter 7.

Haughton and Traylor[12] used a questionnaire to elicit information on continuing education needs of personnel in public health nutrition. Their questionnaire consisted of three parts: professional background and employment status, preference for continuing education formats, and need for particular continuing education topics.

Dietetic education researchers need to be aware of the importance of word usage when developing questionnaires. The accuracy of data collected can be jeopardized when a question's meaning is misinterpreted. Pretesting the questionnaire can help reduce the chance for misinterpretation of questions.

Questionnaires that are distributed through the mail present a measure of uncertainty as to whether an adequate number of responses will be received to represent the population being studied.

Interviews

Touliatos and Compton[13] define an interview as a conversation in which an interviewer tries to obtain information from and sometimes impressions about an interviewee. Interviews vary in the amount of structure imposed and thus are categorized as structured or unstructured. Friebel and co-workers[14] used interviews of clients to obtain information on the effectiveness of students as nutrition counselors.

Dietetic educators using interviews need to consider the possible increased cost involved using this technique and the bias the interviewer can create. Training and using skilled interviewers is expensive, and the time involved is often great. Interviewer training is critical, however, to help reduce bias. When several people serve as interviewers, interrater reliability must be assessed to reduce potential rater bias in results.

Observation

Observation, as a data collection technique, allows researchers to document visual perceptions of behavior as it occurs, rather than rely on self-reports of behavior in tests, questionnaires, and interviews.

Anderson and colleagues[11] indicate that observation data can be collected using ratings, systematic observation, or sequential narratives. They define ratings as subjective assessments made on an established scale. They state that systematic observation instruments include two types of recording systems: sign and category. Sign systems list a large number of variables, and each variable that occurs during a given period of observation is marked. For example, a list of classroom behaviors might include: student asks question, teacher gives directions, and so forth. An observer using a sign system type of observation instrument would check each of the behaviors observed. Behaviors occurring more than once during the observation period are checked only once. Category systems generally include a more restricted number of variables. These variables are recorded continuously as often as they occur to produce an ongoing, moving record of behaviors. In the classroom example just cited, the observer would record continuous behavior, documenting each time the student asks a question, each time the teacher provides direction, and so on. Data collected using the category system of observation would include a sequence of events in the classroom and the frequency of occurrence of particular behaviors. Sequential narratives are a written description of all behaviors that occur during an observation session.

Lewis and associates[15] used observation to collect data on counseling skills of nutrition students. Students were videotaped while conducting diet counseling interviews. Trained observers used a category type of systematic observation to record the number of each counseling behavior exhibited during the session.

The Hawthorne and halo effects are two concerns that face dietetic education researchers who choose to use observation techniques for data collection. The Hawthorne effect refers to changes in behavior that occur when the subjects in an experiment or evaluation are aware of their special status. Students may work more eagerly or teachers teach more enthusiastically, perhaps because they feel that they are specially chosen. To help reduce the Hawthorne effect, researchers often need to minimize the newness of the program under study or find ways to make both the treatment and control groups feel that they are receiving something special. The halo effect occurs when raters allow their general impressions to influence their judgment when documenting observations. Thorough training of observers usually is needed to help reduce the impact of the halo effect.

FUTURE RESEARCH NEEDS

Research in dietetic education is important to the growth and development of the profession of dietetics and is essential if the education of future dietitians is to be effective. A current focus in dietetic practice is the issue of cost effectiveness. Research is needed to determine the educational strategies that will result in preparation of quality entry-level dietitians at the lowest possible cost. Dietetic educators are continually challenged to find methods that help achieve maximum learning by students. Additional research is needed to determine effective educational strategies. Interdisciplinary research projects conducted with education researchers could produce information on why students learn and factors that help motivate students in the learning process.

References

1. The American Dietetic Association: *Accreditation/Approval Manual for Dietetic Education Programs.* Chicago, Ill: The American Dietetic Association; 1987.
2. Chambers MJ. Professional dietetic education in the U.S. *J Am Diet Assoc.* 1978;72:596–599.

3. Questionnaire for the education section. *J Am Diet Assoc.* 1925;1:31.
4. Borg WR, Gall MD. *Educational Research.* 2nd ed. New York, NY: Longman; 1977.
5. Cloninger BJ, Messersmith AM, McEwan CW. Food item inventory instructional simulation using microcomputer. *J Am Diet Assoc.* 1988;88:1090–1093.
6. Deskins BB, Spicher CB. Food science instruction in undergraduate dietetic education. *J Am Diet Assoc.* 1989;89:1250–1253.
7. Moore GW. *Developing and Evaluating Educational Research.* Boston, Mass: Little Brown and Co; 1983.
8. Buros OK, ed. *Mental Measurements Yearbook.* Highland Park, NJ: Gryphon; 1939–1978; 1–8.
9. Buros OK, ed. *Tests in Print II.* Highland Park, NJ: Gryphon; 1974.
10. Miller JL, Shanklin CW. Status of menu item forecasting in dietetic education. *J Am Diet Assoc.* 1988;88:1246–1249.
11. Anderson SB, Ball S, Murphy RT. *Encyclopedia of Educational Evaluation.* San Francisco, Calif: Jossey-Bass Publisher; 1975.
12. Haughton B, Traylor MN. Continuing education needs of personnel in public health nutrition in the eight southeastern states. *J Am Diet Assoc.* 1988; 88:359–363.
13. Touliatos J, Compton NH. *Research Methods in Human Ecology/Home Economics.* Ames, Iowa: Iowa State University Press; 1988.
14. Friebel DM, Sucher K, Lu NC. University wellness program: the effectiveness of students as nutrition counselors. *J Am Diet Assoc.* 1988;88:595–598.
15. Lewis NM, Hay AL, Fox HM. Evaluation of a workshop model for teaching counseling skills to nutrition students. *J Am Diet Assoc.* 1987;87:1544–1556.

19. META-ANALYSIS IN NUTRITION AND DIETETICS

Anne M. Dattilo, PhD, RD

This chapter introduces the topic of meta-analysis with a definition, a summary of its historical background, and a description of specific features. Because meta-analysis is one of many ways to summarize existing data, it is compared with other, more traditional methods of reviewing and combining trial results. Relevant criticisms of meta-analysis are presented with practical suggestions of how the researcher can help increase the reliability and validity of a meta-analysis. Particular attention is directed to the application of meta-analysis with regard to the nutrition literature throughout this discussion.

DEFINITION

Meta-analysis uses the results of many empirical studies to answer specific, quantitative questions.[1] Glass[2] was the first to use the term, which, in its Greek derivation, means an analysis that is more comprehensive.

Glass differentiated primary analysis, secondary analysis, and meta-analysis in a manner that distinguished meta-analysis from other types of data analysis. Primary analysis is the original analysis of data in a research study. The units of analysis are the subjects in the study, and data provided by these subjects are analyzed and presented as summary statistics. Secondary data analysis is typically the reanalysis of data from a primary research project. The goal of secondary data analysis is usually to answer additional questions from the existing data set or to apply advanced statistical procedures to those data. In meta-analysis, the statistical unit is the primary or secondary research study, and its data points are the summary statistics provided by those research studies. Glass, McGaw, and Smith[3] more recently defined meta-analysis as "the attitude of data analysis applied to quantitative summaries of individual experiments." They further explained that "Meta-analysis is not a technique; rather it is a perspective that uses many techniques of measurement and statistical analysis."

HISTORICAL BACKGROUND

Meta-analysis, per se, is not new to the review literature. As early as the 1930s researchers attempted to combine results from agricultural studies. Lush[4] investigated the relationship between the initial weight of steers and their subsequent weight gain. From five studies, he computed an average correlation between baseline and subsequent weight of $r = 0.39$. Lush did not report an overall test of significance to assess the probability that the particular set of correlations with their associated tests of significance could have been obtained if the true value of the correlation in the appropriate population were zero.[5] Methods for testing statistical significance of combined probability levels were being established in the early 1930s by Fisher,[6,7] and Pearson.[8,9] Thus, early meta-analysis included two separate approaches: One focused on estimating the magnitude of the experimental or treatment effect; the other presented the results of combined significance tests to quantify results from studies with similar hypotheses.[10] Both approaches are still used today.

Integrating findings from various research efforts in the biological sciences became popular in the 1970s and 1980s when manuscripts[2,3,5,10–14] advanced the meta-analytical methodology. Sacks, Berrier, Reitman, Ancona-Berk, and Chalmers[15] surveyed the medical literature for papers that pooled results of controlled clinical trials. The 50 journals they searched published a total of 177 meta-analysis papers prior to 1986. Of the 86 papers that met the inclusion criteria, the earliest one cited by Sacks and colleagues was Beecher's, published in 1955, on the results of placebo effects. By that year, most of the groundwork for methodology used in meta-analysis today had been established[16-19]; however, the majority (80%) of the meta-analysis studies reviewed by Sacks and colleagues were published in the 1980s. Thus, meta-analysis has become a popular and acceptable way to summarize results of a number of different studies in the medical literature.

Recently, meta-analyses have been published in the field of nutrition. In the area of coronary heart disease (CHD) risk factor reduction, meta-analysis procedures have been used to assess the effectiveness of weight loss as a treatment for hypertension,[20] determine attributes of successful smoking cessation programs,[21] quantify the effects of exercise on blood lipids,[22,23] and the effects of exercise on weight reduction.[24] In the area of treatment of CHD, meta-analysis has been applied to assess the effects of beta blockade during and after myocardial infarction,[25] examine the usefulness of cardiac rehabilitation after myocardial infarction,[26] compare the effectiveness of coronary artery bypass graft surgery and nonsurgical interventions for coronary artery disease,[27] present the value of exercise[28] and exercise testing in post-myocardial infarction patients,[29] and evaluate the effectiveness of intravenous streptokinase on acute myocardial infarction.[30] In the area of nutrition education, meta-analysis has been used to assess the effectiveness of nutrition education on nutrition knowledge, attitude, and behavior[31,32] and to evaluate the effectiveness of education for patients recovering from surgery and heart attacks.[33] Meta-analytical techniques have also been applied to help determine the relationship of alcohol consumption to risk of breast cancer,[34] define the relationship of breastfeeding to development of atopic disease in infants,[35] assess the effectiveness of perioperative total parenteral nutrition,[36] and describe trends in dietary consumption.[37]

Meta-analysis is most useful when addressing quantitative research questions that are tested with a sample size that is too small to detect a statistically significant effect, or when results of several investigators disagree.[38] Other types of integration and review may be more appropriate to address qualitative aspects of studies that meta-analysis is unable to determine.

SPECIFIC FEATURES

To date, optimal methods for combining and analyzing study findings have not been established.[15,38] However, two separate methods have been used extensively in the meta-analysis literature. As stated previously, one method involves pooling probability levels from independent studies to obtain an overall significance level. The second method involves pooling effect sizes from individual studies to describe the strength of the relationship between two variables of interest.

Axelson, Federline, and Brinberg[31] first used combined significance tests in their meta-analysis to determine whether the set of probability levels from their pool of nine studies could have been obtained if the null hypothesis of no relationship between the variables (nutrition knowledge and dietary intake) were true. Because the overall probability was significant ($P < 0.01$), the authors rejected the hypothesis that there was no relationship between nutrition knowledge and dietary intake. Axelson and co-workers then proceeded to calculate the magnitude (effect size) of the relationship.

Pooling Probability Levels

Although pooling results using combined probability methods is often performed in meta-analysis, pooled probability results are sometimes of limited value, since they do not address the magnitude of effect between variables. However, pooling probabilities is associated with greater power than the narrative review or vote counting method (subsequently described). For example, Axelson and colleagues[31] found a significant relationship between nutrition knowledge and dietary intake for nine studies after combining probability levels from each study. These authors chose the Fisher method[6] of adding z-transformed probability levels (weighted by each study's associated degrees of freedom) to calculate an overall probability. Although the z-transformation is a popular method of combining probability levels, Rosenthal[13] has described eight additional methods from which analysts can choose. In most situations, regardless of the procedure employed, the difference in overall results is slight.[39]

Because six of the nine studies reported nonsignificant correlations in the meta-analysis by Axelson and colleagues,[31] the vote counting method would conclude that no support existed for a relation between the two variables. Relationships were small but consistent, so combining results decreased the chance of concluding that no relationship existed when there was a significant relationship. Therefore, combining significance levels can be of value when the number of studies to be pooled is limited. The increase in power from combining a small number of studies can help highlight subtle effects that individual studies miss.[12] However, when the number of studies increases, the null hypothesis is likely to be rejected simply because of sample size. As Glass and colleagues[3] stated: "For most problems of meta-analysis, the number of studies will be so large and will encompass so many hundreds of subjects that null hypotheses will be rejected routinely."

Reporting results of an effect size along with the combined probability value is advocated by researchers who use combined tests.[14,40] Others do not use combined probability tests in their reviews because testing the significance of combined results does not address the magnitude, direction, and consistency of experimental effects.[10] Thus, estimating and combining effect sizes from studies should be performed and is the preferred method of data amalgamation.

Results of pooling significance levels from a large database of studies can be a misleading, highly significant overall effect, even if treatment effects are small and have little substantive importance. For this reason, some reviewers have relied less on statistical significance tests that report whether the treatment works or not than on the value of the treatment or effect size.

Pooling Effect Sizes

To summarize results from all studies in the meta-analysis in terms of magnitude, some common scale or metric must be established. Individual study findings are measured in terms of an effect size, which is a scale-free way of measuring results. The effect size is most often measured by either the standardized mean estimate of the difference between groups or the correlation between variables. The type of effect size indicator used in a meta-analysis depends on the nature of data provided in studies and the research design used in the studies.

When studies include experimental and control groups, the effect for each treatment can be assessed, relative to the placebo or control group, by calculating the standardized mean difference between the two groups and its confidence interval. Differences in incidence reported as proportions, risk ratios, or odds ratios also have been used to describe the effect size in medical literature.[41] If the overall effect size measurement is the difference between the experimental group mean and control group mean expressed in standard deviation units, the overall effect size is expressed as a standardized score and can be interpreted as a z score. In a normal distribution, the mean + one standard deviation encompasses 68% of the population; of the remaining 32%, one-half, or 16%, will be on the right tail. For example, if the mean effect of a medication versus a placebo on hyperactivity results in mean effect size of −1.00, the conclusion would be that the average patient taking the medication exhibits a level of hyperactivity one standard deviation below that of the average patient on the placebo. With the aid of standardized tables and assuming normality, 16% of the patients in the placebo group are less hyperactive than the average of those taking the drug.[2] Although confidence intervals around the mean effect size are not always reported in meta-analysis, this indicator of random error is very useful when interpreting results.

Johnson and Johnson[32] used the standardized mean difference in their meta-analysis comparing nutrition behavior of subjects participating in a nutrition education program (experimental group) to those who did not participate (control group). The average effect size reported was 0.47, meaning that, in terms of nutrition behavior, subjects receiving nutrition education were at 0.47 standard deviation units above the mean of the group not receiving nutrition education. The authors concluded that nutrition education participants (score of the average person in the experimental group) ate nutritionally at the 69th percentile of the control (exceeded that of 69% of people in the control group). If the effect size were −0.47, the average person in the experimental group exceeded that of only 31% of people in the control group. Standard deviations, instead of confidence intervals, were reported by these authors to help the reader assess variation in results.

When control groups are absent, or when variables are scaled in intervals, the correlation coefficient is used as the index of effect size. The correlation coefficient is a scale-free measure of the relationship between variables, so it can be used as an index of effect magnitude.[10] The goal of correlational meta-analyses, such as standardized mean difference meta-analyses, is to identify one common effect size that can best describe results of all studies reviewed. To achieve this goal, correlation coefficients must be obtained from each study. The Pearson product moment correlation coefficient (r) is the most common effect size indicator of correlational studies.

Interpreting the overall effect size when correlation coefficients have been averaged is more familiar to many readers than interpreting effect sizes that have been calculated by the standardized mean difference methods. Cohen[42] applied general descriptive terms to small (r = 0.10), medium (r = 0.30), and large (r = 0.50) effect sizes. Although these guidelines are somewhat arbitrary, they can be helpful in interpreting the magnitude of the overall effect.[39]

Another way to interpret the mean effect size is by comparing correlations for different sub-groups in the meta-analysis. For example, Tran, Weltman, Glass, and Mood[23] reported correlations between number of hours in an exercise training program and changes in the total cholesterol/high-density lipoprotein-cholesterol (HDL-C) ratio. The relationship was large (r = 0.62, $P < 0.01$)

for men and small ($r = 0.09$, not significant) for women. Assuming the relationship was linear, men apparently responded more favorably to increased hours of exercise training in terms of the total cholesterol/HDL-C ratio than women.

Comparing correlations can also be used when reviewing results of different hypotheses within the same meta-analysis. Axelson et al[31] used correlational meta-analysis in their report of the relationship between nutrition knowledge and dietary intake and food and nutrition-related attitudes and dietary intake. Although estimates of the effect sizes of these relationships were relatively small ($r = 0.10$ and $r = 0.18$, respectively), the relationship between attitudes and dietary intake was slightly stronger.

Correlation coefficients are frequently reported in meta-analysis. Because they only describe the strength of the relationship between variables, correlation coefficients are often limited in practical situations. In contrast, regression coefficients provide insight into the actual amount of change predicted in a treatment or condition. Although linear regression techniques can be applied to meta-analysis, Hedges and Olkin[10] reported that unless all studies included in the meta-analysis have the same sample size and the same population correlation, the individual "error" variances can differ greatly. Therefore, assumptions of ordinary regression analysis may be violated in meta-analysis. Thus, Hedges and Olkin presented methods analogous to ordinary regression analyses that weight each study by its number of subjects and that are useful when calculating regression coefficients.

TRADITIONAL METHODS OF RESEARCH SYNTHESIS

Although meta-analysis is gaining popularity, more common approaches used to summarize findings from empirical studies are the narrative review and vote-counting method. These methods present and aggregate results from several studies to help resolve ambiguity; however, they have limitations. Neither method describes the strength or size of the effect of an intervention. In addition, the accumulation of information presented in a narrative review article is typically unsystematic[12] and statistical methods used in vote-counting are unsound.[12,39,43–44] The vote-counting method of research summation has a different approach from the narrative method; it forces the reviewer to be quantitative. Vote counting is used when a reviewer is interested in assessing whether the majority of studies reviewed finds a treatment effective. However, results from a vote count do not indicate the degree of effectiveness.

Components of traditional methods of research synthesis are described in the following section.

Narrative Review

The traditional narrative review has a number of shortcomings in providing a comprehensive and accurate means of extracting important information from study results. This type of data summation simply inspects and describes findings without clear methodology for data aggregation. If a large number of studies is read, the reviewer must remember individual findings from many studies to establish a common conclusion. Thus, Glass and associates[3] state, "Contemporary research reviewing should be more technical and statistical than it is narrative. . . .The findings of multiple studies should be regarded as a complex data set, no more comprehensible without statistical analysis than would hundreds of data points in one study."

Cooper and Rosenthal[45] have shown that even when the number of studies reviewed is as small as seven, reviewers who use narrative methods to reach an overall conclusion and reviewers who use quantitative methods of meta-analysis may reach different conclusions. These researchers randomly assigned 41 graduate students and faculty members to two groups. Members of each group worked independently. Both groups reviewed the same seven papers addressing gender differences in task persistence and were asked to test the null hypothesis of no gender difference in task persistence.

Participants in one group were provided detailed instructions on how to combine significance levels to obtain an overall test of significance for the seven studies through meta-analysis. Participants in the other group were assigned to the traditional procedure condition and were asked to use any procedure they would normally use when conducting a review of literature. Although the seven studies clearly showed that females were significantly more task persistent than males, 73% of the traditional review participants found no gender relationship compared with only 32% of the meta-analysis reviewers. These results indicated that traditional methods of reviewing used by participants in this experiment were susceptible to type II errors (failing to reject null hypotheses that are false). If a relationship does exist in a given review, the traditional narrative review therefore may not detect it.

Traditional review articles typically have no established criteria for inclusion or elimination of references, and protocol has not been defined for determining what findings from the original research papers should be included. Large numbers of studies may be excluded, and the fact that these studies influence final conclusions is overlooked. Bias by the author of such a review could easily result.[3]

Jackson,[46] interested in potential problems with the narrative review, critiqued 36 review articles randomly sampled from leading journals in the social sciences. He reported that analysis and discussion sections of review papers often focused on only a part of the full set of studies the authors found. Typically, the subsets of studies were not representative of the entire samples, and no information was provided on how the subsets were chosen. For example, only 3% of the review articles appeared to have used existing indexes or thorough attempts to secure available literature, and only 22% of the reviewers reported on a "fair" sample of studies, as judged by Jackson's coders. Half of the articles used references from studies that promoted a research proposition; studies that disagreed were ignored. Jackson concluded that reviewers usually provide such scanty detail about their methods of review that validity of the conclusions cannot be assessed by the reader.

Another common finding of review articles is that they conclude by calling for more research in the particular area to resolve "conflicting results."[11] Since most reviews report at least some conflicting findings,[46] Light and Pillemer[12] suggested that variation between studies be examined to determine if differences in outcome were due to random sampling variation around a single population parameter, or if a cluster of population parameters existed. Examining variation systematically may shed light on why conflicting results exist. The narrative review paper typically does not address this variation.

Although many negative aspects of traditional narrative reviews have been presented, narrative reviews do not by definition contain flaws.[44] An effective narrative review with explicit detail of methods and analytic procedures can provide qualitative information of value.

Vote Counting

Methods for performing a vote count of the pool of studies collected are relatively simple. Study results are grouped in terms of significantly positive findings, significantly negative findings, or nonsignificant outcomes. The number of studies in each category is tallied. The category of the three with the most votes is assumed to provide the best estimate of direction for the relationship between independent and dependent variables.[47]

The vote counting method has been criticized to the extent that some writers recommend that it not be used because of its lack of statistical accuracy.[39] For example, the vote count gives no information about sample sizes in various studies. Because large samples produce more statistically significant findings than do smaller samples, results are likely to be biased.[12] In addition, when both sample size and treatment effect are small, but consistent in one direction, the vote count does not identify an overall significant effect.[43] Another criticism of the method is that the procedure disregards the quality of studies and the practical significance of statistically significant findings.[12] Finally, vote counting neglects important information about the strength, magnitude, and relationships among variables.[2]

The effect size, a feature of meta-analysis previously discussed, is often reported with results from the vote count. For example, Johnson and Johnson[32] provided both voting results and effect sizes in their review on the effectiveness of nutrition education programs on knowledge, attitude, and behavior change. The authors noted that vote counting provided only a rough estimate of what could be identified by more advanced statistical techniques.

ISSUES IN META-ANALYSIS

Meta-analysis has advantages over traditional methods of research integration and can be used alone or in conjunction with traditional methods. Instead of simply reporting that variation in studies exists, as is typical for traditional narrative methods, meta-analysis explains the variation by identifying study characteristics that influence or interact with the relationship between the dependent and independent variables. Not only are statistical findings of many studies analyzed, as should occur in traditional methods, but the sample size and unique features of each individual study are assessed before making final conclusions.[38] Although the use of meta-analysis is likely to become a standard practice for future literature reviews,[48] several criticisms of its reliability and validity have been identified.

Reliability Issues

Reliability, in general, refers to consistency of measurement. Consistency in locating and selecting articles are reliability issues that must be addressed. The procedures for locating articles to be included in the meta-analysis must be consistent, and the collection must be comprehensive. Through systematic and thorough search procedures that are explicitly outlined in the methodology, the analyst can attempt to attain reliability.

Locating studies. Studies are usually found through indexes that cite and abstract information from primary research studies. Journals, dissertations and theses, government reports, papers from scholarly meetings, as well as review periodicals (nutrition abstracts and reviews) are potential sources of studies.[3] Automated computer searches are now popular because of their speed in identifying relevant literature. However, caution is extended to the reviewer who relies solely on this method to ascertain studies. Sacks and colleagues[15] recommend not using computer searches as the only means to collect studies because a number of potential studies lack the primary descriptors, or indexing terms, used to search the database. Tran and Weltman[22] reported that only 35% of the final 95 studies collected for their meta-analysis were located by computer searches. Similarly, Louis[1] found only six papers of the 27 he included in a meta-analysis of public health literature through an automated search. Therefore, in addition to searching the automated bibliographic systems, hand searching of journals, discussions with professionals and researchers working in the interest area, and the individual analyst's knowledge of the literature should be called upon to secure the best representation of available studies. Nevertheless, every study performed in a given area probably will not be uncovered. In addition, the analyst may choose to select only studies published in peer-reviewed journals for the meta-analysis.

Selecting inclusion criteria.   The issue of whether to include unpublished studies in a meta-analysis is not resolved. Some analysts choose to include unpublished studies (dissertations, abstracts, or papers presented at meetings) in their pool of studies,[31, 32] whereas others argue that the quality of these studies is lower than those published in peer-reviewed or refereed journals and choose to include only formally published works.[1, 15, 22, 23, 38]

Glass and associates[3] reported two examples in which unpublished studies had equal or better designs than comparable published studies and concluded that excluding unpublished studies in a meta-analysis may produce misleading results. In addition, they reported the relationship between the source of publication and findings for 11 different meta-analyses in social psychology. The authors concluded that in all nine cases in which a direct comparison could be made, effects from primary research studies published in journals were larger than findings reported in unpublished theses or dissertations. Similar findings were reported by Devine and Cook[49] in their meta-analysis of the effects of psycho-educational intervention on length of hospital stay; effect sizes of dissertations were consistently less than effects calculated from journals or books. However, others report that unpublished papers (eg, abstracts) lack methodologic rigor and present larger effects than studies published as journal articles.[38]

Abstracts presented at professional meetings or published in abstract form have been included in some meta-analyses. However, Goldman and Loscalzo[50] followed a group of cardiology papers submitted to national scientific meetings (published in abstract form) for three years to determine which abstracts were published in peer-reviewed journals. Only half of the published abstracts were ultimately published as full-length articles. Relman,[51] in an editorial addressing reliability of abstracts, suggested that the remaining papers followed by Goldman and Loscalzo were so flawed that they were either never submitted for publication or rejected by the peer-review process. In addition, published abstracts without subsequent publication as papers have been shown to report larger effects than studies published as papers.[38] The decision and rationale for the type of manuscript included in the database of studies for meta-analysis should be clearly indicated by the analyst.

Because one source of manuscript may report greater effects than another form, Glass et al[3] recommend that the meta-analyst collect all literature addressing the hypotheses and analyze it separately by mode of publication. However, this practice may result in the inclusion of data from the same study more than once. If, for example, a dissertation's findings are later published, only one, the dissertation or published article should be included in the final meta-analysis. Similarly, a review article or book chapter may include data from several primary research articles. Each primary research finding should be included only once in the final analyses and in its highest scientific form. If all forms of literature are included in the pool of studies, it may be impossible to ascertain that data from a given study are not represented more than once. For this reason, most meta-analyses report only studies found in journals. In addition, if a large number of studies are reported in journals, the assumption that the large number of studies are a true representation of all research results seems reasonable. However, Glass and collegues[3] reported that studies with significant results are published more often than nonsignificant studies.

A chronological trend in research findings that is not realized by the reviewer may also bias meta-analyses results. Often, as a matter of convenience, researchers restrict publication inclusion to a specific number of years. This practice is cautioned. Glass and associates[3] reported that the correlation between date of publication and effect size for six meta-analyses was 0.13, suggesting that more recently published studies had a greater effect than older studies. They further constructed a linear regression equation relating date of publication to effect size. These calculations indicated that studies published in 1975 showed a 0.22 average effect size advantage over experiments dated 1965. Glass and associates therefore suggest that reviewers avoid arbitrarily limiting inclusion dates.

Fail-safe N. Rosenthal[13] addressed the potential problem that studies published are a positively biased sample of all studies actually conducted: "The extreme view of this problem, the file drawer problem, is that the journals are filled with the 5% of the studies that show type I errors, while the file drawers back at the lab are filled with the 95% of the studies that show nonsignificant (eg, $P > 0.05$) results." There is no definitive solution to the problem of publications only presenting positive results; however, Rosenthal[13] reported a formula given as:

$$X = K [K\bar{Z}^2 - 2.706]/2.706$$

where K is the number of studies combined, Z is the mean Z value from the pooled probability value obtained from the K studies, and X is the number of filed or unretrieved studies, or the "fail-safe N."

The fail-safe N is used to estimate the number of unpublished studies with negative results necessary to change a statistically significant result into an insignificant overall finding. If the number of filed or unretrieved studies is very large, concern that publication bias may influence results is unlikely. For example, Rosenthal and Rubin[14] reported that in a review of 345 studies, 65 123 unpublished studies showing no significant relationship between variables would have to be locked in file drawers to overturn the combined significance of the 345 published studies. Although it appears unlikely that more than 65 000 studies on any topic would have been performed, computing a fail-safe N is a useful procedure to estimate the impact that unpublished studies could have on conclusions drawn from the studies used in a meta-analysis. Thus, the fail-safe N can provide the reader with information about how many additional studies would be needed to negate the effects reported.

Coding study findings. In addition to consistency in locating and selecting studies for the meta-analysis, the act of coding information from the studies has been an issue in reliability. Inconsistencies in coding study findings can occur if different coders do not judge study characteristics in the same way, or if methods for coding varies.[3] Intercoder reliability can be enhanced by pilot-testing coding forms, making necessary changes, and training coders to use the code book and coding forms. Intercoder reliability then can be readily assessed[52] and the coefficient reported in the results of the meta-analysis.

Studies with multiple findings. A decrease in reliability of effect sizes can result if researchers do not address non-independence of effects from the same study. Since the unit of analysis for most meta-analysis is the finding, not the study, studies that report multiple findings (eg, results for male subjects and female subjects, values at ten weeks and three months after treatment) have more effect sizes (ie, more weight) than those that report only one finding. When including multiple effect sizes from the same group of subjects, there is no easy solution to the question of how many independent units of information exist when studies are pooled. One approach to increasing the independence of effects is to use the entire study as the unit of analysis, rather than individual findings. This method increases the independence of the data, but it severely limits the use of available data. Glass and colleagues[3] suggest two practical solutions to address the number of unknown independent units in the larger data set.

The first is the method used by Tran and associates.[22,23] Their "risky" solution assumes that each finding is independent of the others. Inferential calculations could be applied to the data, and the results (means, correlations, and regression coefficients) could be reported as long as a qualifying statement of the independence assumption is included. The risky solution is a problem when the number of findings per study is large, and the pool of studies is small. The other, more complex method to address interdependencies in large data sets utilizes Tukey's jackknife method,[53] which allows the analyst to determine if a transformation of the data set is necessary, and if the transformation applied is suitable. Glass and colleagues[3] applied Tukey's jackknife procedure to the 108 different comparisons found from analyzing 14 studies that addressed the effect of class size on achievement. When interdependencies were considered, the confidence intervals for regression coefficients were more than 350% wider than when the data were assumed to be independent.

Studies with varying sample sizes. An additional decrease in reliability of effect sizes can result if researchers do not explain how studies with different sample sizes are handled. By assigning equal weight to studies with differing sample sizes, small samples that may be unrepresentative of a greater population contribute as much weight to the results of a meta-analysis as studies with large numbers of subjects. Thus, weighting schemes for studies with differing sample sizes have been suggested by Hedges and Olkin,[10] Hunter et al,[11] Rosenthal,[5,13] and Wolf.[39]

Hunter et al[11] found that a weighted average (each correlation weighted by the number of subjects in the study) is superior to the unweighted average in all but one situation. While coding data on 13 studies located for one meta-analysis, the authors found one study with a sample size of 15 000. The other 12 studies had sample sizes of 500 or less. If the weighted average were used, the one large study would have more than 30 times the weight given to any other study. Therefore, the authors recommend performing two separate analyses in such cases. A first analysis would include the large sample study, and a second analysis would exclude it. Because Hunter and co-workers have no solution if the two analyses show major differences, and eliminating a study with a large sample size is not appropriate, investigators are encouraged to report both the mean weighted and unweighted correlation for all studies.[32]

Although most meta-analysis methodologists suggest weighting study findings by sample size,[5,10,11,13,39] Tran and associates[23] chose not to use weighting schemes. These authors found no significant correlation between sample size and effect size, concluding that "weighting the studies by sample size would give undue emphasis to arbitrary choices of sample sizes and to researchers with greater ambition or resources." The nonsignificant correlation found by the authors could have resulted if the majority of the studies used in their meta-analyses had similar sample sizes. However, in many meta-analyses, sample size from studies can vary widely, so performing both weighted and unweighted analyses is preferred.

Validity Issues

Validity of a meta-analysis refers to adequacy of reported information and clarity of definitions of variables. While coding study characteristics, the coder must exercise judgment to ascertain certain characteristics. If variables have standardized measurements (eg, age, body weight, serum lipids), validity is less of a problem than if variables have many methods of measurement (eg, an attitude scale that can differ from study to study).

Study quality. Study quality is another area that has been suggested to influence validity of final results. Many reviewers choose to eliminate studies with results that have been biased due to methodologic flaws[46] or poor research design. Although using data from studies lacking methodologic rigor can influence internal validity of the final meta-analysis, this issue can be addressed by coding and accounting for study quality or features of studies thought to influence study quality in the model.

Hovell[20] reviewed and rated study quality for 21 intervention studies assessing effects of weight reduction on hypertension. Although the point system Hovell used appears somewhat arbitrary and subjective, and it was not validated, a thorough explanation of the scale was provided so the reader could assess appropriateness. Hovell allowed a total of 18 points for studies with ideal research design, and 17 points for studies that met ideal blood pressure measurement criteria. For example, four points were awarded to a study that included a control group, three points for random allocation of participants to groups, two points for repeated measures of blood pressure within each visit, and one point if trained personnel in blood pressure measurement were identified. Results indicated that only four studies earned a score of nine or better in terms of research design. Thus, if studies with methodologic weakness were eliminated from the pool of 21 studies that Hovell collected, his review of the effects of weight reduction on hypertension would consist of a limited number of studies.

Quality should be assessed for each study included in a meta-analysis, but not all methodologic inadequacies or weak designs cause biased results. For example, Glass and colleagues[3] reported the relationship between design quality (high, medium, and low) and effect size for twelve different meta-analyses. They concluded that in general, no more than a 0.1 standard deviation unit was found between studies of high validity and low validity. Similarly, Stock, Okin, Haring, and Witter[54] found no relationship between research design and study results for their meta-analysis on age differences in subjective well-being. Straw[55] also found no difference in the effects of deinstitutionalization on mental health from studies of different quality. Generally, all manuscripts from an a priori pool (eg, only peer-reviewed published papers, or all published works) should be included in the analyses, unless obvious evidence of bias from methodologic problems is present[46] or it is clear that the authors have made an error in reporting results. It is prudent, however, to examine characteristics of studies that could influence study quality.

Individually coding study characteristics thought to influence study quality has advantages over arbitrarily rating study quality. To date, no system has been developed to rate "good" studies and "lesser quality" studies systematically. Results can be erroneous if the scoring system used to rate study quality has not been validated. For these reasons, the analyst should code individually study characteristics that could potentially influence results (eg, if a control group was included in a study, if subjects were free of disease or not taking medications). These variables could be entered in regression analysis to determine how study variables influence results.[48]

Journal quality. In addition to coding study characteristics that may influence study quality, journals that provided studies for meta-analysis can also be coded to indicate "journal quality." Journal quality may not necessarily be an indicator of study quality. However, the practice of reporting the number of studies from each journal used in the meta-analysis would allow readers to assess which journals contribute the most studies.

Combining "different" studies. The final issue in this chapter is perhaps the most common criticism of meta-analysis and the largest threat to external and construct validity. Combining many different studies has raised concern, but Glass and colleagues[3] argue that averaging data from different persons is no different from aggregating data from different studies. "These persons are as different and as much like apples and oranges in their way as studies are different from each other." Thus, combining results from studies by the use of meta-analysis is not so different theoretically from combining results from individual subjects in primary research. However, to ensure that the studies collected for a meta-analysis can be combined and to decrease the threat to validity, several procedures have been identified. First, researchers should ascertain that only studies addressing similar hypotheses are considered for any particular meta-analysis. Second, grouping studies together a priori, according to similar coding characteristics and testing for homogeneity, can help decrease the chance of combining studies that are more dissimilar than alike. Third, regressing study characteristics on effect sizes can determine variables that significantly influence overall results and should not be arbitrarily combined. By using procedures to determine which studies can logically and statistically be combined, the researcher will not fall victim to combining "apples with oranges."

META-ANALYSIS METHODOLOGY

Methodology to perform meta-analyses has been described in detail by many.* However, procedures described by Glass and colleagues[3] are perhaps the most often used for measuring findings. Many statisticians have provided details of their procedures that vary from the Glassian method,[10,11,13] but these methods, as does the method of Glass and colleagues,[3] include the sequence of

*References 2,3,10,12,13,15,18,38,39, 41,43–47

searching the literature for manuscripts (studies), specifying inclusion or exclusion criteria, recording study characteristics, and pooling and analyzing appropriate findings. Readers are referred to aforementioned references to choose the most appropriate method for their data before performing a meta-analysis.

SUMMARY

In response to the inadequacy of the traditional review process, reviewers have applied more quantitative procedures to independent study findings to achieve conclusions that are meaningful and more reliable than traditional methods of research review. These procedures, known collectively as meta-analysis, offer several advantages over other forms of reviewing, particularly when a large volume of literature is being examined. Thus, meta-analysis is becoming more popular as the preferred way of reporting summary findings in the areas of public health and clinical research.[1,15,38] However, meta-analysis has not gone unchallenged. The criticisms directed at the process have served the useful purpose of forcing meta-analysts to examine threats to reliability and validity and general procedures for meta-analysis. If reliability and validity issues are considered by the reviewer and if acceptable procedures are used, meta-analysis is a viable approach to combining trial results and can produce objective, repeatable conclusions.

References

1. Louis T. Findings for public health from meta-analyses. *Annu Rev Public Health.* 1985;6:1–20.
2. Glass G. Primary, secondary, and meta-analysis of research. *Educ Researcher.* 1976;6:3–8.
3. Glass G, McGaw B, Smith M. *Meta-analysis of Social Research.* Beverly Hills, Calif: Sage; 1981.
4. Lush JL. Predicting gains in feeder cattle and pigs. *J Agric Res.* 1931; 42:853–881.
5. Rosenthal R. *Meta-analytic Procedures for Social Research.* Beverly Hills, Calif: Sage; 1984.
6. Fisher RA. *Statistical Methods for Research Workers.* 4th ed. London, England: Oliver and Boyd; 1932.
7. Fisher RA. *Statistical Methods for Research Workers.* 7th ed. London, England: Oliver and Boyd; 1938.
8. Pearson K. Appendix to Dr. Elderton's paper on "The Lanarkshire milk experiment." *Ann Eugen.* 1933;5:337–338.
9. Pearson K. On a method of determining whether a sample of size n supposed to have been drawn from a parent population having a known probability integral has probably been drawn at random. *Biomed.* 1933;25:379–410.
10. Hedges L, Olkin I. *Statistical Methods for Meta-analysis.* Orlando, Fla: Academic Press Inc; 1985.
11. Hunter J, Schmidt F, Jackson G. Meta-analysis. In: *Cumulating Research Findings Across Studies.* Beverly Hills, Calif: Sage; 1982.
12. Light R, Pillemer D. *Summing Up: The Science of Reviewing Research.* Cambridge, Mass: Harvard University Press; 1984.
13. Rosenthal R. *Judgment Studies: Design, Analysis, and Meta-analysis.* Cambridge, Mass: Cambridge University Press, 1987.
14. Rosenthal R, Rubin D. Interpersonal expectancy effects: the first 345 studies. *Behav Brain.* 1978;3:377–415.
15. Sacks H, Berrier J, Reitman D, Ancona-Berk V, Chalmers T. Meta-analyses of randomized controlled trials. *N Engl J Med.* 1987;316:450–455.
16. Cochran WG. Problems arising in the analysis of a series of similar experiments. *J R Stat Soc.* 1937;Suppl 4 (1):102–118.
17. Cochran WG. The comparison of different scales of measurement for the experimental results. *Ann Math Stat.* 1943;14:205–216.
18. Mosteller F, Bush R. *Selected Quantitative Techniques.* Cambridge, Mass: Addison-Wesley; 1954.

19. Stouffer S, Suchman E, DeVinney L, Star S, Williams R. *The American Soldier: Adjustment During Army Life.* Princeton, NJ: Princeton University Press; 1949;1.
20. Hovell M. The experimental evidence for weight-loss treatment of essential hypertension: a critical review. *Am J Public Health.* 1982;72:359–368.
21. Kottke T. Attributes of successful smoking cessation interventions in medical practice: A meta-analysis of 39 controlled trials. *JAMA.* 1988;259:2882–2889.
22. Tran Z, Weltman A. Differential effects of exercise on serum lipid and lipoprotein levels seen with changes in body weight. *JAMA.* 1985;254:919–924.
23. Tran Z, Weltman A, Glass G, Mood D. The effects of exercise on blood lipids and lipoproteins: a meta-analysis of studies. *Med Sci Sports Exerc.* 1983;15:393–402.
24. Epstein L, Wing R. Aerobic exercise and weight. *Addict Behav.* 1980;5:371–388.
25. Yusuf S, Peto R, Lewis J, Collins R, Sleight P. Beta blockade during and after myocardial infarction: an overview of the randomized trials. *Prog Cardiovasc Dis.* 1985;27:335–371.
26. Oldridge N, Guyatt G, Fischer M, Rimm A. Cardiac rehabilitation after myocardial infarction: combined experience of randomized clinical trials. *JAMA.* 1988;260:945–950.
27. Wortman P, Yeaton W. Synthesis of results in controlled trials of coronary bypass graft surgery. In: Light RJ; ed. *Evaluation Studies Review Annual.* Beverly Hills, Calif: Sage; 1983:536–551.
28. LeMura L, von Duvillard S, Bacharach D. Central versus peripheral adaptations for the enhancement of functional capacity in cardiac patients: a meta-analytic review. *J Cardiopul Rehab.* 1990;10:217–223.
29. Froelicher V, Perdue S, Pewen W, Risch M. Application of meta-analysis using an electronic spread sheet to exercise testing in patients after myocardial infarction. *Am J Med.* 1987;83:1045–1054.
30. Stampfer M, Goldhaber S, Yusuf S, Peto R, Hennekens C. Effect of intravenous streptokinase on acute myocardial infarction: pooled results from randomized trials. *N Engl J Med.* 1982;307:1180–1182.
31. Axelson M, Federline T, Brinberg D. A meta-analysis of food- and nutrition-related research. *J Nutr Educ.* 1985;17:51–54.
32. Johnson D, Johnson R. A meta-analysis and synthesis of nutrition education research. *J Nutr Educ.* 1985;17(suppl.):s11–s27.
33. Mumford E, Schlesinger H, Glass G. The effects of psychological intervention on recovery from surgery and heart attacks: an analysis of the literature. *Am J Public Health.* 1985;72:141–151.
34. Longnecker M, Berlin J, Orza M, Chalmers T. A meta-analysis of alcohol consumption in relation to risk of breast cancer. *JAMA.* 1988;260:652–656.
35. Kramer M. Does breast feeding help protect against atopic disease? Biology, methodology, and a golden jubilee of controversy. *J Pediatr.* 1988;112:181–190.
36. Detsky A, Baker J, O'Rourke K, Goel V. Perioperative parenteral nutrition: a meta-analysis. *Ann Intern Med.* 1987;107:195–203.
37. Stephen A, Wald N. Trends in individual consumption of dietary fat in the United States, 1920–1984. *Am J Clin Nutr.* 1990;52:457–469.
38. L'abbe K, Detsky A, O'Rourke K. Meta-analysis in clinical research. *Ann Intern Med.* 1987;107:224–233.
39. Wolf F. *Meta-analysis: Quantitative Methods for Research Synthesis.* Beverly Hills, Calif: Sage; 1986.
40. Rosenthal R. Combining results of independent studies. *Psychol Bull.* 1978;85:185–193.
41. Thacker SB. Meta-analysis: a quantitative approach to research integration. *JAMA.* 1988;259:1685–1689.
42. Cohen J. *Statistical Power Analysis for the Behavioral Sciences.* New York, NY: Academic Press; 1977.
43. Hedges L, Olkin I. Vote-counting methods in research synthesis. *Psychol Bull.* 1980;88:359–369.
44. Light R, Pillemer D. Numbers and narrative: combining their strengths in research reviews. *Harvard Educ Rev.* 1982;52:1–26.
45. Cooper HM, Rosenthal R. Statistical versus traditional procedures for summarizing research findings. *Psychol Bull.* 1980;87:442–449.
46. Jackson G. Methods for integrative reviews. *R Educ Res.* 1980;50:438–460.
47. Light R, Smith P. Accumulating evidence: procedures for resolving contradictions among different studies. *Harvard Educ Rev.* 1971;41:429–471.

48. Strube M, Hartman D. Meta-analysis: techniques, applications, and functions. *J Consult Clin Psychol.* 1983;51:14–27.
49. Devine E, Cook T. A meta-analytic analysis of effects of psychoeducational interventions of length of post-surgical hospital stay. *Nurs Res.* 1983;32:267–274.
50. Goldman L, Loscalzo A. Fate of cardiology research originally published in abstract form. *N Engl J Med.* 1980;303:255–259.
51. Relman A. News reports of medical meetings: how reliable are abstracts? *N Engl J Med.* 1980;303:277–278. Letter.
52. Tinsley HE, Weiss DJ. Interrater reliability and agreement of subjective judgements. *J Couns Psyc.* 1975;22:358–376.
53. Mosteller F, Tukey J. Data analysis, including statistics. In: Lindzey G, Aronson E, eds. *Handbook of Social Psychology.* Reading, Mass: Addison-Wesley; 1968.
54. Stock W, Okin M, Haring M, Witter R. Age differences in subjective well-being: a meta-analysis. In: Light RJ, ed. *Evaluation Studies Review Annual.* Beverly Hills, Calif: Sage; 1983:279–302.
55. Straw R. Deinstitutionalization in mental health: a meta-analysis. In: Light RJ, ed. *Evaluation Studies Review Annual.* Beverly Hills, Calif: Sage; 1983:253–278.

PART 6
USEFUL NUMBERS
IN RESEARCH

Balancing available resources and powerful research design challenges all investigators. For research to be beneficial, a sample size adequate to answer the research question and statistical analysis appropriate to evaluate the resulting data are critical. Chapters 20 and 21 address these two issues.

In determining sample size, a researcher must set the levels of two parameters: α, the desired statistical significance level, and β, the power to detect the magnitude of anticipated difference. A type I error, known also as an α error or false positive, occurs when the researcher assumes that there is a difference or effect when none actually exists. A type I error is customarily set at 5% or $P = 0.05$. In this example, the probability of correctly finding that there is no difference or effect is $1 - \alpha$, ie, 95% or $P = 0.95$.

A type II error, known also as β error or false negative, occurs when one assumes that there is no difference or effect when there really is one. A type II error usually is set at 20%, ie, $P = 0.20$. The power to find a real difference is $1 - \beta$, ie, 80% or $P = 0.80$. As sample size increases, the power to find a true effect increases. Increasing sample size also decreases the likelihood of a type II error.

Chapter 20 discusses various formulas to estimate sample size. The appropriate formula to select is based on the type of data to be analyzed (eg, continuous or proportion) and the research design (eg, sampling method). Economic constraints may require adjustment of the desired power and proposed significance level; however, these two terms cannot be modified drastically without jeopardizing the usefulness of the projected research.

Once the data are collected, the researcher should look at them thoughtfully. Chapter 21 illustrates the process of devising various data plots during data analysis to enable ready visual inspection. If the data do not follow a normal distribution, it is wise to consider transforming the data (eg, into logarithms) or using nonparametric statistical methods. Although an investigator may graph and inspect the data in many different plots, none of the initial plots may be necessary when the research is reported or published.

Plot the data, develop summary statistics, estimate the magnitude of the data comparisons, and assess the differences by statistical analysis. Summary statistics, which include means, frequencies, range, and standard deviations

(SDs), are useful in describing data sets. The SD needs to be differentiated clearly from the standard error of the mean (SE). The SD indicates the distribution, spread, or variation around the mean; the SE indicates the precision of the measure. Because SE is always a smaller number than SD (SE is derived by dividing the SD by the square root of the size of the sample), people may be tempted to report SE, thinking that it connotes sharper control. The SD and SE are different statistics and should be used knowledgeably.

Table 21.1 categorizes statistical methods appropriate for evaluating differences between groups. During the design phase, before data collection, the statistical tests by which the data will be analyzed are determined on the basis of four elements: the nature of the research question (comparative or relational), the scale of measurement of the data to be collected (discrete or continuous), the relationship between samples (dependent or independent), and the number of samples to be evaluated (one, two, or multiple). Multiple comparisons, or multiplicity, raises statistical problems in that the more comparisons that are made, the more likely it is that false positives will be "detected." If the significance level is set at 5%, one expects that, by chance alone, 1 out of 20 comparisons will appear to be significant (see chapter 2). For example, if one compares the intake of 15 nutrients with 12 serum levels one will find that, by chance, approximately 9 of the 180 comparisons appear to be statistically significant. The mistaken appearance of statistical significance from multiple comparisons has been referred to as the "runaway P value."

A wise investigator uses statistics to evaluate whether the observed differences are significant, then further evaluates whether the differences make a difference. As Thomas Carlyle said, "A judicious man looks at statistics, not to get knowledge, but to save himself from having ignorance foisted on him."

ERM, Editor

20. ESTIMATING SAMPLE SIZE

Carrie L. Cheney, PhD, RD, and Carol J. Boushey, MPH, RD

Sample selection, discussed in chapters 8 and 9, and sample size are two determinants of whether an investigation is worthwhile. An otherwise excellent study can fail to detect an important effect just because the sample size is too small. Results of such studies serve to confuse the issue under investigation; worse, they can lead to misleading or patently wrong conclusions.

The process of estimating the required sample size involves several steps and can be technically complex; it is wise to seek the help of a knowledgeable statistician. An understanding of the basic elements of estimating the sample size, which this chapter will provide, will facilitate interaction with a statistician. This chapter will highlight the issues underlying the logic of sample size calculations, outline the general procedure that is common to all situations, describe the procedures specific to common research situations, and provide references for further information.

THE LOGIC OF SAMPLE SIZE CALCULATIONS

Statistics allows the investigator to estimate the unknown. By use of statistics, characteristics of a population can be estimated based on observations of a sample drawn from it. The size of the sample largely determines how accurate or precise the estimates from the sample are; the larger the sample, the more information about the population and the more precise the estimate. Uncertainty always exists. The investigator, however, can specify in advance the amount of uncertainty that is acceptable for the study and perform appropriate sample size calculations.

Two hypotheses, the research hypothesis and the null hypothesis, provide the framework for the logic of sample size calculations. Before an investigation is undertaken, a research hypothesis that serves as the basis of the investigation is formulated. The null hypothesis, ie, that there is no difference or effect, serves as a standard of comparison. Statistical analysis is conducted to determine whether the results of the study are consistent with the underlying null hypothesis. If the results do not demonstrate the presence of a difference or an effect, it is concluded that the data fail to refute the null hypothesis.

When drawing conclusions from statistical results, there are four possible outcomes, two correct and two incorrect (*Table 20.1*). First, one can correctly conclude there is no difference or effect ($1 - \alpha$; for convenience in sample size calculations, it is assumed that failure to reject the null hypothesis is the same as concluding that the null hypothesis is true; however, this is not appropriate when interpreting results). Second, one can conclude that there is a difference or effect when there is none (α, false positive, type I error). Third, one can conclude that there is no difference or effect when there is one (β, false negative, type II error). Finally, one can conclude that there is a difference or effect, which is truly present ($1 - \beta$, power). All four possible outcomes are expressed statistically as probabilities.

		Truth About Study Hypothesis	
		True (alternate, H_1)	**False** (null, H_0)
Statistical Test Results About Hypothesis	**True** (reject H_o)	Correct ($1 - \beta$, power)	False positive (type I error, α error)
	False (do not reject H_o)	False negative (type II error, β error)	Correct ($1 - \alpha$)

The type I error, or α error, is also known as the significance level of the study; its complement, $1 - \alpha$, is the correct conclusion if the null hypothesis is true. By convention, α is usually set at 5%, or $P = 0.05$. This means that the maximum acceptable risk of drawing a false positive conclusion is 5%. Obviously, the smaller the α, the lower the risk of drawing a false positive conclusion. The investigator specifies the α level during the planning of the study and compares the resulting P value with α at the end of the study. If the observed P value is less than α, the result is considered to be statistically significant.

The type II error, or β error, expresses the probability of missing a difference; and its complement is power, or $1 - \beta$. If the null hypothesis is not true and a difference or effect exists, the β probability quantifies the risk of missing that difference and power quantifies the chance of finding it. As β decreases, power increases. The investigator specifies β during the planning of the study, which then determines power. For example, if the risk of missing a difference is set at 20% ($P = 0.20$), the chance that the study would find a real difference would be 80% ($P = 0.80$).

The probability that, if a true effect exists, a study will detect it (ie, power) largely depends on the sample size. Increasing the sample size increases the power. At the same time, increasing the sample size decreases the risk of a false negative conclusion (ie, β or type II error) because the ability to detect a true difference is increased.

The power of a study also depends to some degree on the true magnitude of difference or effect under study. For any given power, a large difference can be detected with a smaller sample size than can a small difference. Accordingly, for any given sample size, the study will be more likely to detect a large difference than a small difference. The investigator determines in advance the magnitude of difference or effect that is important for the study to be able to detect.

The general relationship among sample size, power, and the magnitude of the difference or effect sought can be expressed as[1]:

$$\text{Sample size (n)} > 2 \left[\frac{(\alpha \text{ error} + \beta \text{ error}) \times \text{SD}}{|\text{Difference}|} \right]^2$$

where mathematically the α and β errors are converted to the standardized normal deviates (Z values) for the probabilities, the SD equals the estimated standard deviation, and the difference is the absolute value of its magnitude. For example, a change in low-density lipoprotein cholesterol (LDL-C) levels from 5.19 mmol/L to 4.87 mmol/L would be a difference of -0.32 mmol/L or an absolute difference of 0.32 mmol/L.

Because of this relationship, if the sample size is not restricted, the investigator will want to determine the sample size required to ensure a high probability of detecting a meaningful difference or effect of XX magnitude. If, on the other hand, the sample size is limited, ie, predetermined, the investigator can use sample size calculations to determine the probability (power, $1 - \beta$) that the study will be able to detect a meaningful difference. In practice, the final determination of the size of the research project will be a judicious balance of power and economics.

GENERAL PROCEDURE FOR SAMPLE SIZE CALCULATIONS

Sample size estimates are based on a number of assumptions about the conditions of the study. Since it is not possible for an investigator to know in advance what the conditions of the study will be, the calculations provide only an estimate. The general procedure for calculating the required sample size involves seven steps.

Step 1. Choose the main end point of interest and the method by which it is to be measured. A series of sample size calculations may be performed if there is more than a single important end point for the study. In such cases, the largest estimated sample size is generally used.

Step 2. Choose the statistical test that is appropriate for the data and the research question. It is best to consult with a statistician at this point (see chapter 21).

Step 3: Specify the magnitude of the difference or effect that is meaningful to detect. The magnitude of the difference or effect selected should be practical, ie, an important difference in practice. Additionally, it should be sufficiently small that a negative study outcome (ie, no significant difference) would be assurance that if a true difference existed, it would be too small to be of practical importance.

Step 4. Estimate the expected variability, ie, the estimated SD. Preferably, this value comes from a pilot study conducted earlier, but it can also come from published research results. Lacking either of these, a "best guess" must be made.

Step 5. Specify the maximum acceptable risk of a false positive conclusion (α, type I error). Alterations in α concomitantly alter power and β. As α is lowered, power decreases and β increases; as α is increased, power increases and β decreases. By convention, the α probability is set at 0.05, although the situation may warrant setting a lower or higher risk. The seriousness of a false positive conclusion determines whether the maximum acceptable risk should be set lower. Only under rare circumstances is α set greater than 0.05, because to do so can compromise the ability of the results to be convincing. An increased α would be warranted, however, in circumstances in which there are serious consequences of a false negative conclusion (β error), and it is desired to decrease β without increasing the sample size beyond what is feasible.

Another consideration in choosing α is whether the statistical test is to be one-tailed or two-tailed (see chapter 21). A one-tailed α is more liberal than a two-tailed α, as it tests for a difference in only one direction. The more conservative approach of applying a two-tailed significance test enables the investigator to test for a difference in either direction from the null and is generally preferred.

Step 6. Specify the probability of successfully detecting the difference or effect, if it exists (power, $1 - \beta$). Alternatively, the probability of a false negative conclusion can be specified (β, type II error). By convention, power is usually set at 0.80 to 0.90 and β is set at 0.20 to 0.10, respectively. Again, the seriousness of a false negative conclusion guides the decision.

Step 7. Apply the appropriate calculations (see the following examples).

It may be that the estimated sample size is larger than what is feasible under the actual circumstances and with available resources. If this is the case, the power of the study should be calculated according to the number of subjects that is feasible with available resources. The procedure for calculating the power of a study with a fixed sample size prior to undertaking it is similar to that just given. Steps 1 through 7 should be performed, substituting the fixed sample size for power in step 6 and solving for power instead of sample size in step 7.

Research design often requires a compromise of the ideal and the feasible; the goal of design is a practical and economic balance between power and sample size. However, in deciding to compromise power, the investigation must recognize that the ability of the study to accomplish its objective is also compromised. A study may not be worth doing if there is a low probability of detecting a meaningful effect.

SAMPLE SIZE DETERMINATION FOR SPECIFIC RESEARCH SITUATIONS

Continuous Data

Paired observations. A paired t test is usually used in an investigation in which a continuous response measure is observed before and after the subject receives a treatment, or in which observations in two groups are linked by pairing. In this instance, the sample size formula accounts for the correlation between the measurements within the pairs.[2,3]

An example might be a study to assess whether a particular intervention will decrease dietary cholesterol intake as measured by three-day food records (step 1). For one sample, before and after study design, an experimental effect can be tested with a paired t test (step 2). Using the data of Cohen and associates,[4] it can be determined that a change of -75 mg would be meaningful and practical (step 3). Further, the SD of the difference (SD_{diff}) can be estimated (step 4) as 158.9 mg, according to the study of Van Horn and co-workers,[5] which used three-day food records.

In advance, α is specified as 0.05 with a two-tailed test (step 5). The decision is made to set power or $1 - \beta$ at 0.80, making β 0.20 (step 6). The appropriate calculations (step 7) can now be applied. The sample size needed to conduct a test with significance-level α and power, $1 - \beta$, is:

(Formula 20.1) $\qquad n = \left[\dfrac{(Z_{1-\beta} + Z_{1-\alpha}) \times SD_{diff}}{|\mu_1 - \mu_0|} \right]^2$

The quantities $Z_{1-\beta}$ and $Z_{1-\alpha}$ are values from the standard normal distribution analogous to α and β. *Table 20.2* gives selected values of $Z_{1-\beta}$ and $Z_{1-\alpha}$

corresponding to commonly used values of α and β. From above, $SD_{diff} = 158.9$ mg and $\mu_1 - \mu_0 = 75$ mg. Therefore, using formula 20.1, the sample size for a two-sided test can be estimated as follows:

$$n = \left[\frac{(Z_{1-\beta} + Z_{1-\alpha/2}) \times SD_{diff}}{|\mu_1 - \mu_0|} \right]^2$$

$$= \left[\frac{(0.84 + 1.96) \times 158.9}{75} \right]^2$$

$$= \left[\frac{444.92}{75} \right]^2$$

$$= \mathbf{35.2} \text{ or } \mathbf{36} \text{ subjects}$$

Table 20.2
Unit Normal Deviates Z_α and Z_β for Selected Values of α and β

α or β	Two-sided test* $Z_{1-\alpha/2}$	$Z_{1-\beta}$
0.01	2.58	2.33
0.025	2.24	1.96
0.05	1.96	1.64
0.10	1.64	1.28
0.20	1.28	0.84
0.30	1.04	0.52

* If using a one-sided test, the $Z_{1-\alpha}$ values would be the same as in the $Z_{1-\beta}$ column.

If the investigators also planned to measure the difference in other nutrients, eg, saturated fat intake, these calculations would be repeated for each nutrient of interest, and the final sample size would correspond to the calculation with the highest n. Finally, when they recruited subjects, the investigators would enroll extra participants to allow for attrition during the intervention without compromising the study's power.

Tables are available by which sample size and power can be estimated for a variety of differences and levels of α and β errors.[2,6] A computer program is also available.[7]

The examples in this section use continuous variables; for discrete variables, the formulas would be slightly different[8] and are discussed later. Chapter 21 clarifies the issue of continuous versus discrete variables.

Independent groups. Study designs addressing nutrition questions usually involve comparison of two samples. Investigations often are planned to observe the response measures on subjects who receive either of two treatments, typically an experimental treatment and a control treatment. The response variable, eg, HDL-C, is measured on a continuous scale. A difference of a specified magnitude or greater is set at a level thought to be important with a particular power. The comparison is usually made by t test for independent samples.

An example might involve members of the dietetics department of a health maintenance organization (HMO), who are concerned that the agency's current screening criteria for anemia using the hemoglobin value may need to be revised. The article by Nordenberg and colleagues[9] suggests that hemoglobin cutoff values should be adjusted upward for smokers. The HMO collects detailed smoking information on each new enrollee and determines hemoglobin value as well, so an investigation is planned to determine whether women smokers and nonsmokers between the ages of 18 and 44 years have significantly different hemoglobin values. One of the study components involves comparing the mean hemoglobin values of a random sample of smokers to a random sample of nonsmokers.

In this case, the main end point of interest is hemoglobin, a continuous variable (step 1). To compare the means of the two randomly selected groups, an independent t test can be used (step 2). The results reported by Nordenberg and colleagues[9] indicate that the mean hemoglobin value among female smokers is 137 g/L and 133 g/L among female nonsmokers. The calculated difference of interest is 4 g/L (step 3). A standard error of 0.4 g/L for smokers and 0.5 g/L for nonsmokers was reported.[9] By converting these values (step 4) to their corresponding SDs (standard error = $SD/\sqrt{n}$), setting α at the conventional 0.05 (step 5) and power at 90% (step 6), and applying the appropriate formula, the sample size for the two groups can be determined. The formula for a two-sided test is[8]:

(Formula 20.2) $$n = \frac{(SD_1^2 + SD_2^2)(Z_{1-\beta} + Z_{1-\alpha/2})^2}{(\bar{x}_2 - \bar{x}_1)^2}$$

The values for $Z_{1-\beta}$ and $Z_{1-\alpha/2}$ can be found in Table 20.2. The SDs for smokers and nonsmokers are 12.37 and 17.37, respectively. The difference of interest, $(x_2 - x_1)$, is 4 g/L. According to formula 20.2, the sample size is:

$$n = \frac{(17.37^2 + 12.37^2)(1.28 + 1.96)^2}{(-4)^2}$$

$$= \frac{(454.7338)(10.4976)}{16}$$

$$= \mathbf{298} \text{ in each group (596 total)}$$

However, the funding is limited to 175 subjects in each group (350 total). This is a common occurrence. As a consequence of various constraints, a sample size analysis often begins with a fixed value for n. In this case, the resulting power $(1 - \beta)$ can be determined by rearranging formula 20.2 and solving for $Z_{1-\beta}$:

(Formula 20.3) $$Z_{1-\beta} = \sqrt{\frac{(\bar{x}_2 - \bar{x}_1)^2 \cdot n}{(SD_1^2 + SD_2^2)}} - Z_{1-\alpha/2}$$

Using all of the values determined previously, but substituting 175 for n, the study power is calculated as:

$$Z_{1-\beta} = \sqrt{\frac{(4)^2 \cdot 175}{(17.37^2 + 12.37^2)}} - 1.96$$

$$= \sqrt{6.157} - 1.96$$

$$= 2.48 - 1.96$$

$$= \mathbf{0.52}$$

Table 20.2 indicates that 0.52 corresponds with $\beta = 0.30$, so $1 - \beta = 0.70$, or 70% power. The investigators conclude that the 175-subject sample size will provide adequate power and continue with plans for the study.

Because the actual formula for calculating sample size based on the t test can be solved using computational iterative methods, tables have been constructed for use.[2,6] These tables provide sample sizes necessary to detect a range of differences with varying degrees of power. Additional tables indicate the power provided by various sample sizes and magnitudes of differences, and the text that accompanies them describes their use in detail.[2] An even simpler method to compute sample size and power for the t test can be found in a computer program offered by Dupont and Plummer.[7]

Three or more independent groups. Studies that compare a continuous response measure in more than two groups are usually analyzed by analysis of variance rather than several t tests. Based on analysis of variance, Day and Graham[10] provide a nomogram to estimate the required sample size when comparing three or more treatment groups.

More complex designs. Nutrition studies commonly employ designs, such as prospective cohort or retrospective case-control designs, that evaluate the association of a risk factor with some outcome of interest. The measure of association estimated from these studies is the relative risk or odds ratio. The procedures appropriate for the prospective cohort study are given by Phillips and Pocock[11] and for the case-control study by Lubin, Gail, and Ershow.[12]

Reliability studies. Reliability studies, eg, of the reliability of methods of assessing dietary intake, are also common in nutrition and dietetics. In these studies, reliability is often estimated by the coefficient of intraclass correlation from an analysis of variance. Sample size requirements for reliability studies are discussed by Donner and Eliasziw,[13] who also provide power contours to guide in the planning.

Proportions

Independent groups. In an investigation in which a dichotomous or categorical response measure is observed in two independent groups, the frequencies of response are compared between groups, usually by the χ^2 test in a two-way contingency table. As with the procedure for the t test, the investigator must guess about an unknown quantity, in this case, one of the proportions. The investigator then is asked, as usual, to specify the smallest difference from this amount that is important to detect and the α and β errors that are acceptable. With these quantities, the investigator can estimate the required sample size.

For the example of anemia (hemoglobin < 120 g/L) among smokers and nonsmokers, a two-way contingency table based on the data reported by Nordenberg and colleagues[9] can be constructed (*Table 20.3*). The proportions can be quantified, eg, $46/956 = 4.8\%$ prevalence of anemia among smokers. The prevalence of anemia among nonsmokers is 8.4%, therefore the difference of interest could be 3.6, or any value specified as meaningful in the population.

Table 20.3
Two-way Contingency Table

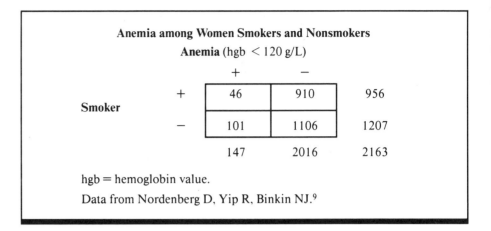

Anemia among Women Smokers and Nonsmokers

		Anemia (hgb < 120 g/L)		
		+	−	
Smoker	+	46	910	956
	−	101	1106	1207
		147	2016	2163

hgb = hemoglobin value.

Data from Nordenberg D, Yip R, Binkin NJ.[9]

Although formulas are available to calculate sample size,[3,14,15] a simpler and perhaps more informative method is to use graphs[16,17] or tables.[18,19] Tables and graphs have the advantage of providing at a glance the required sample sizes for several combinations of proportions and differences. The computer program by Dupont and Plummer[7] also performs the required calculations.

An example using available tables might be a trial planned to assess the efficacy of vitamin C in preventing the common cold. The subjects, employees in a large machinery plant, have agreed to be assigned randomly to receive a vitamin C supplement or a placebo daily for the duration of the winter season. A previous survey has shown that the usual incidence of colds during the winter season is 50%. The investigators think that a reduction in the incidence by half (ie, to 25%) would result in a meaningful economic benefit to the company and the employees. The investigators adhere to convention and set α at 0.05. Because a number of trials have shown negative results (with questionable statistical power), the investigators also wish to be reasonably certain to avoid a false negative conclusion and to have sufficient power for the results to be conclusive, so they set β at 0.10, giving 90% power. Using the tables provided by Fleiss,[18] they find a sample size of 85 per group, or a total of 170, is needed for a two-tailed test of the difference in proportions in this study.

After discussions with the company administration, the investigators are told that funds are available to support a study of only 120 subjects, or 60 per group. Referring to the tables by Fleiss,[18] they find that 60 subjects per group will provide power of 75% at an α of 0.05. The investigators decide that this level of power is acceptable and proceed with plans for the study.

Paired observations. An investigation that employs a matched design, pairing observation from a case with observation from a control (ie, matched case-control study) is analyzed in a manner that accounts for pairing, such as McNemar's test for paired studies.[20] Procedures for sample size determination are provided by several authors,[18,20,21] and a computer program is offered by Dupont and Plummer.[7]

More complex designs. When the investigation involves more than two groups and more than one response measure, the analysis, and thus the sample size determination, become more complex. The analysis generally utilizes some form of the χ^2 test in a multi-way contingency table. Lachin[22] provides the statistical rationale and methods for determining the required sample size for such studies for the statistically inclined investigator; those who are less mathematically inclined should consult a statistician.

A related class of studies common in nutrition epidemiology are those of more than two risk factors that are dichotomous measures, such as cohort or case-control studies of the association of several risk factors with a chronic disease. Clinical trials can also evaluate more than two treatments simultaneously. Studies of this type generally employ discrete multivariate analysis methods (eg, multivariate contingency tables and unconditional logistic models). A general method for sample size determination in this class of study is described by Greenland.[23] A modified method is applied to prospective studies by Phillips and Pocock[11] and to cohort and case-control studies by Lemeshow and associates.[24] Again, investigators who are unfamiliar with these techniques should consult a statistician.

Performance characteristics of laboratory tests. It is frequently of interest in dietetics to employ tests to classify persons or to screen them for certain characteristics or risks. The use of anthropometrics to assess nutritional status and screen for patients at risk of malnutrition at hospital admission is one example. Tests are often compared with one another to determine the performance characteristics and relative usefulness in classifying persons, especially when one test is more expensive or labor-intensive. The important performance characteristics are the positive and negative predictive values (described in chapter 6), two proportions that determine the practical usefulness of tests.[25,26] Power and sample size requirements of studies of this nature are presented by Arkin and Wachtel.[26]

References

1. Armitage P. *Statistical Methods in Medical Research.* London, England: Blackwell Scientific Publications; 1971:186.
2. Dixon WJ, Massey FJ Jr. *Introduction to Statistical Analysis.* 3rd ed. New York, NY: McGraw-Hill Book Co; 1969:269.
3. Lachin JM. Introduction to sample size determination and power analysis for clinical trials. *Controlled Clin Trials.* 1981;2:93.
4. Cohen NL, Laus MJ, Stutzman NC, Swicker RC. Dietary change in participants of the better eating for better health course. *J Am Diet Assoc.* 1991;91:345.
5. Van Horn L, Moag-Stahlberg A, Liu K, et al. Effects of serum lipids of adding instant oats to usual American diets. *Am J Public Health.* 1991;81:183.
6. Pearson ES, Hartley HO. *Biometrika tables for statisticians.* 3rd ed. Cambridge, England: Cambridge University Press; 1970;1.
7. Dupont WD, Plummer WD Jr. Power and sample size calculations: a review and computer program. *Controlled Clin Trials.* 1990;11:116.
8. Rosner B. *Fundamentals of Biostatistics.* 2nd ed. Boston, Mass: Duxbury Press; 1986:264,322.
9. Nordenberg D, Yip R, Binkin NJ. The effect of cigarette smoking on hemoglobin levels and anemia screening. *JAMA.* 1990;264:1556.
10. Day SJ, Graham DF. Sample size and power for comparing two or more treatment groups in clinical trials. *Br Med J.* 1989;299:663.
11. Phillips AN, Pocock SJ. Sample size requirements for prospective studies, with examples for coronary heart disease. *J Clin Epidemiol.* 1989;42:639.
12. Lubin JH, Gail MH, Ershow AG. Sample size and power for case-control studies when exposures are continuous. *Stat Med.* 1988;7:363.
13. Donner A, Eliasziw M. Sample size requirements for reliability studies. *Stat Med.* 1987;6:441.
14. Casagrande JT, Pike MC, Smith PG. An improved approximate formula for calculation sample sizes for comparing two binomial distributions. *Biometrics.* 1978;34:483.
15. Fleiss JL, Tytun A, Ury HK. A simple approximation for calculating sample sizes for comparing independent proportions. *Biometrics.* 1980;36:343.
16. Feigl P. A graphical aid for determining sample size when comparing two independent proportions. *Biometrics.* 1978;34:111.

17. Aleong J, Bartlett DE. Improved graphs for calculating sample sizes when comparing two independent binomial distributions. *Biometrics.* 1979;35:875.
18. Fleiss JL. *Statistical Methods for Rates and Proportions.* 2nd ed. New York, NY: John Wiley and Sons; 1981:260.
19. Cohen J. *Statistical Power Analysis for the Behavioral Sciences.* 2nd ed. New York, NY: Academic Press; 1977.
20. Schlesselman JJ. *Case-control Studies: Design, Conduct, Analysis.* New York, NY: Oxford University Press; 1982:160,207.
21. Fleiss JL, Levin B. Sample size determination in studies with matched pairs. *J Clin Epidemiol.* 1988;41:727.
22. Lachin JM. Sample size determinations for r × c comparative trials. *Biometrics.* 1977;33:315.
23. Greenland S. Power, sample size and smallest detectable effect determination for multivariate studies. *Stat Med.* 1985;4:117.
24. Lemeshow S, Hosmer DW Jr, Klar J. Sample size requirements for studies estimating odds ratios or relative risks. *Stat Med.* 1988;7:759.
25. Weiss NS. *Clinical Epidemiology: The Study of the Outcome of Illness.* New York, NY: Oxford University Press; 1986:14.
26. Arkin CF, Wachtel MS. How many patients are necessary to assess test performance? *JAMA.* 1990;263:275.

Additional Readings

Arkin CF. The t-test and clinical relevance. Is your B error showing? *Am J Clin Pathol.* 1981;76:416–420.

Detsky AS, Sackett DL. When was a 'negative' clinical trial big enough? *Arch Intern Med.* 1985;145:709–712.

Diamond GA, Forrester JS. Clinical trials and statistical verdicts: probable grounds for appeal. *Ann Intern Med.* 1983;98:385–394.

Ellenberg SS. Determining sample sizes for clinical trials. *Oncology.* 1989;3:39–46.

Hall JC. A method for the rapid assessment of sample size in dietary studies. *Am J Clin Nutr.* 1983;37:473–477.

Young MJ, Bresnitz EA, Strom BL. Sample size nomograms for interpreting negative clinical studies. *Ann Intern Med.* 1983;99:248–251.

21. STATISTICAL APPLICATIONS

Carrie L. Cheney, PhD, RD

For the nonstatistician, the process of selecting the statistical method to apply to research data can be a challenge. Seeking guidance from a statistician during the planning of the research project and as necessary throughout the research effort is a wise course of action. To facilitate communication with a statistician, the investigator should be familiar with the fundamentals of statistics and their applications. This chapter reviews the fundamentals of statistical analysis, outlines the general procedure involved, provides suggestions for analysis of several common research situations, and illustrates the procedure with a detailed example of applying statistical methods to a typical study design. References are provided throughout and readers are encouraged to use them, especially for the technical aspects of statistical calculations, which are not presented here.

FUNDAMENTALS

Four elements of the study design help guide the selection of statistical method. These elements are: the research question, the scale of measurement in which the data are collected, the relationship among samples, and the number of samples to be evaluated. Additional considerations relate to characteristics of the statistical test and include the test's assumptions about the normal distribution, frequently referred to as the Gaussian distribution, and whether the test should be applied as a one-sided or two-sided test of significance.

The Research Question

Most, if not all, research questions, as applied to research in dietetics, can be categorized into one of two main categories of questions: *comparative* or *relational*. In operational terms, the research is concerned with drawing comparisons or examining relationships. The distinction is largely a result of the sampling method and study design chosen. The statistical methods for these two types of questions are not the same because the purposes of the analyses differ. The comparative question asks the statistical analysis to determine if differences exist; the relational question asks the statistical analysis to determine whether associations exist.

Examples of comparative research question. Does vitamin C supplementation elevate serum oxalate levels in patients with renal disease? In a hypothetical study designed to answer such a question, patients could be randomized to receive either the standard vitamin preparation that includes vitamin C (the one currently in use in the clinic) or a similar vitamin preparation that excludes vitamin C. The analysis evaluates the difference, particularly the amount of increase, in serum oxalate levels between patients who receive vitamin C supplementation and patients who do not receive vitamin C supplementation.

Example of relational research question. Is vitamin C supplementation associated with an increased risk of hyperoxalemia among patients with renal

This work was supported in part by grant CA18029 awarded by the National Cancer Institute, USDHHS to the Clinical Nutrition Program, Clinical Research Division, Fred Hutchinson Cancer Research Center, Seattle, Wash.

disease? In a study designed to answer this type of question, all patients in a given clinic could be examined to determine serum oxalate levels and interviewed about use of vitamin C supplements. The analysis evaluates whether vitamin C supplement use is associated with the presence of hyperoxalemia.

The Scale of Measurement (Type of Data Collected)

The measurements collected in research are referred to as *variables*. Variables can be classified in a number of ways that are useful for determining the method of data analysis to use. Variables that are not inherently numerical in nature—ie, for which only a few possible values exist, as would be the case for sex—have a distribution that is *discrete*. If the distribution is *continuous*, the variables have numerical meaning, as would be the case for blood pressure. The statistical methods used for discrete variables differ from those used for continuous variables.

Discrete variables. Although the symbol used to represent discrete information may be a number, these data are categorical in nature, ie, they represent or name categories. A discrete datum may be further classified by whether it is nonordered, termed *nominal*, or ordered, termed *ordinal*. Nominal data correspond to a limited number of categories that have no ordered meaning. Nominal variables that fit into two categories, such as present and absent, are termed *binary*. Ordinal data are ordered by categories, but the space between the categories is undefined. Treatment group may be considered ordinal if the different treatments differ by dosage of a particular supplement. Examples of these measures are:

Binary	Gender (female, male)
	Disease status (present, absent)
Nominal	Race (several categories, no order)
Ordinal	Clinical stage of cancer (ordered 1 through 4)

Continuous variables. Continuous variables are those that have a numerical value (numerical "category"), and the space between the values is defined and can be measured. Continuous data fit into a theoretically unlimited number of categories with equal spaces between the categories. Common examples of continuous data are height, weight, and energy intake.

The Relationship Among Samples

Independent samples. The assumption underlying many statistical tests is that the measures among samples are independent. Samples are independent when the data points in one sample are unrelated to the data points in the second sample. An investigator may be interested in the relationship between smoking and hemoglobin level in women between the ages of 18 and 44 years. If the investigator identifies a group of smokers and a group of nonsmokers from a prepaid health plan and measures their hemoglobin levels, the two samples would be completely independent, since the data are obtained from unrelated groups of women.

Dependent samples. Measures in samples that are related are dependent, ie, they are inherently correlated. There are a number of situations in research that produce related measures, and thus do not meet the assumption of independence.

Pairing and matching.   Samples can be related by pairing or matching in the study design. An example of a common study design that utilizes pairing is the crossover trial, a study that uses subjects as their own controls. In a crossover trial, an initial observation is compared with a second observation measured on the same subject after the completion of some intervention by the investigator.

Related observations are also obtained when the subjects are matched. In the usual matched study, each subject in one group is matched with a subject in another group by one or more factors, such as age and gender. Specially designed statistical tests that account for the pairing and its resulting dependence among measures must be used. Examples of such tests are the paired *t* test and the sign test, described by standard statistics textbooks.

Serial measures.   Besides matching and pairing, another situation giving rise to dependent measurements is the practice of obtaining repeated or serial measures on individual subjects. It is common to repeat measurements of a variable at several points in time and to evaluate the change from baseline or how the measurement varies over time. If more than one group is studied, the variation over time must also be compared between groups.

The dependence inherent in serial measures is not widely appreciated in the nutrition literature. Such studies are frequently analyzed by applying *t* tests at each time period. Because the measures are related, this procedure is not appropriate. This approach also may present the problem of multiplicity (see the following section on The Number of Samples). A simple approach to the analysis described by Matthews and associates[1] is a two-stage method that summarizes the observations of the individual responses over time, then analyzes the summary measure by standard techniques. Another method would be to use repeated measures analysis of variance to determine whether groups differ in their responses over time. Investigators who are not familiar with this procedure should consult a statistician.

Replicate measurements.   Replicate measures, or several measurements taken without regard to time, are also related observations. Analysis of variance can be used for replicate measurements of a continuous variable, provided the number of observations is the same for each subject. If this is not the case, the analysis is more complex, and statistical advice should be obtained.[2] The distribution-free Friedman test is useful to analyze several related discrete observations or continuous data that are not normally distributed (see the section on Assumption of Normality).

The Number of Samples

Statistical tests are designed to compare one sample, two samples, or more than two samples. Tests are so designed because, as the number of groups increases, the number of possible pair-wise comparisons increases. For two groups, only one comparison is possible; for three groups, three comparisons are possible; for four groups, six pair-wise comparisons are possible, and for five groups, ten comparisons may be made. The chances of finding a spurious significant result increases as the number of tests applied to a single set of data increases, giving rise to the statistical problem of *multiple comparisons* or *multiplicity*.

More than two groups.   In the multiplicity situation, the level of statistical significance, or α level, increases dramatically with the number of groups compared. Instead of the chances of a false positive result at the conventional 5% level (ie, $\alpha = 0.05$), the chance of a false positive "significant" result is greater, almost 15% in the case of three groups (three comparisons) and up to 40% in the case of five groups (ten comparisons).[3] Clearly, the possibility for mistaken conclusions is great.

For this reason, the common procedure of using the t test to examine each pair in such studies is not appropriate, because the t test does not account for multiplicity present in the study design. Multiple comparisons techniques are described by Godfrey[3] and detailed in standard statistics texts. In general, when the number of samples being compared is more than two, the appropriate statistical procedure is to first determine whether an overall difference is present using a test designed to do so, such as analysis of variance. After finding that a statistically significant difference does exist, the appropriate multiple comparison technique should be applied to determine which individual pairs of samples differ. Examples of multiple comparisons methods are the Bonferroni, Scheffé, Tukey, Newman-Keuls, and Duncan.

Unrestrained significance testing. Multiplicity is also present in a situation in which group comparisons are done on a large number of variables, as is common in nutrition research. In fact, inappropriate methods for multiple comparisons, particularly the unrestrained, repeated use of t tests, are frequently seen in nutrition literature and are no doubt responsible for a number of the claims of statistically significant results.[4]

To avoid this problem, the conventional α level should be applied only to those tests that address the research questions. Results of significance tests applied to the hypotheses that serve as the basis of the study should carry the greatest weight.[2] If other tests are performed, they should be regarded as exploratory, and a more conservative α level should be used. The chances of spurious false positive results' occurring can be reduced by adjusting downward the criterion of statistical significance. This can be done by use of a technique such as the Bonferroni, in which the α level is made more conservative by dividing it by the number of comparisons.[5,6] For example, if 20 comparisons were made, the significance level would be $0.05/20 = 0.0025$, instead of the conventional 0.05.

Other Considerations

Assumption of normality. The validity of many statistical tests depends on the assumptions that the data are from a normal distribution and that the variability within groups is similar. Tests that depend on these assumptions are termed *parametric* and are, to some degree, sensitive to violations of those assumptions. Violating these assumptions does not necessarily rule out the use of parametric statistical methods, but the nonstatistician usually does not know the consequences of doing so. In general, parametric statistical procedures applied to data that form a skewed distribution can yield misleading results.[6] When parametric assumptions are clearly not met, it is better to be cautious and choose a method that accounts for the violations. There are two common options for doing so: transformations and nonparametric methods.

Transformations. One option is to transform the data to induce normality in the distribution, then apply the statistical test to the transformed data.[7] A data set that has extreme observations may be transformed to an approximately normal distribution by scale transformation, such as a logarithmic conversion (eg, natural or log base 10). Plotting the transformed data using a histogram to determine whether the transformation is appropriate, resulting in an approximately normal distribution. The drawback of this option is that interpretation of the results may not be straightforward.

Nonparametric methods. The second option is to use a nonparametric or distribution-free statistical method. Nonparametric statistical tests do not depend on the normal distribution, thus are valid with skewed data or with data that are collected in categorical form. These tests are easy to apply, and most require minimal calculation. The major disadvantage is that nonparametric tests are usually somewhat less powerful than their parametric counterparts, especially if the assumptions for the parametric test are met and the parametric method can be applied. Nonparametric tests generally are less sensitive in finding effects and produce wider confidence intervals. However, nonparametric statistical methods are useful and should be considered when the sample size is small, when the distribution is skewed, or when categorical data are used. Siegel[8] provides details on the use of nonparametric methods.

One-sided and two-sided significance tests. Departures from the mean (or other parameter of interest) can occur in two possible directions, either above or below it, or in the observed direction and its opposite. A one-sided significance test evaluates departures in only one direction, whereas a two-sided test evaluates departures in both directions.

In the majority of situations, the two-sided test should be used. A one-sided test is justified only in those instances in which the difference is expected to be in a specified direction (stated in advance), and a difference in the opposite direction is either not possible or of no interest. Because one-sided tests are less stringent, they are suspect if the results are marginally significant and the conclusions would change if a two-sided test were applied.[9]

GENERAL PROCEDURE FOR STATISTICAL ANALYSIS

Whether the research question is comparative or relational, the investigator first describes the data, then makes inferences about the population from which the sample was drawn. This is performed statistically by use of descriptive statistics, followed by the application of inferential statistical tests. The procedure involves three steps: summarize, estimate, and assess statistical significance.

First, the observations are summarized using a summary statistic or set of statistics, eg, the mean, frequency, or range of the observations in the sample(s). Summary statistics show the distribution of experiences or characteristics and provides information about the characteristics of the underlying population from which the sample was drawn.

Second, the magnitude of the comparison or relationship from the observations is estimated, eg, how large the difference is, how strong the association. The estimate provides information about the clinical or practical importance of the difference or association. A small difference may be of no consequence, whereas a large difference may make a major impact.

Third, the answer is assessed by determining its statistical significance, ie, how likely it is that the observed difference or association would be obtained if no difference or association exists. The assessment provides information about the probability that the answer is due to chance alone, rather than to a true condition.

Step 1: Statistical Summaries

Plot first. Regardless of the type of data collected, the process of summarizing observations is best approached by plotting the data first, then summarizing it numerically. For comparative questions, a frequency distribution of the data should be constructed and its shape examined. For relational questions, a scatterplot of the two variables of interest should be constructed (see A Hypothetical Clinical Example).

Summarize the plot. From the shape of the distribution or plot, the correct summary statistic to use can be evident. The idea of summarizing is to convey concisely and accurately the characteristics of the shape of the distribution curve or scatterplot.

Discrete observations. For discrete variables, nominal or ordinal data, the frequency distribution can be summarized simply as a single number: the frequency. The frequency describes the distribution of the group completely. Often the frequency is presented as a proportion of the total observations. If the sample size is sufficient (≥ 100), a percentage can be presented, along with the numerator and denominator from which the percentage is derived. Differences between groups can be expressed simply as the difference between the group frequencies or group proportions.

Continuous observations. Statistical summaries of continuous variables are more complex than those of discrete variables. The frequency distribution or histogram forms a shape, usually approximating a curve. It is clear from examining the shape of the distribution that a single number does not describe any curve adequately. In this case, the distribution of the observations is better described by at least two numbers, one describing the curve's height (central location; eg, mean or median) and another describing its width (variation; eg, standard deviation or range).

Standard deviation. The shape of the distribution determines the appropriate summary statistic. If the distribution is generally normal, with a shape approximating a normal bell-shaped curve, it can be summarized by the mean and standard deviation (SD). A normal distribution has the convenient property that 95% of the sample observations lie within the mean $\pm$ 2 SD. If the distribution is asymmetrical or skewed, as is common in nutrition research, the mean and SD are less accurate summary statistics. For skewed distributions, more than two summary statistics may be necessary. The median and the range are helpful additional summaries, as are the values of the 5th and 95th percentiles.

Step 2: Estimate

Statistical procedures are concerned with estimates and uncertainties. Because it is rarely feasible for an entire population to be measured, it is generally agreed that characteristics about populations cannot be determined directly, but must be estimated from samples drawn from the population. The summary statistics, ie, mean, median, correlation coefficient, relative risk, and so on, are single-value or *point estimates* derived from samples.

Because a point estimate varies to some extent even among samples drawn from the same population, it is useful to quantify the "precision" of the estimate in some manner. Precision is measured statistically by calculating the standard error and the confidence interval.

Standard error. If a number of random samples of sufficient size (usually $n > 30$) were taken from a population, the sample means would determine a normal distribution. The height or center of the distribution of sample means—the mean of the means—would be near the true population mean. The width of the distribution—the SD of the means—expresses the variation among the sample means. As with any normal distributions, 95% of all the sample means are within 2 SDs of the population mean.

The standard deviation of the means is estimated from the sample by the *standard error of the mean* (SEM) or the *standard error* (SE). The SE is calculated by dividing the sample SD by the square root of the sample size. Consequently, the SE is inversely related to the sample size, a convenient property of a measure of precision. As the sample size increases, the SE decreases; ie, as the amount of information about the population increases, the variation in the estimate of the mean, although not the mean itself, decreases.

A clarification about the difference between the SD and SE is in order. The SD is used to describe the variation between individual subjects in a sample, while the SE is used to describe the uncertainty in a sample estimate about a population parameter, such as a mean.[10] They are not used interchangeably. When describing a sample distribution, the SD is a more useful statistic than the SE. However, when comparing differences between samples, the SE is helpful. The SE allows probability statements about the population mean (or other estimated parameter) to be made. That is, given the sample data, how likely is it that the population parameter is the value estimated by the sample? This question is best answered by using the SE to calculate a range of probable values, the confidence interval.

Confidence interval. The confidence interval (CI) is the estimated range within which it is likely (eg, with 95% probability) that the point estimate (eg, the true mean, difference, correlation coefficient) exists. Because the CI is calculated using the SE derived from the study sample, it is dependent in part both on the variation in the factor of interest and on the sample size. The CI is also dependent on the degree of confidence assigned to the results, conventionally placed at the 95% level (ie, $\alpha = 0.05$). Mathematically, the CI is generally expressed as:

(Formula 21.1)

$$CI = \text{Point estimate} \pm \text{"confidence } (1 - \alpha) \text{ level"} \times SE$$

The CI shows the range, from the smallest to the largest values of that parameter, that is consistent with the sample data. It is presented alone with the point estimate. A wide CI indicates that the sample's point estimate (eg, mean, correlation coefficient) lacks precision and the true value could actually be any one of a large range of values. A narrow CI indicates that the sample's point estimate is relatively precise and the true value is likely to be one of a few possible values. The width of the CI is inversely related to the sample size, indicating that as the amount of information about the population increases, the precision in the estimate increases.

The CI provides additional information about magnitude that is useful for interpreting results; eg, by how much did the diet alter the hemoglobin levels? What was the increase in risk associated with cholesterol intake? Instead of offering a single value, the point estimate, by which to interpret the magnitude of a difference or association, the CI offers a range of values that are plausible, given the data in hand. This information is especially helpful when evaluating the practical importance of results. The use of the CI is illustrated in the Hypothetical Clinical Example. Gardner and Altman[10] provide an excellent review of the importance of the CI in reporting and interpreting study results and show methods for calculating the CI for a number of situations.

Step 3: Assess Statistical Significance

Since statistical procedures are concerned with uncertainties, an investigator makes assumptions—hypotheses—about the underlying populations prior to initiating the study. The investigator then tests the hypotheses using the research observations. Formally, the hypotheses are known as the *statistical hypothesis* and the *working hypothesis.*

The research question generates the statistical hypothesis. The statistical hypothesis defines the distributions in the populations under study. For example: A parenteral amino acid solution rich in branched-chain amino acids enhances nitrogen retention, as compared with a standard parenteral solution.

The null hypothesis is the working hypothesis. The null hypothesis states that there is no difference or no relationship among the factors under investigation, there is no difference in the distributions in the study populations. In an investigation of a parenteral amino acid solution rich in branched-chain amino acids and its effect on nitrogen retention, the null hypothesis (H_0) would be that the branched-chain solution has the same effect on nitrogen retention as a standard amino acid solution. The study or alternative hypothesis (H_1) would be that the branched-chain solution enhances nitrogen retention as compared with a standard amino acid solution.

Hypothesis testing. Because the two hypotheses assume different characteristics about the underlying population distributions, the hypothesis-testing procedure employs statistical tests to compare the expected distribution, defined by the null hypothesis, with the observed distribution, estimated by the study results. The statistical test assesses statistical significance (ie, the probability or P value) that the results are consistent with the null hypothesis. The question the statistical significance test asks is: How likely is it to observe the values for the distribution characteristics given by the sample if the null hypothesis is true?

Results yielding a P value that is less than α indicate that the study data provide evidence to reject the null hypothesis and to support an alternative hypothesis. Results yielding a P value that is greater than α indicate that the study was unable to detect evidence that is contrary to the null hypothesis.

Interpretation. Caution and common sense must guide the use and interpretation of statistical probability values. Although statistical significance is important to assess, it is not the primary result of a data analysis. Statistical hypothesis testing is used to determine whether results are consistent or not consistent with the null hypothesis and, as noted by Rothman and others, artificially classifies results into a dichotomous outcome: significant or not significant.[10-12] This answer is not adequate as a guide for decisions in many practical situations. It completely ignores the size of any effect that was observed and whether the study was able (ie, had sufficient power) to detect statistically significant results. A finding of statistically nonsignificant does not mean the findings are insignificant. Likewise, a finding of statistically significant results does not mean the findings are meaningful.

Significance values must be interpreted in relation to other aspects of the study, including design characteristics, sample size, missing values, biases in sampling and measurement, and compliance to study requirements and treatment, if given. In addition, the size of the differences or effects must be considered when interpreting results. The CI provides the information about size and it, along with P values and point estimates, should be presented in order for a meaningful conclusion to be drawn.

ANSWERING THE RESEARCH QUESTION

This section describes in general terms how the three-step process just outlined would be applied to several of the most common research situations. Because readers are most familiar with studies of differences, these applications are presented in a simple outline form that will serve as a ready reference for future use. Methods used for evaluating associations are provided in a more detailed narrative form. The reader is urged to use these descriptions and suggested applications as a foundation for further study of the topic; to refer to the references given to determine whether a suggested statistical method is appropriate for the application at hand; and, when possible, to consult with a statistician. An example illustrating both comparative and relational applications follows in the Hypothetical Clinical Example.

Comparisons and Differences

When comparing differences between samples or groups, the statistical method selected may be determined by the variable type, eg, binary, ordinal, continuous. Suggested statistical methods for evaluating these differences are outlined in *Table 21.1*.

Relationships and Associations

Relationships are summarized by a variety of procedures. If the data are discrete, frequency plots that are cross-classified by categories can be used. Such plots are summarized simply by constructing contingency tables (2×2 table or multi-way) of the cross-category frequencies; see Table 20.3 for an example of a 2×2 table. The association between variables in a 2×2 table, ie, the hypothesis that the rows are independent from the columns, can be assessed statistically by the χ^2 statistic, described by Rimm and colleagues,[6] Fleiss,[13] and standard statistics texts.

As previously noted, the statistical assessment of the association is not adequate by itself. It conveys no information about the degree of association or its practical importance, and since the P value is dependent in part on the sample size, an association of little strength may be statistically significant if the sample is large enough. For this reason, it is important also to estimate a measure of the strength of the association.

Discrete data. The strength of the association among binary variables can be measured by various methods, depending on the type of study design. For behavioral and educational studies, the ϕ coefficient is popular despite its deficiencies. Calculated from a 2×2 table, the ϕ coefficient is interpretable as a correlation coefficient ranging from -1 to $+1$ with values near zero indicating little or no association between the two variables. However, Fleiss[13] cautions that the ϕ coefficient has serious deficiencies and should be avoided in areas of research in which it must be possible to compare findings among investigations.

Table 21.1
Suggested Statistical Methods
for Evaluating Differences
Between Samples or Groups

Sampling Situation	Variable Type	Hypothesis	Summarize	Estimate	Assess	References
Two independent samples	Binary	Proportions are equal	Frequency table (2 × 2 table)	Difference in proportions with its CI*	χ^2	6 (pp237–256); 10; 13 (pp 19–30)
	Ordinal	Medians are equal	Median, interquartile range	Difference in medians with its CI	Mann-Whitney Test, Wilcoxon rank sum test	6 (pp 272–276); 23; 24
	Continuous	Means are equal	Mean SD†	Difference in means with its CI	Independent t test	6 (pp 213–216); 10
Several independent samples	Binary	All proportions are equal	Group frequencies (contingency table)	Difference in proportions; pair-wise CI from multiple comparisons	Global χ^2 followed by multiple comparisons analysis	13 (pp 138–143)
	Binary, but groups are ordered	Proportions are equal	Group frequencies (contingency table)	Difference in proportions	Bartholomew's test	13 (pp 147–149)
	Ordinal	All medians are equal	Medians, interquartile range	Difference in medians	Kruskal-Wallis (Jonckheere), nonparametric test	24
	Continuous	All means are equal	Group means, SDs	Difference in means; pair-wise CI after multiple comparisons analysis	One-way analysis of variance followed by multiple comparisons methods	3; 6 (pp 222–228)
Crossover, measures taken at two times in a single group	Nominal or ordinal	Medians of time periods do not differ	Medians, interquartile range	CI for median change	Wilcoxon sign rank test	6 (pp 277–279); 24
	Continuous	Means of time periods do not differ	Means, SD	Difference in means with its CI	Paired t test	6 (pp 218–220)
Two independent groups, change in measures taken at two times, eg, before and after treatment	Binary	Proportion improved is equal	Group frequencies (2 × 2 table)	Difference in proportions with its CI	Normal approximation to binomial or χ^2 test; matched study–McNemar's test	10; 13 (pp 100–103, 112–119)
	Continuous	Change in measures is equal	Mean, SD of changes	Difference in mean change with its CI	t test of mean changes, or analysis of covariance (see Hypothetical Clinical Example)	20–22
Two independent groups, serial measures, difference in the response over time	Continuous	Response over time is equal	Plot response over time to determine how it changes over time (peaked or growth curves) then select appropriate summary	If appropriate, difference with its CI	t test of mean difference (from summary), or repeated measures analysis of variance, or multivariate analysis of variance	1, 25

* CI = confidence interval

† SD = standard deviation

Fortunately, better measures of association exist. Two of the most useful measures are the relative risk and the odds ratio. The relative risk is used when the investigation is a cohort analysis, and the odds ratio is appropriate for investigations that are of case-control design. Both measures describe the degree of association between an antecedent factor and an outcome event, such as morbidity,[14] thus, both are important in observational analytical studies that evaluate potentially causal relationships. Methods for calculating and interpreting the relative risk and the odds ratio are discussed in chapter 8. Readers are also referred to Fleiss[13] for details on deriving the CIs for both measures and for assessing statistical significance.

Continuous data. The relationships among continuous variables are commonly explored by scatterplot and summarized with linear regression or correlation coefficients. Although they are related, regression and correlation analysis are used for different purposes and thus are interpreted differently. Linear regression expresses the relationship between two variables by a mathematical model describing a straight line. The correlation coefficient measures the degree of linear association between the two variables. Regression analysis is used most commonly to quantify the association between two variables and to make predictions based on the linear relationship. The correlation coefficient is used to measure the strength of the linear association and provides little other descriptive information.

The first step in regression or correlation analysis is to plot the data. In regression analysis, a scatterplot is constructed with the dependent (predicted) variable on the vertical axis (Y) and the independent (predictor) variable on the horizontal axis (X). The plot will help determine whether a straight line model is appropriate for the data. In both regression or correlation analysis, any outlying observations can seriously affect the analysis, and a scatterplot assists in detecting these observations. If the scatterplot appears to be nonlinear, methods other than linear regression should be used.

Regression analysis. After plotting the data, the regression equation to summarize the plot is calculated. This is particularly useful when an investigator wishes to predict one variable from another. The regression equation summarizes the straight line relationship between two variables by the equation $Y = A + BX$. The equation is expressed conceptually as:

Predicted variable $=$ Intercept $+$ (Slope $\times$ Predictor variable)

The equation provides coefficients for the intercept (a), slope (B), and the correlation. The intercept is the estimated value of Y when $X = 0$. The slope describes the average value of Y at each value of X and is thus dependent on the units in which X and Y are measured. Because of this, the slope can be used to predict the change in Y that is associated with each unit change in X. Both the intercept and slope have error terms (variances) that are used to calculate additional significance tests and CIs.

The correlation coefficient has a special interpretation in regression analysis. When squared (R^2), it expresses the proportion of the variation in Y that is explained by the linear regression with X. This interpretation is different from that of the correlation coefficient (r), which will be covered later.

In addition to the coefficients, the degree to which the data points cluster around the regression line is also important to quantify. The difference between the actual observed value of Y and the value predicted by the regression equation is known as the *residual (Figure 21.1),* thus the quantity of interest is the *residual variance.* The residual variance measures the amount by which the actual values of Y differ from the predicted values. A good regression equation minimizes the residual variance.

Figure 21.1
The difference between the
observed values of Y and the
fitted regression line (predicted
values of Y).

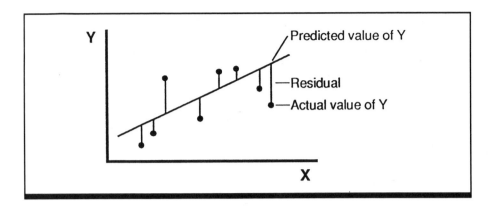

It is important to verify, at least roughly, that the regression equation accurately summarizes the data.[15] Briefly, the procedure involves examining the residuals by plotting them on the X axis with the predicted values on the Y axis and determining whether a pattern exists. A relatively accurate regression equation exhibits no distinctive pattern, whereas a less-accurate equation shows a systematic trend, such as a V-shaped spread. The regression equation requires further refinement if a trend is detected. Details on residual analysis are provided by Kleinbaum, Kupper, and Muller[16] and Godfrey[15]; the procedure usually is done by computer analysis.

The important summary statistics of regression analysis are the regression equation, the coefficients and variances of the slope and intercept, the variance of the residuals, and the proportion of the variation in the dependent variable explained by the regression equation (R^2).

Correlation. The *product moment*, or *linear correlation coefficient* (r), is a measure of the strength of the linear association between two variables. It is dependent on the slope and the sample size and does not depend on the units of measurements of the original observations. The correlation coefficient ranges from −1 to +1. When the correlation coefficient is zero, the slope of the regression line is also zero. A value of either −1 or +1 indicates that the data approximate a straight line and that the slope of the line is not zero. A positive coefficient indicates a positive relationship: that Y increases as X increases. A negative coefficient indicates the opposite, a negative or an inverse relationship in which X increases as Y decreases.

The correlation coefficient can be useful in indicating whether Y is related to X, but it provides no other quantitative information to describe the linear relationship. It does not describe the amount of change in Y that occurs for each unit change in X as did the previously described coefficients in the regression equation. Further, because of its dependence on the slope and variance, the correlation coefficient can be influenced by both the steepness of the line and the degree to which the data points cluster about the regression line. Because it does not distinguish between these two components, it is difficult to interpret the correlation coefficient correctly when presented alone.[17] A large value can be misleading. For example, it is possible for a correlation coefficient to be large simply because the axes are scaled in such a way that the slope is steep. For this reason, interpretation of the correlation coefficient is better done when paired with a plot of the data or with the regression equation, including the slope and variances. The purpose of the analysis determines which to include. If the purpose of the analysis is predicting Y, regression analysis is used; if the purpose is determining whether a linear relationship is present, correlation analysis is used.

Correlation analysis assumes that the observations are independent. Observations of X and Y are taken on each subject, but each subject contributes only one X-Y pair. A common error in correlation analysis is to compute correlation coefficients on data that are related. The most frequently seen example is the correlation analysis of serial measurements.[6] For example, if serum magnesium and magnesium intake are measured on each subject at several points in time, it is not valid to pool all the data to calculate the correlation coefficient for the relationship between magnesium intake and serum magnesium. This procedure is not appropriate because measurements taken on the same person are related.

Correlation for discrete variables. A scatterplot also can be used for ordinal or ordered categorical data. Unlike continuous data, however, nominal and ordinal data should not be analyzed by the usual product moment correlation. Data of these types are better summarized with a distribution-free correlation procedure, such as the Spearman or Kendall correlation coefficients.

A HYPOTHETICAL CLINICAL EXAMPLE

Application of the statistical methods just described can be demonstrated using a study undertaken to determine whether the use of a glucose polymer could enhance magnesium absorption as determined by serum magnesium levels. (Charuhas and co-workers[18] reported such a study, and their results are modified here for the purposes of illustration.) The subjects were 40 patients with hypomagnesemia who required daily magnesium supplementation until their serum magnesium levels were normal. The patients were randomized into two groups ($n_1 = 20$, $n_2 = 20$) to receive their magnesium supplementation with either a solution containing glucose polymer or a placebo solution that was identical in appearance and taste. The effectiveness of the glucose polymer was determined by measuring the patients' serum magnesium levels after seven days of treatment and comparing the increase in serum magnesium of the patients receiving glucose polymer with that of the patients receiving placebo. The hypothetical raw data are presented in *Table 21.2.*

Table 21.2
Example Study Data on Serum
Magnesium Levels

Subject	Baseline (mmol/L)	Final (mmol/L)	Change* (mmol/L)	% Change
Placebo group				
1	0.51	0.56	0.05	10.6
2	0.55	0.58	0.03	4.5
3	0.59	0.62	0.03	4.9
4	0.54	0.60	0.06	11.5
5	0.59	0.64	0.05	8.3
6	0.55	0.61	0.06	11.2
7	0.55	0.59	0.04	8.3
8	0.56	0.59	0.03	5.9
9	0.50	0.58	0.08	14.8
10	0.57	0.60	0.03	5.8
11	0.59	0.64	0.05	8.3
12	0.50	0.59	0.09	17.2
13	0.52	0.57	0.05	10.2
14	0.58	0.62	0.04	7.8
15	0.55	0.61	0.06	10.4
16	0.54	0.58	0.04	8.4
17	0.53	0.60	0.07	12.4
18	0.56	0.61	0.05	9.6
19	0.58	0.62	0.04	6.4
20	0.60	0.69	0.09	14.4
mean =	0.55	0.60	0.05	9.5
SD =	0.031	0.029	0.017	3.40
Glucose polymer group				
1	0.59	0.62	0.03	4.2
2	0.52	0.58	0.06	11.1
3	0.51	0.59	0.08	15.2
4	0.58	0.67	0.09	15.7
5	0.60	0.65	0.05	8.2
6	0.52	0.61	0.09	17.5
7	0.51	0.62	0.11	22.0
8	0.54	0.64	0.10	19.2
9	0.58	0.66	0.08	13.4
10	0.56	0.65	0.09	15.3
11	0.52	0.64	0.12	22.0
12	0.56	0.67	0.11	19.1
13	0.58	0.68	0.10	17.0
14	0.58	0.69	0.11	19.3
15	0.51	0.63	0.12	22.4
16	0.55	0.64	0.09	17.3
17	0.59	0.69	0.10	17.6
18	0.53	0.62	0.09	17.8
19	0.57	0.64	0.07	12.9
20	0.57	0.67	0.10	17.4
mean =	0.55	0.64	0.09	16.2
SD =	0.031	0.030	0.023	4.57

* Change = final value − baseline value

Comparison of Proportions

A number of approaches to the analysis of this study are possible. The calculations, figures, and tables that follow are useful in assessing the data, but for the most part, would not be submitted for publication. A simple method would be to describe the proportion of patients in the two groups whose serum magnesium levels improved to at least 0.65 mmol/L:

Treatment	Response No. Improved (no./n)	Total n
Glucose polymer	9 (0.45)	20
Placebo	1 (0.05)	20
Overall	10 (0.25)	40

The simple difference in the proportions is calculated in this instance as:

$$\text{Difference} = (9/20) - (1/20)$$
$$= 8/20 \text{ or } 0.40 \text{ or } 40\%$$

Confidence intervals for differences between two proportions can be constructed similarly to those for continuous variables (see Formula 21.1), using as the SE:

(Formula 21.2)
$$SE_{\text{difference}} = \sqrt{\frac{P_1 Q_1}{n_1} + \frac{P_2 Q_2}{n_2}}$$

where P_1 = proportion improved in group 1
$Q_1 = 1 - P_1$
P_2 = proportion improved in group 2
$Q_2 = 1 - P_2$

This procedure is useful for samples of sufficient size, say 50 per group, and with proportions within the range 0.1 to 0.9.[10] Smaller sample sizes require more accurate but complex procedures; a statistician should be consulted. Readers are referred to Gardner and Altman[10] and Fleiss[13] for details and examples of the usual procedure. Since the example data do not meet the size requirement, a CI is not constructed.

To assess statistical significance, the usual approach when the sample size is large would be to apply the Z test (normal approximation to the binomial distribution) or the χ^2 test, described in standard statistics texts and Fleiss.[13] However, if an expected frequency is small (ie, ≤ 5), the χ^2 test may not be accurate.[6]

Treatment	Response Improved (serum magnesuim level ≥ 0.65 mmol/L)		
	+	−	Total
Glucose polymer	9	11	20
Placebo	1	19	20
Total	10	30	40

To compute the expected frequencies for the glucose polymer response trial, refer to *Table 21.3*, which gives the observed values for these data. The row totals are 20 and 20; the column totals are 10 and 30; and the grand total is 40. Thus,

E_{11} = expected number of units in the (1,1) cell
= 20(10)/40 = 5

E_{12} = expected number of units in the (1,2) cell
= 20(30)/40 = 15

E_{21} = expected number of units in the (2,1) cell
= 20(10)/40 = 5

E_{22} = expected number of units in the (2,2) cell
= 20(30)/40 = 15

Because the expected frequency of two cells is small (≤ 5), a more accurate significance test is given by use of the Fisher's exact test. Although the assumptions of this test—that all marginal frequencies are fixed—is rarely met in nutrition research, it is commonly used for studies in which two of the marginal frequencies are fixed, as in the case of this study (ie, $n_1 = n_2 = 20$). Details of Fisher's test for 2×2 tables is given by Matthews and Farewell[19] and others[6,13]; in addition, computer programs are available to complete this test. When applied to this table as a two-tailed test, the P value is 0.008.

The statistically significant result indicates that it is unlikely that a difference of this magnitude (40%) would be observed if there were no true difference in the underlying populations. The magnitude, 40%, implies that of every 100 patients given placebo (in whom an improvement of 5% is expected), an additional 40% would be expected to achieve serum magnesium levels of at least 0.65 mmol/L within one week had they been given glucose polymer instead.

This degree of improvement was considered important by the clinic staff, who concluded that glucose polymer is superior to the standard therapy (placebo) as an adjunct to magnesium supplementation in the treatment of patients with hypomagnesemia.

Analysis of Continuous Variables

Another approach to the analysis would be to evaluate the response as a continuous variable. First, the baseline magnesium levels are summarized by graphing them using a histogram and the shape of the curve is examined (*Figure 21.2*). The histogram helps assess whether the two groups are similar in the distribution of baseline measures. The distributions of the two groups are also similar, indicating that randomization was successful in making the two groups comparable in this baseline measure. The distributions appear to be approximately bell-shaped, indicating that parametric statistical methods are appropriate for these data. If this had not been the case, nonparametric methods would be preferable to use.

Figure 21.2
Histogram of baseline
magnesium measurements
(n = 20 subjects per group).

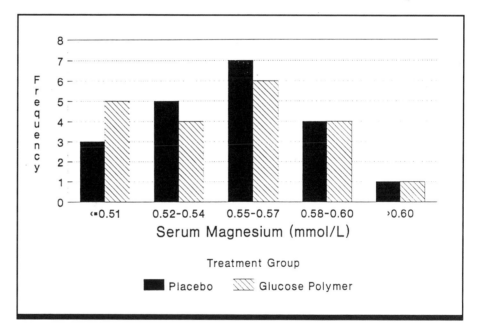

The comparison of interest is the magnitude of increase in serum magnesium. A histogram of the final serum magnesium values by group is shown in *Figure 21.3*.

Figure 21.3
Histogram of final serum
magnesium measurements
(n = 20 subjects per group).

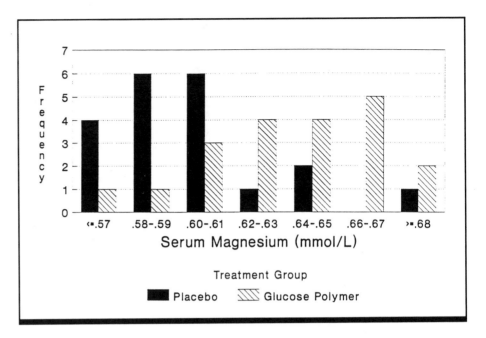

A simple analysis of the difference in group means of the final serum magnesium measurement by an independent t-test may be misleading, ie, 0.60 versus 0.64 in Table 21.2. This is because the final measurement may be related to the initial measurement. For example, the final value for patients with low baseline levels may be lower than that for patients with higher baseline levels. It is best to plot (scatterplot) the final measure with the baseline measure to determine whether they are related.[20] As is evident in the scatterplot of these data (*Figure 21.4*), this is the case:

Figure 21.4
Scatterplot of the final measurement with the baseline measurement.

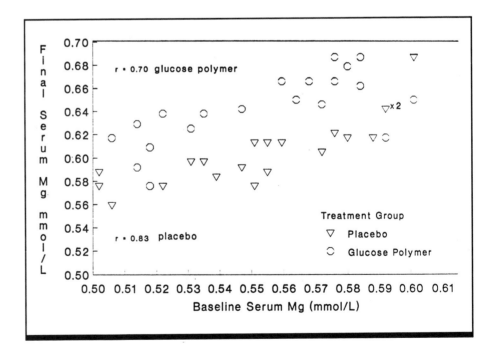

The final measurement of serum magnesium is linearly related to the baseline measurement. The correlation coefficients (r) are also indicative of the relationship; r = 0.70 (P = 0.0006) and r = 0.83 (P = 0.0001) for the glucose polymer and placebo groups, respectively. Because the purpose was to determine whether a linear relationship existed, the correlation coefficient was adequate when presented along with the scatterplot.

When the two measurements are related, some adjustment for the baseline measurement is necessary. This is most commonly achieved by computing the change value, the difference between the final and first measurements, then applying statistical methods to this value. The difference computed for each subject is shown in Table 21.2, and a histogram for these values is presented in *Figure 21.5.*

Figure 21.5
Histogram of change in serum magnesium from baseline to final value (n = 20 subjects per group).

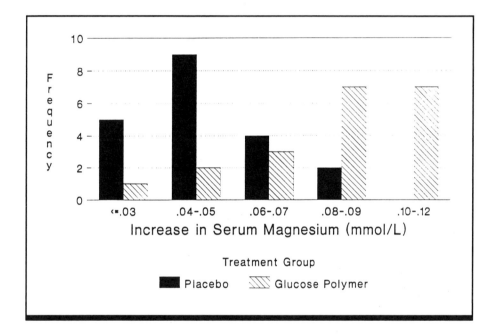

In some situations, investigators may be tempted to use percentage change instead of the value of the change between the two measures. The choice between change and percentage change is not an arbitrary one. Kaiser[20] provides guidance on choosing between the two values. Briefly, change and percentage change versus the baseline for each treatment group are plotted, and the one that shows little dependence on the baseline value is chosen.[20] The scatterplots for the study data are shown in *Figures 21.6* and *21.7.*

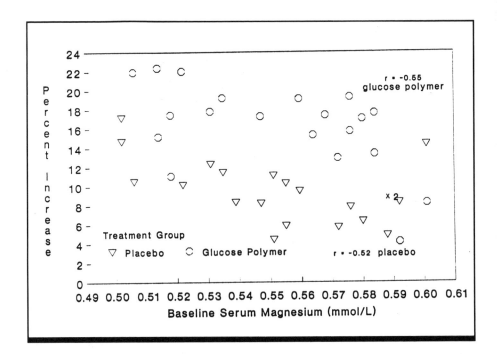

Figure 21.6
Scatterplot of percentage change in serum magnesium and baseline measurement.

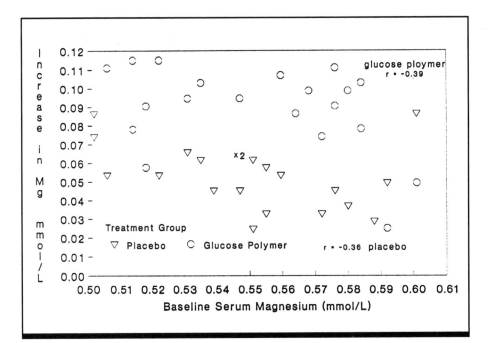

Figure 21.7
Scatterplot of the change and baseline measurements.

Useful Numbers

The scatterplots and r values shown in Figures 21.6 and 21.7 indicate that the value of change is less dependent on the initial values than percentage change, so it is this value that should be compared between groups. The CI for the difference in the mean change is computed and its statistical significance by the usual t test assessed. Results are as follows:

Increase in Initial Serum Magnesium Measure (mmol/L)

	Mean	SD	SE
Placebo	0.05	0.017	0.004
Glucose polymer	0.09	0.023	0.005
Difference	0.04	0.0206*	0.0065*

* Pooled SD, SE

From the standard tables of the t distribution, the value of Student's t at $\alpha = 0.05$ and 38 degrees of freedom (df) is 2.021. The 95% CI of the difference between the means can be calculated using Formula 21.1:

$$95\% \text{ CI} = \text{Difference} \pm t \times (\text{SE difference})$$
$$= 0.04 \pm 2.021 \times 0.0065$$
$$= 0.027, 0.053 \text{ or } (0.03, 0.05)$$

The pooled variance is used since the sample variances are similar. (As a general rule, variances may be considered to be similar if the ratio of the sample variances is < 2.)[6] The statistical significance test for the hypothesis that the mean change is the same for both groups is given by the standard two-tailed Student's t test; which results in:

$$t = 5.652 \text{ and } P < 0.0001$$

These results provide evidence to reject the null hypothesis and to conclude that the mean change in serum magnesium differs between the groups. The size of the difference is estimated from the study to be 0.04 mmol/L, although the data are consistent with a difference of as little as 0.03 mmol/L and as large a difference as 0.05 mmol/L. Whether this is a clinically meaningful difference is a matter of judgment by the investigators and the readers.

Analysis of Covariance

Although the t test of the difference between initial and follow-up measures among groups is the most common approach to analyzing data from a study of this type, another method of analysis should be considered here as well. Analysis of covariance is generally a more efficient statistical significance test than the t test when the response measure is related to the initial measure, as are these data.[20-22] Briefly, analysis of covariance involves computing the linear regression of the final measure data (dependent) versus the initial measure data (independent) and testing the difference between groups by comparing the distance between the regression lines.[21] The procedure, described for medical investigators by Egger and associates,[21] produces a parallel-lines analysis of covariance model by first testing whether the slopes of the regression lines for the two groups are equal and then, if the slopes are not significantly different, testing whether the intercepts of the two lines differ (*Figure 21.8*).

Figure 21.8
Plot of serum magnesium values
for completing analysis of
covariance.

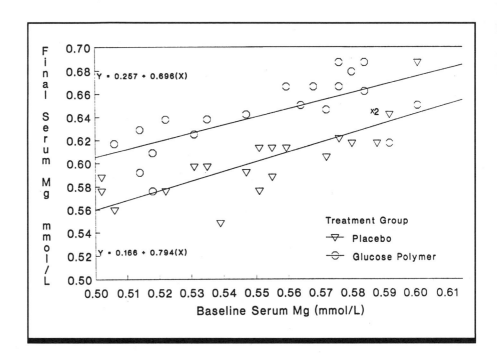

This procedure warrants consideration and may at times be preferred to the more common analysis previously described. Readers are referred to Egger and associates[21] for details regarding its use and misuse, although readers who are unfamiliar with analysis of covariance also should consult a statistician.

Analysis of covariance is applied to these data to illustrate this powerful technique. The text by Kleinbaum, Kupper, and Muller[16] is a presentation of the topic with an emphasis on application rather than theory and is particularly helpful for the nonstatistician investigator.

The results of analysis of covariance for the example study data are shown in *Table 21.4*. Three questions are relevant to the analysis, and three regression models are constructed from these data to provide the components for answering the questions. The regression coefficients, β_1, β_2, and β_3 are associated with the independent variables: baseline serum magnesium (X), treatment group indicator (Z), and an interaction variable (XZ) that is a product of the other two variables. This can be shown by the following equation:

$$Y = \beta_o + \beta_1 X + \beta_2 Z + \beta_3 XZ + \text{Error term}$$

The first question: Is the relationship between the initial value and the final value the same for both groups? This is answered by determining if the lines are parallel or nearly so, because if they are not, another method of analysis would be necessary (statistical advice is recommended). A test of the hypothesis that the regression coefficient β_3 is equal to zero assesses whether the regression lines are parallel. The testing procedure is detailed in reference 16. The results, as shown in *Table 21.5A* (F = 0.22; 2,36 df; $P > 0.10$) indicate that there is no evidence to show that the two lines are not parallel. Figure 21.8 also shows the lines appear to be parallel.

Table 21.4
Analysis of Covariance Results for Example Data

Source	df *	Sum of Squares	Mean Square†	F Value‡
Regression (X)§	1	0.019762	0.019762	27.38
Residual	38	0.027418	0.000722	
Regression (X,Z)‖	2	0.033357	0.016679	44.60
Residual	37	0.013823	0.000374	
Regression (X, Z, XZ)¶	3	0.033443	0.011148	29.18
Residual	36	0.013737	0.000382	

* df = degrees of freedom

† mean square = (sum of squares/df)

‡ F value = (regression mean square/residual mean square)

§ where X = initial serum magnesium value (mmol/L)

‖ where Z = 0 if placebo group, 1 if glucose polymer group

¶ where XZ = interaction term X × Z (ie, 0 for placebo, initial serum magnesium for glucose polymer group)

Table 21.5
ANOVA Tables for Analysis of Covariance Models (Using Results From Table 21.4)

Source		df *	Sum of Squares	Mean Square	F Value
A. With the Interaction Variable					
Regression	(X,Z)	2	0.033357	0.016679	43.66
	(XZ∣X,Z)	1	0.000086	0.000086	0.22
Residual		36	0.013737	0.000382	
Total		39	0.047180		
B. For Coincident Lines					
Regression	(X)	1	0.019762	0.019762	51.73
	(Z,XZ∣X)	2	0.013681	0.006841	17.91
Residual		36	0.013737	0.000382	
Total		39	0.047180		
C. For Difference of Means Between Groups					
Regression	(X)	1	0.019762	0.019762	52.84
	(Z∣X)	1	0.013595	0.013595	36.35
Residual		37	0.013823	0.000374	
Total		39	0.047180		

*df = degrees of freedom

Second, are both the slopes and intercepts the same in the groups? It is important at this step to determine whether the two lines are actually the same line. The test of the hypothesis that both regression coefficients β_2 and β_3 equal zero assesses whether the lines are coincident. The results in Table 21.5B (F = 17.91; 1,36 df; $P < 0.001$) provide strong evidence that the two lines are not coincident.

Third, is there a difference in the mean scores? The first and second questions indicate that the lines are parallel but not coincident, so the logical next step is to determine whether the distance between the lines is large enough to provide evidence of a difference between them. The test of the hypothesis that the regression coefficient β_2 equals zero is a measure of the distance and determines whether there is a difference in means between the groups. The results in Table 21.5C (F = 36.35; 1,37 df; $P < 0.001$) indicate that the means of the placebo and glucose polymer groups are significantly different. These results confirm those of the t test and reject the null hypothesis at the $< 1\%$ level.

As with all methods of analysis, assessing statistical significance is only one part of data analysis in analysis of covariance; estimating the size of the difference is also important. Analysis of covariance is a linear regression procedure, so it produces coefficients that express the linear relationship of the variables of interest. The parameters resulting from analysis of covariance are (omitting XZ and its related regression coefficient, β_3):

Parameter

Variable	Coefficient	Estimate	SE Estimate
Intercept	β_0	0.193257	0.056963
Initial Mg	β_1	0.744974	0.102725
Group	β_2	0.036873	0.006112

In the example study, the coefficient of interest is β_2, or the coefficient associated with the group variable. The β_2 coefficient estimates the difference between the two mean scores after removing (in part) the influence of the initial magnesium value. Analysis of covariance estimates the difference to be 0.037 mmol/L, close to the estimate (0.04 mmol/L) from the simple analysis using the mean change values. The confidence interval can also be computed in the usual way from the SE of the coefficient:

$$95\% \text{ CI for } \beta_2 = 0.036873 \pm 1.96 (0.06112)$$
$$= 0.0249, 0.0488 \text{ or } (0.03, 0.05)$$

These results are nearly identical to those derived by the previous method and would be interpreted in the same way. The benefit, however, of using analysis of covariance is that it can be a more efficient analysis than the t test (as indicated by the narrower CI) when the initial and final measurements are linearly related and the sample size is sufficient (approximately > 20).[21,22]

It is useful to consider the conclusions possible if the significance test resulted in a statistically nonsignificant P value. As Rothman[11] pointed out in 1978, the CI becomes key to the interpretation in such a case. The CI shows the readers the range of values that are plausible, given the data in hand. If the CI were to range from -0.02 to 0.10, the interval includes 0, which corresponds to a nonsignificant P value. However, most of the values extend into the range of increased mean values. The CI shows that, although the data are consistent with no real difference, the data are also consistent with an increase in serum magnesium levels that generally suggests a favorable result of the treatment. A more meaningful interpretation of the data is possible when the CI is reported along with the P value. Readers then have the information to consider whether the position of the interval warrants a conclusion other than "not significant." In reporting the results, a simple tabular presentation of descriptive statistics and a statement of the analysis of covariance statistics (F value, df, and P value) are sufficient.

CONCLUSION

This chapter has focused on the area of statistics that deals with analyzing and drawing conclusions from data. The field of nutrition and dietetics offers many opportunities to carry out research. This introduction to statistical methods is intended to enhance the investigator's skills in this area, as well as facilitate communication with statisticians in planning and completing research projects. Numerous references were cited to encourage further reading in this topic and provide guidance for developing a resource library. The basic steps discussed in this chapter will help with the many decisions that need to be made in approaching and executing successful research.

References

1. Matthews JNS, Altman DG, Campbell MJ, Royston P. Analysis of serial measurements in medical research. *Br Med J.* 300:230, 1990.
2. Altman DG, Gore SM, Gardner MJ, Pocock SJ. Statistical guidelines for contributors to medical journals. *Br Med J.* 1983;286:1489.
3. Godfrey K. Comparing the means of several groups. *N Engl J Med.* 1985;313:1450.
4. Ried M, Hall JC. Multiple statistical comparisons in nutritional research. *Am J Clin Nutr.* 1984;40:183.
5. Tukey JW. Some thoughts on clinical trials, especially problems of multiplicity. *Science.* 1977;198:679.
6. Rimm AA, Hartz AJ, Kalbfleisch JH, Anderson AJ, Hoffmann RG. *Basic Biostatistics in Medicine and Epidemiology.* New York, NY: Appleton-Century-Crofts; 1980.
7. Gore SM. Assessing methods—transforming the data. *Br Med J.* 1981;283:548.
8. Siegel S. *Nonparametric Statistics for the Behavioral Sciences.* New York, NY: McGraw-Hill; 1956.
9. McKinney WP, Young MJ, Hartz A, Bi-Fong Lee M. The inexact use of Fisher's exact test in six major medical journals. *JAMA.* 1989;261:3430.
10. Gardner MJ, Altman DG. Confidence intervals rather than P values: estimation rather than hypothesis testing. *Br Med J.* 1986;292:746.
11. Rothman KJ. A show of confidence. *N Engl J Med.* 1978;299:1362.
12. Poole C, Lanes S, Rothman KJ. Analyzing data from ordered categories. *N Engl J Med.* 1984;311:1382.
13. Fleiss JL. *Statistical Methods For Rates and Proportions.* 2nd ed. New York, NY: John Wiley and Sons; 1981.
14. Cornfield J. A method of estimating comparative rates from clinical data. Applications to cancer of the lung, breast and cervix. *J Natl Cancer Inst.* 1951;11:1269.
15. Godfrey K. Simple linear regression in medical research. *N Engl J Med.* 1985;313:1629.
16. Kleinbaum DG, Kupper LL, Muller KE. *Applied Regression Analysis and Other Multivariable Methods.* 2nd ed. Boston, Mass: PWS-Kent Publishing Co; 1988.
17. O'Brien PC, Shampo MA, Anderson CF. Statistics in nutrition. Part 4: regression. *Nutr Intl.* 1986;2:331.
18. Charuhas PM, Cheney CL, Aker SN, Stern JM, Barale KV. Effect of glucose polymer on serum magnesium in adult allogeneic marrow transplant recipients. *FASEB.* 1989;3:A1071. Abstract.
19. Matthews DE, Farewell VT. *Using and Understanding Medical Statistics.* New York, NY: Karger; 1985.
20. Kaiser L. Adjusting for baseline: change or percentage change? *Stat Med.* 1989;8:1183.

21. Egger MJ, Coleman ML, Ward JR, Reading JL, Williams HJ. Uses and abuses of analysis of covariance in clinical trials. *Controlled Clin Trials.* 1985;6:12.

22. Samuels ML. Use of analysis of covariance in clinical trials: a clarification. *Controlled Clin Trials.* 1986;7:325.

23. Moses LE, Emerson JD, Hosselini H. Analyzing data from ordered categories. *N Engl J Med.* 1984;311:442.

24. Forrest M, Anderson B. Ordinal scale and statistics in medical research. *Br Med J.* 1986;292:537.

25. Morrison DF. *Multivariate Statistical Methods.* 2nd ed. New York, NY: McGraw-Hill Book Co; 1976.

PART 7
PRESENTATION OF
RESEARCH DATA

The exuberance of completing one's research fuels the next step: communicating one's findings effectively and ethically. The three chapters that follow guide researchers in preparing presentations, in devising effective tables and graphs, and in addressing issues related to research journals and peer review. The perspectives of reviewers, as the guardians of scientific literature, and readers, as the ultimate recipient and user, are also addressed.

Original research can be presented in many ways: technical reports (interim, summary, and evaluation reports), abstracts (to introduce a report, to summarize projects, and to submit for presentation consideration), posters at technical and scientific meetings, oral presentations, video and film presentations, and manuscripts prepared for publication in professional and research journals. The specific format needs to fit the purpose and the type of presentation. All presentations benefit by thoughtful clear organization.

Oral presentations (chapter 22) are frequently orchestrated with supportive slides and overhead transparencies. These visual materials are designed to aid, not distract, the listener. They should be readable from anywhere in the room; thus, they should be simple and composed of large letters and large numbers. Although slides should be intelligible by themselves, they lose effectiveness if they contain long titles, elaborate footnotes, or multiple data columns acceptable in tables for written reports. Slides must be visually strong; two or more may be needed to support oral presentation of material that would be summarized in a single written table. A useful guide for preparing effective slides recommended by the Federation of American Societies for Experimental Biology is to present no more that 42 characters and spaces horizontally and no more than 14 lines (including double-spaced lines) vertically.

Visibility is equally important in poster presentations. The difficult part is to arrange the material so that people standing behind others can read readily. It is customary to lead the eye from top to bottom, moving from the left to the right panels. Within this construct, the most important material should be placed at or above eye level, where it is easiest to read. Although all the information is of interest to the people attending poster sessions, the abstract, key data, and conclusions and recommendations are particularly favored.

Chapter 23 gives excellent suggestions to aid in illustrating research effectively. The decision whether to devise a table or a graph depends on what is to be presented and the intended audience. The investigator's purpose is to inform. Consider several formats and revise for clarity. Order your information logically, such as from highest to lowest or from most recent to least recent. Avoid acronyms uncommon to readers. Assure consistency of scale within the various tables and within the text. All tables and graphs should be intelligible by themselves: Is the number of samples indicated? Are key characteristics of the subjects stated? Are the units of measurement indicated clearly?

Chapter 24 takes the outlooks of the writer, the reviewer, and the reader. The writer's goal is to communicate logically, clearly, accurately, and ethically. In designing the research and in presenting the findings, the researcher is advised to secure consultation from a statistician. Issues related to responsible authorship are delineated clearly (see also chapter 2). The reviewer plays a prominent role in maintaining the quality of the scientific literature. Peer review is a serious business and a professional responsibility. As peers, reviewers need to respect the work of their colleagues and to maintain its confidentiality. Thoughtful, conscientious review gives clear, constructive direction.

The third critical corner of the presentation triangle is the reader. Guidance is given to aid readers in developing skills appropriate to evaluate the scientific literature critically. Understanding basic statistics (chapter 21) speeds interpretation of scientific articles. Suggestions are made to enhance efficiency in reading the vast scientific literature: look at the title and the list of authors; determine the article's intent; and read the abstract, methods, results, discussion, and recommendations. The skilled reader avoids overgeneralizing the findings by assessing the research design, sample selection, and data collected. Only if the study controls well the many variables of the research may its findings be generalized to a population other than the specific study sample. The triangular support—the researcher, reviewer, and reader—form a strong base for research.

ERM, Editor

22. TECHNIQUES AND APPROACHES FOR PRESENTING RESEARCH DATA

Ronni Chernoff, PhD, RD

Conceiving, designing, conducting, and analyzing research studies and data provide answers to previously unanswered questions and give a sense of accomplishment to investigators and their colleagues. In previous chapters, the skills needed to plan, implement, and evaluate research have been discussed. The link between the work completed and the audience with whom it needs to be shared is the essence of research data presentation. There are as many methods for presenting research information as there are audiences to whom to present it.[1] The method chosen to share the results of a research project should be matched carefully to the intended audience, and the same research results may be presented in many different ways to suit the interests of different audiences. The varied techniques and approaches that can be used to present the findings from research projects will be discussed.

TECHNICAL REPORTS

Dietitians are called upon, with increasing frequency, to present research or technical information within their organizations. The current focus on justifying expenditures, new programs, resource utilization, and research projects requires both oral and written presentations of data including, among others, cost benefits and recovery, production figures, anticipated income, and expected outcomes.

Technical papers also may be reports to grant or contract agencies (federal or state agencies, foundations, professional organizations, pharmaceutical or nutrition companies, academic institutions, or others) on the progress or outcomes of grants and contracts. Usually when a proposal or contract to do work is written, there are requirements for periodic progress reports. Information on progress, completion, and evaluation of the project is often a requirement of the commitment to perform the work.

Writing clear, concise, and thorough technical reports, whether the audience is within an organization or external to it is a challenge.[2] The process may not allow for great creativity, but it does provide excellent opportunities to hone writing skills and to learn how to present data clearly, concisely, and in a straightforward manner. Technical reports should be written in direct, precise terms for their audience, setting out the purpose and objectives of the project, what was done, why it was done, how it was done, what was accomplished, and what outcomes were measured.[2] In evaluation reports, the implications of the outcomes are discussed thoroughly, relating results to the purpose of the project and how the results can be applied to future projects or activities.

Interim Reports

Written reports generally have a clearly defined structure; reports usually follow the outline of the original grant or proposal, and many granting agencies provide forms or guidelines to follow. Interim reports chart progress to date and are written at specified points in the course of the research or project. An interim report starts with a summary or abstract that describes the study under way. It should recap the rationale for the project, what the target outcomes are for subject accrual, what interventions are being used, what data are being collected, or what progress has been made toward accomplishing feasibility studies or marketing goals. If impediments to achieving goals or difficulties with planned interventions have been encountered, an interim report is a reasonable place to explain the problems and discuss alternative plans to achieving the project's goals.

Graphs and figures that chart advancement toward achieving goals may be an effective way to present progress visually.[3] This technique may serve to depict how the study or project has progressed and may help determine mid-course corrections.

Interim reports should be well-structured, concise, clear, and focused. Their purpose is to restate the objectives of the research study or project, review the methods used to collect and analyze data, describe the progress made toward the stated objectives, and discuss the problems encountered and the solutions attempted. The conclusion of an interim report should summarize what has been stated and project future accomplishments and achievement of the study objectives.

Summary Reports

Summary reports follow the same format as interim reports; however, they can be used to present completed projects or studies. They should recap the study or project objectives, review the data collection methods, describe the data analysis methodology, and report the results. A discussion section can be used to recount problems, difficulties, or unplanned occurrences and report the solutions that corrected or resolved them. Summary reports are required at the completion of a contract or grant and often are needed when a project is concluded. If a researcher prepares interim reports conscientiously, summary reports will be fairly easy to write.

Evaluation Reports

Evaluation reports have an added dimension to summary reports: They must include a section of analytic discussion to interpret the results. This section transcends presentation of data, discussing implications and evaluating results. The impact of the outcomes should be analyzed, and the application of the results interpreted within the context of the objectives of the study. Evaluation reports are challenging to write because they go beyond presentation of facts, requiring analysis and evaluation.

ABSTRACTS

Abstracts often serve as the introduction to technical reports and manuscripts. They may also stand alone as concise publications of work conducted or of oral presentations that cannot be published verbatim. Abstracts are also succinct summaries of research that are used as the basis of short paper or poster presentations. In addition, they can be used to summarize briefly the content of formal papers in tables of contents or as succinct descriptions in computerized or printed literature summations.[4]

Abstracts have all the basic components of longer manuscripts, reduced to include only essential information. Abstracts usually are limited by space (*Figure 22.1*) or the number of words allowed, so every word must contribute to the clarity of the message. The reader should understand what was done, how it was done, and what the results were from reading an abstract.

Presentation of Research Data

Figure 22.1
Abstract application form.

Abstracts must be submitted on this form, and postmarked no later than April 5, 1991. All accepted papers will be printed exactly as submitted. Abstracts must conform to the guidelines listed on the reverse side.

Presentation Preference
(check only one)
☐ Poster Session
☐ Original Contribution
   (research only)

I agree to change presentation preference as recommended by reviewers.
☐ Yes
☐ No

Classification of Abstract
(check only one)
☐ Clinical Nutrition Practice
   and Research
☐ Community Dietetics
   Practice and Research
☐ Food Management Practice
   and Research
☐ Dietetic Education Practice
   and Research
☐ Quality Assurance/Quality
   Improvement
☐ Nutrition Education/Public
   Relations

Mail original and 5 copies of this two sided application to:
Program Coordinator
Department of Meetings
The American Dietetic
   Association
216 West Jackson Blvd.
Suite 800
Chicago, IL 60606-6995   .

Do not fold or staple papers for mailing

Example

THE EFFECT OF PRE-OPERATIVE TOTAL PARENTAL NUTRITION ON SURGERY OUTCOMES. MT Younathan, PhD, RD, and C.C. Grimes, MS, RD, School of Home Economics, Louisiana State University, Baton Rouge, LA
   The effect of pre-operative total parenteral nutrition (TPN) on length of hospitalization, morbidity and/or mortality was studied in a retrospective analysis of seventy . . .

Entire abstract must be typed within the borders

Organization

Abstracts, as with longer manuscripts, should contain a brief introduction that states the purpose of the work, a description of the methodology used, a report of the results, and a succinct statement of conclusion. Occasionally a brief table may be included, but most authors prefer to use the space to present written information; tables often consume a lot of space. There is no need for references to be included in an abstract. Abbreviations can be used if they are defined or commonly used. If the abstract is being prepared for a journal or scientific meeting, guidelines for authors usually specify the abbreviations that are acceptable.

Writing abstracts is not easy. It often takes many drafts before the abstract is the correct length for the space or word allowance. The first draft of an abstract should be focused on writing the information to be presented. Extraneous words can be edited, and abbreviations can be devised for recurrent terms. Usually abbreviations that are most useful describe the study groups or treatment methods; for example, "long-term tube-fed patient group" may be abbreviated as "LTF." Usual abbreviations may include mg, dL, kg, mmol, cm, hr, and other frequently used terms of measure.

It is wise to allow sufficient time before an abstract is due so that colleagues can read it and suggest changes, and for the author to gain some perspective on it. Writing an abstract is an intellectual challenge similar to completing a crossword puzzle. The right words will fit into the space allocated. Writing abstracts takes some skill, but when they are mastered they give the author some measure of satisfaction for having chosen the best words according to the designated limits.

Submitting Abstracts

Abstracts are published as a summary of work accomplished and can be cited as a publication. Submissions should be clean, clear, and camera-ready since they frequently are printed just as they are submitted, photo-offset directly from the abstract form. The blue-line border commonly used does not copy or photograph.

POSTERS

Many professional organizations support both short oral presentations and poster sessions. The presentation of posters is different from that of short oral presentations.[4] Posters are more visual than abstracts and allow for more interaction between the author or presenter and the audience. Posters that address the same or similar themes are presented during a specified period.

When an abstract is accepted for a poster session, the organizing institution provides guidelines for preparation.[5] Posters are mounted on boards that are usually 4 ft high by 6 ft wide; they are made from soft materials so they can be mounted using pushpins. Posters should be constructed from lightweight cardboard or other materials that are easily transported, since the author will have to carry them from home to the meeting site.

Before a poster session, the elements should be laid out on the floor or a conference table in a space that approximates the size of the poster board and marked for sequence and spacing. Having colleagues review the material and ask questions is a reasonable rehearsal.

A poster should follow the outline of the abstract by presenting the purpose of the research; the subjects, materials, and methods used; the results with data; and the conclusions. Posters can be illustrated with graphs, tables, figures, photographs, and illustrations. There should be visual interest; a poster that consists of only print material will not be very interesting to the viewer. If possible, color should be used, and the layout should direct the viewer's eye through the information starting at the introduction and ending with the conclusions. A title board, often put together in segments, should run across the top of the poster. It should include the paper title, authors, and their affiliations. The title should be large enough to be seen from 40 ft and each panel should be clearly legible from 2 ft. Examples of a poster are shown in *Figure 22.2.*

Figure 22.2
Tips for preparing posters.

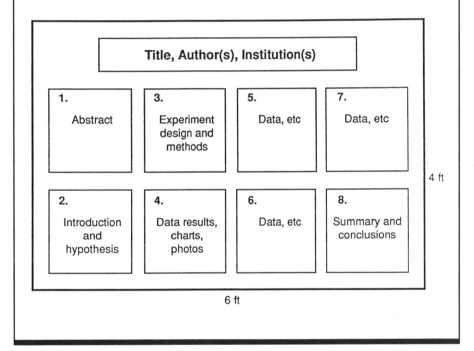

1. Remember that your illustrations and information will be viewed from a distance of 3 feet or more; all lettering should be at least ½ inch high, if possible.
2. Illustrations, charts, graphs, and photos used may be similar to those you would use in making slides, although the lettering should be large and easy to read. The format should be kept as simple as possible.
3. Do not mount artrwork or lettering on heavy board that may be difficult to keep pinned to the tackboard. Please do not write or paint on the tackboards.
4. Be sure that all items, including your title sign, will fit in an area 4 feet high by 6 feet wide.
5. A sample poster layout is shown below.

ORAL PRESENTATIONS

One of the first steps in preparing an oral presentation is to analyze the anticipated audience.[6] Presenting data at a scientific gathering minimizes the effort needed to define the character and needs of the audience. By being at the meeting and participating in the organization's activities, attendees have a common interest. Most organizations exist as special interest groups to disseminate content- or profession-specific information, so the audience for a poster or short paper session will have been defined by the forum in which the data is to be presented.

Organization

An oral presentation of abstracted data provides an opportunity to elaborate on the details of the research. A brief review of the literature, providing a rationale for the research being presented, helps engage the listeners in the presentation. If they understand the study rationale and importance, they will listen more carefully to the information being offered. They will want to know about subject selection criteria, data collection methods, data analysis methods, results of the study, and what conclusions can be drawn from the information presented to them. Too much data overwhelms listeners; therefore, significant results should be the focus of an oral presentation. The data in their entirety can be presented in a published manuscript. If the oral presentation is based on a submitted abstract, the abstract should serve as an outline for the organization of the presentation.

Planning and Preparation

Owing to the time required to plan a scientific meeting, where most research data are presented, an author will have advance notice that he or she needs to prepare a talk. Notification of acceptance for a scientific paper or poster session is usually sent three months or more before the meeting dates. An expanded outline of the presentation should be constructed from the material that has already been prepared. An analysis of appropriate visuals or illustrations should be made; consideration of research data that will be clearer if it is graphically displayed will help an author decide what should be described verbally and what will benefit from some visual presentation. Usually relationships between variables will be clearer if they are graphically displayed, as will the impact of an intervention on an important variable. Major points in an oral presentation can be put on slides. Poster presentations should tell the whole story of the research being described, and the author should be available to answer questions and elaborate on theory, method, rationale, results, and conclusions for the interested observer.

When the presenter has a firm idea of what background information and research data are to be presented, note cards can be prepared for the major points and slides or poster illustrations can be made. Oral presentations can be written and rehearsed, but the presenter should be familiar enough with the study and its findings that his or her speech is conversational and not read. A certain spontaneity in presentation is more engaging for the audience and demonstrates confidence on the part of the speaker.[6,7] It is wise for the presenter to rehearse the presentation several times prior to the actual event to coordinate slides with verbal descriptions.

Developing Visual Materials

Both short paper (abstract) and poster presentations are visual events, and strong visual support must be developed. For oral presentations, the visual support should highlight important points, present complex data, and elucidate relationships among variables. Various techniques can be used to effectively present information visually.[6]

Overhead projectors and transparencies. Several options for visual materials can be used effectively in oral presentations. One method is transparencies displayed by an overhead projector. An effective use is to develop sequential transparencies that can overlay each other to demonstrate progressive or multiple relationships. Figures, graphs, tables, and other illustrative material should be centered on the transparency with wide margins to avoid distortion during projection. Print should be large so that it can be read easily from the back of the room. The print used should be clear and have high contrast with the background, which is frequently white. There should not be too many words or too much data on a transparency or it will be difficult to read. Legends on graphs, tables, and figures should be easy to read. The rules provided for the development of graphics in chapter 23 should be followed for transparencies.

It may be difficult to use an overhead projector with transparencies for short paper presentations because transparencies have to be placed and replaced manually. Often short paper presentations are held in large auditoriums where the presenter is at a podium, and there may be some distance between the podium and the overhead projector. This data presentation with overhead projectors may be more appropriate in a small room, with a more interactive type of lecture or workshop.

Slides. Slides frequently are used as visual support for short paper research presentations, and they offer the most effective visual support for an oral presentation of research data. Slides can visually demonstrate the relationships among variables and make complex data more comprehensible by displaying them graphically. Slides can be used to make specific points and, as mentioned, effectively show data, although the most difficult and least successful slides are those that contain rows and columns of data that are illegible to everyone, including the speaker.

Effective slides are an adjunct to the verbal presentation of research data. The title of the presentation, the study design, a succinct description of subject selection and exclusion criteria, a description of the research methods, an explanation of the statistical analyses used, the data results, and the conclusions drawn can be put on slides. Lists can be highlighted with bullets and key phrases. Slides do not have to be written in complete sentences and can be effective if they contain trigger words, which may serve as headings for persons who are taking notes.

Slides can be made in varying degrees of technical sophistication. They can be made by typing the message in a space that approximates the dimensions of a standard slide. For this purpose, a typewriter that uses a film ribbon and a simple typeface will produce the most legible slides; the darker and sharper the typed version, the clearer the slide. One idea is to place a piece of carbon paper face-up behind the page so that the carbon image comes out on the back of the typed page, making the contrast between type and paper greater. Graphs, figures, and illustrations should be drawn with india ink on plain, nonerasable paper, preferably by a graphics artist. Most academic institutions have instructional media departments that provide support for making scientific presentation graphics. Recently, many investigators have started to use computer graphics packages to construct figures, graphs, and tables. Dot-matrix printers make copies that produce fuzzy slides; laser printers yield the sharpest images. Paper images have to be photographed, and the best copy will produce the best slides. Color also can be used effectively to accentuate differences among groups or variables and make data more comprehensible. Guidelines for slide production are listed in *Table 22.1.*

Table 22.1
Guidelines For Preparing Slides

- A horizontal format, using a ratio of 2 units of height for 3 units of width (ie, 6 cm x 9 cm), makes the best slides.
- Capital letters in a bold, simple typeface are easiest to read.
- Illustrations, graphs, and figures should be drawn in india ink on a white background.
- Use a simple design: do not put too much information on one slide.
- Do not exceed 50 spaces (including letters, spaces, and punctuation) per horizontal line.
- Do not exceed 7–10 lines of lettering or numbers per slide.
- Use maximum contrast between lettering and background: black on white, black on light yellow, white on blue.
- Limit each slide to one idea, even if it takes several slides to make your point.
- Allow an adequate margin on all sides.
- Legends on graphs, tables, and figures should be clear and legible.
- Color can be used to highlight points or accent different data sets.
- Complicated data can be supported with handouts.
- Proofread all material to avoid misspellings, which are distracting.
- Place a red dot or number on the lower left-hand corner of the slide when you hold it so that you can read it.
- Important features on an x-ray or photomicrograph should be pointed out with arrows or other symbols.
- Illustrations and photographs should be easily recognizable.

Giving an oral presentation of research data using slides as visual support requires some practice. A presenter should allow sufficient time for slides preparation so that he or she can rehearse the synchronization between slides and oral presentation. Most meeting facilities have remote-control slide advancement so that the train of verbal description does not have to be interrupted by asking an audiovisual support person for the next slide.

Videotape and film. Videotapes and film can be used effectively as adjuncts to oral presentations. They are, however, expensive methods of audiovisual support. Certainly for a brief abstract presentation, videotapes and films can effectively demonstrate procedures or depict events that require motion. A few brief minutes of film can save thousands of words of explanation. For example, a cine film (filmed using an x-ray device) of subclavian catheter placement is more effective in illustrating a procedure than any number of verbal explanations. The impact of vitamin deficiency on altered gaits in chickens or an exercise regimen in stroke rehabilitation will be remembered better if seen by the learner.

The use of videotape or film also can be impressive when used as part of a poster presentation, since it attracts attention and can run continuously. However, the decision to use film should be made with serious consideration of its cost versus its usefulness in making a point, describing an intervention, or demonstrating results. Films and videotapes are expensive to produce and require special equipment to project. The relative contribution that a film will make to a presentation should be very high to justify the extra cost and effort involved in using this technology to present data. It should be used because it is necessary to show activity or movement that cannot be conveyed through slides or still photographs.

Handout materials. Printed handout material is a useful, inexpensive adjunct to a short oral presentation or poster presentation. The short paper or poster abstract is published in a program book or supplement to the organization's official publication, so it is not necessary to duplicate it for handout material. An expanded summary can be written and provided as handout material at a poster session. Other effective ways to supplement an oral presentation with handouts include a bibliography or reference list on the topic; reproductions of complex slides; elucidation of metabolic pathways, examples of questionnaires or survey instruments; product comparisons; an outline of the presentation; a list of definitions of abbreviations or unfamiliar terminology; sources of equipment; ordering forms for pamphlets or other resource materials; and other information that would be too time-consuming or complex to describe verbally.

Printed material should be legible, neat, and attractive with adequate margins, appropriate headings, and easy-to-read typeface. Colored paper can be used to distinguish among different handouts or to make one page of a handout more noticeable. The same rules about maximum contrast between type and background colors applies to printed handout materials too. Black print on a light background is the most commonly used combination. Grammatical conventions and correct spelling should be checked carefully, and drawings or illustrations should be simple, clear, and well-labeled.

At poster sessions, handouts are effective in that they later serve to remind the observer of the poster after the meeting or session is over. They may also be saved for future reference for prospective, new research studies.

Oration Techniques

Being in front of a large crowd of people can be very anxiety-producing for many people. One way to reduce the anxiety and give a cohesive, coherent presentation is to rehearse it so that it becomes familiar and comfortable.[6,7] It may help to write out the talk so that it is possible to make a good estimate of the length when it is read. However, one of the most important rules of oral presentation is: *Do not read a speech.* Writing it down helps to organize it, to ensure that all the major points are included, and to make notes from which to actually talk. A draft prepared for oral delivery is different from a draft prepared for a technical report or manuscript.

Speaking well in public requires a great deal of practice and development of self-confidence. Experience and rehearsal are factors that make this process easier. Practicing a speech in front of a mirror, before a friend, before colleagues, or into a tape recorder can help make it feel comfortable. A researcher who presents his or her own research should be the most confident. The literature has been reviewed, the work has been conducted, the data have been analyzed, the results have been assessed, the implications have been discussed, the abstract has been written and accepted for presentation. No one knows the work better than the researcher; it just takes some practice to present research well.

Techniques for securing the interest of the audience include displaying a high level of enthusiasm for the topic, introducing conversational vocal inflections, pacing of the presentation so that it is not too fast or too slow, and appearing relaxed. Speaking in a monotone and appearing nervous distracts the audience from the message. Some eye contact with the audience should be attempted, rather than looking only at notes or talking to a spot on the wall.

It is important to stay within the time limits established. Many organizations provide timers on the podium with a green light that turns yellow when there are five minutes left, and red when there is no time left. If appropriate, time should be left for a question or two. If there is no time for questions, the presenter should remain available after the session so that members of the audience can ask questions.

Giving any type of oral presentation can be uncomfortable, but with practice, preparation, planning, and good visual support, giving a talk to an audience of interested colleagues can be educational and fun for everyone.

PUBLISHING A RESEARCH PAPER

Having had an opportunity to present data in a brief published form, such as an abstract, and to present it orally as a short paper, the researcher may be ready to write a paper for publication consideration by a peer-reviewed journal. This is the most difficult step in the continuum of presenting research data. Writing for publication is time-consuming, repetitive, and demands commitment to producing a quality product. Nevertheless, writing for publication can be the most satisfying experience in the research process.[8,9]

Selecting the Journal

Selecting the journal that might publish the paper should be one of the first steps in getting ready to write.[8] Journals have specific readerships defined by profession or subject interest; if an abstract or poster has been presented at a professional meeting, the official publication of the professional organization might be the first choice. There may be other journals that address the same topic areas that might also be considered.

Selecting the journal to which the "as yet unwritten" paper will be submitted may seem premature, but there are advantages to making this decision before anything has been written. Many journals, such as the *Journal of The American Dietetic Association*, have several different types of articles with different formats. These may include research reports, short papers, case studies, continuing education articles, literature reviews, and others. Choosing the format to use to present information determines how the paper should be developed. Every journal has its own set of guidelines for its authors, and these may vary depending on the type of article that is being submitted.

Reading the journal's most current guidelines for authors is an important step, which may save considerable time in manuscript preparation. Margins, page numbering, heading and subheading rules, acceptable abbreviations, line spacing, punctuation guidelines, bibliographic style, number of copies needed for submission, rules for figures and tables, and manuscript length are indicated in the guidelines provided. It is much easier to start with proper directions than it is to reformat a manuscript after it is written and revised.

Planning an Article

The first step in planning an article is to decide on the set of data to be published.[9] Often research studies generate more data than can or should be presented in one paper. If the research data have been reported in abstract form, the focus may already have been identified. The paper to be written will address one main theme, which will make it easier to develop thoroughly. If data are

Presentation of Research Data

sufficient, additional articles may be considered; having one manuscript completed provides a basic structure and some important information in already written form.

The next step after selecting the data that will be used for the article is to outline it in broad terms.[1,9] As previously mentioned, the guidelines for authors for the selected journal may provide a broad structural outline for the paper. If this information is not specifically given in the guidelines, reviewing a few issues of the selected journal can reveal how published papers are organized. Most journals have a preferred format that includes the following sections: introduction, methods, results, and discussion.

The introduction should include the presentation of the problem, a concise review of pertinent literature, the investigators' hypothesis, and the motivation for conducting the research being reported. The introduction should tell the reader the purpose of the study, why it was conducted, and describe its scientific context.

The methods section tells the reader how the study was done. It should describe the subject groups and their selection, the research design, the methods or instruments used to collect data, and the data analysis methods used.

The results part of the paper includes the outcomes of the study without interpretation; it also may include the final numbers of completed subjects, reasons for subject drop-out or loss, a description of the variables, and the data collected. The results should be described objectively with an explanation of the statistical analyses.

The discussion segment is where the author interprets the data.[10] Results are compared and contrasted with similar research done by others or associated with previous work performed by the author of the present paper. The implications and applications of the reported research can be explored in this part of the paper.

An outline, following the selected journal's format, is the most logical way to approach the planning of the paper. It can be filled in with phrases and notes of what should be covered under each major heading. As ideas come and are notated, the first draft will start. A well-developed outline makes it easier to write a thorough, organized, comprehensive paper.

During this phase of development, the author might develop a working title for the paper, which should help to focus on the main theme of the paper. A title should be informative, brief, and to the point; some journals restrict the number of characters allowed. Such a limitation is noted in the guidelines for authors.

Writing the Article

The first draft serves to get everything down on paper and is probably the most difficult of all the stages of writing. Notes of references to be used, ideas for tables and figures, possible placement of tables and figures, and headings and subheadings can be penciled in when the first draft is completed.[9] After the first draft is completed, the manuscript should be put away for a few days. An author needs some distance from the first draft to give a clearer perspective on the paper and some time to reflect on what has been written and to allow new ideas to percolate.

After a few days, the author can read the first draft with a fresh, objective view of the paper. It is a good idea to reread the journal's guidelines for authors to review the appropriate sections, length, and bibliographic style. Writing style should be examined and the paper evaluated for appropriate paragraph breaks, one-paragraph sentences, misplaced modifiers, dangling participles, and other grammatical transgressions. Logical sequence of paragraphs, development of themes, relevance of cited literature, and inclusion of pertinent data can be assessed.

A second draft offers an opportunity to evaluate whether each of the paper's sections provides adequate information to explain to the reader why the research was undertaken, how it was conducted, what was accomplished, and what implications and applications can be derived from the outcomes reported. Tables and figures should be drafted at this stage with consideration given to the contribution each will make to the final product.[3] Data described in the text of the paper do not need to be repeated in tables, and some information described in the text may be better presented in a table format. References should be inserted into the text and the bibliography written following the journal's preferred style. Word processing spelling checks, or a careful reading of the draft to correct for spelling errors should be done at this point.

After the second draft is completed to the author's satisfaction, it is time to have the paper read by co-authors and colleagues. The paper is being written for others to read, and having it read first by friendly eyes should be minimally stressful. Criticism should be assumed to be constructive, serving to improve the clarity and quality of the paper. Co-authors want their names on work that reflects excellence, so they will offer suggestions that will make the paper better. It is important to remember that writing is an iterative process, and that published journal articles often have gone through multiple revisions and rewriting. Nothing that appears in print is a first or even second draft of a manuscript. The paper should be regarded as a work in progress.

Future drafts of the manuscript, integrating suggestions from co-authors and colleagues, should serve to refine and polish the paper. A final manuscript should tell a clear, concise, cohesive, complete story; it should have a beginning, a middle, and an end. Each section should flow into the next, explaining the why, what, where, how, and who of the research being reported. The final manuscript should be well-written, avoiding jargon, demonstrating consistency in language, grammar, and verb tense.

Experienced authors know that writing research reports or articles for publication does not get easier with time. The advantage of experience comes in knowing what to expect when starting the process of writing, and helping to accept constructive criticism with equanimity.

Submitting the Article

Preparing the article for submission means giving some attention to the details of publishing. Reference style should be checked, as should the completeness of each citation. Pages should be numbered and page numbers should be in the designated position (eg, lower-left corner, upper-left corner). Figure legends often are required to be on a separate page; figures should be drawn in india ink on white paper or produced by a laser or other high-resolution printer. All symbols used on tables and figures should have easily spotted explanations in footnotes.[3]

Many journals provide a checklist for the author to ascertain that everything required for submission is included with the manuscript. All the required paperwork should be reviewed for completeness. If a figure that appeared elsewhere is to be used, written permission to reprint it from the copyright holder must accompany the article. Journal articles usually contain original figures; using already published figures is a more frequent occurrence in publications such as book chapters.

Each journal requires an original and several copies of the manuscript. In peer-reviewed journals, two or more reviewers read and critique each paper and they each need a copy of the paper.

A letter of transmission to the editor of the journal should accompany the package consisting of an original manuscript, correct number of copies, glossy prints of figures, permissions to reprint, and other documents, such as copyright release forms, as required by the journal. Letters of transmission initiate a dialogue between author and editor and are an accepted courtesy.

Peer Review

Having a paper read by two or more content or practice experts can be very valuable. These experts read the manuscript for scientific accuracy, clarity, completeness, and contribution of new knowledge. Their criticism and comments are designed to make the paper clearer and more complete. They ask questions and make suggestions that are designed to help the author see what is missing or unclear. Depending on the journal, articles may be reviewed anonymously. Reviewers are rarely made known to the authors, but some journals allow the reviewers to know who the authors are. After the review process, revisions often have to be made and the paper resubmitted before it is accepted for publication. This process may take several months. In publishing, patience is definitely a virtue.

Between Acceptance and Publication

There usually is a lag of several months between final acceptance of the article and publication. During this period, the manuscript is copy edited for style, grammar, and conventions specific to the journal. A copy of the edited manuscript is returned to the author with the typeset version of the paper. It is important that these galley proofs be read carefully for typographical errors. Publishers often require that galleys be returned quickly, sometimes within 48 hours, so that publishing deadlines can be met. Depending on the publication, two sets of galleys may be sent so that the author can keep one. Typeset tables also need to be compared carefully against the original manuscript to ensure that numbers have not been transposed and that columns and rows have been maintained and headings properly aligned.

During this time, permissions to reprint figures can be secured if not yet accomplished. Additional figures or graphic materials may need to be produced in camera-ready form. The final details of publication are addressed to ensure a polished product. Many journals will provide a copy of the issue prior to its mailing date for the author.

Issues of Authorship

Issues of authorship are among the most difficult to resolve in publishing. However these issues are decided, they should be decided before papers are written. This topic is discussed in chapters 2 and 24.

SUMMARY

There is a great deal to be gained by participating in research and by presenting the research data in public forums, whether verbally or in print. Research in nutrition and dietetics can contribute to the discovery of new knowledge that can make positive changes in the health of Americans. The difficult, potentially tortuous process of presenting research data to interested colleagues can be well worth the effort, resulting in personal satisfaction, career advancement, and professional pride.

References

1. Teel CS. Completing the research process: presentations and publications. *J Neurosci Nurs.* 1990;22:125–127.
2. Steinbaugh ML. Writing technical reports. In: Chernoff R, ed. *Communicating as Professionals.* Chicago, Ill: The American Dietetic Association; 1986:9–13.
3. Perkin J. Developing tables, graphs, and figures. In: Chernoff R, ed. *Communicating as Professionals.* Chicago, Ill: The American Dietetic Association; 1986:29–33.
4. Flynn MA. Writing brief communications. In: Chernoff R, ed. *Communicating as Professionals.* Chicago, Ill: The American Dietetic Association; 1986:35–38.
5. Morra ME. How to plan and carry out your poster session. *Oncol Nurs Forum.* 1984;11:52.
6. Kris-Etherton PM. Developing oral presentations. In: Chernoff R, ed. *Communicating as Professionals.* Chicago, Ill: The American Dietetic Association; 1986:50–55.
7. Lucas SF. *The Art of Public Speaking.* 2nd ed. New York, NY: Random House; 1986.
8. Beare PG. Essentials of writing for publication. *J Ophthal Nurs Tech.* 1988;7:56–58.
9. Chernoff R. Writing journal articles. In: Chernoff R, ed. *Communicating as Professionals.* Chicago, Ill: The American Dietetic Association; 1986:3–7.
10. Zellmer WA. How to write a research report for publication. *Am J Hosp Pharm.* 1981;38:545.

23. ILLUSTRATING THE RESULTS OF RESEARCH

Carol West Suitor, DSc, RD

The effective presentation of research results poses a challenge to even the most experienced investigator. This paper addresses the use of illustrations to enhance communication of research results. Included are tables, graphs, distribution maps, photographs, and algorithms. Emphasis is placed on the most widely used types of illustrations—tables and graphs—primarily as they are used in published works. The usefulness of illustrations in enhancing text (especially for textbooks and readers) has been the subject of considerable study[1-4]; however, an extensive search of the literature reveals that relatively little research has been directed to the types of illustrations used in reporting research results.

PURPOSES OF ILLUSTRATIONS

Illustrations are used to make information more understandable, depict relationships, add needed emphasis, or allow presentation of important, exact data in a clear and compact form. Types of illustrations and their functions are presented in *Box 1*.

Box 1
Functions of Different Types of Illustrations

Type	Function
Table	Representation of exact data in compact form
Graph	Display of trends or relationships in quickly interpretable form
Distribution map	Display of the location of data
Photograph	Accurate representation of the appearance of the subject (eg, a clinically observable disorder, microorganisms, newly developed equipment)
Algorithm, flow chart	Display of the steps in a procedure that lead to one or more outcomes
Other diagrams	Simplified representation of the subject

In a set of guidelines for statistical reporting in medical journals, Bailar and Mosteller[5] state: "Restrict tables and figures to those needed to explain the argument of the paper and to assess its support. Use graphs as an alternative to tables with many entries; do not duplicate data in graphs and tables." These noted statisticians argue for economy in presentation as a method of increasing the chance that an article will be read. Regardless of the type of illustration used, it should contain enough information to be understandable without referring to the text.

Illustrations for published works, posters, slides, or transparencies should be prepared differently. Although all types of illustration are suitable for inclusion in research articles if they fulfill one of the purposes given above, many are unsuitable for display in a poster or on a screen unless they are greatly simplified. Guidelines for preparing materials for posters[6-8] and slides[9-11] focus on simplicity and clarity.

MESSAGES TO BE CONVEYED

In deciding on illustrations for research articles, investigators need to focus on the messages they wish to convey concerning the data, both overall and by each illustration. Different kinds of illustrations send different messages and serve different functions, as described below. Thus, it is inappropriate to use different methods for illustrating similar data sets just to introduce variety in an article.

ILLUSTRATIONS AS A SET

The number of illustrations included in a research article should be kept to a minimum so that the reader can easily comprehend the article's overall message and the data that support it. More extensive illustration may be appropriate for monographs, technical reports, and some types of scientific books.

Consistency adds clarity. Scientific journals therefore specify a style for tables and require its use. However, many do not have rigid specifications for graphs and other figures. Because these journals reproduce the figures submitted with the manuscript, authors are advised to give special attention to consistency, accuracy, and scale when preparing a set of figures. Consistent use of symbols is recommended, along with similar proportions and style. For example, when preparing a series of graphs comparing food use by Mexican Americans and Puerto Ricans, these ethnic groups should be represented by consistent symbols in line graphs or types of fill in bar graphs. More suggestions for achieving consistency among graphs are given in the Guidelines for Preparing Useful Graphs.

When deciding on the order in which comparison groups are to be presented, as in tables or bar graphs, it is often undesirable to be consistent. Instead, the order of presentation ordinarily should be determined by the message to be conveyed. This is illustrated in *Figure 23.1* on pages 392 and 393. The preferred order appears in Figures 23.1C and E because this order makes it easy to compare the relative rankings of the different groups. (The category "Other" remains at the end because it includes many different groups with low individual rankings.)

GUIDELINES FOR PREPARING USEFUL TABLES

Many style manuals, such as the *Chicago Manual of Style,*[14] give extensive guidelines for preparing tables, but these manuals tend to deal only superficially with substantive issues relating to handling data. Day[15] provides a number of examples of poorly designed and well-executed tables. Colton[16] and Ehrenberg[17] (both statisticians) and Clark[16] (a noted editor) present complementary suggestions for making the data in tables more comprehensible. Many of these suggestions are listed in *Box 2*.

Essential Categories of Information

Clark specifies the categories of information that should be included in a table to provide a complete picture of the data.[18] She recommends organizing information before actually preparing a table by producing a descriptor set using the categories in the far left-hand column of *Box 3*. This box includes examples of Clark's approach, using a hypothetical data set. Missing from the list is identification of the sample size, which is necessary for interpretation of the generalizability of the data.

(Text continues on page 394.)

Box 2
Tips for Clear Tables

Provide complete information

- Label clearly, making sure to include a label for the stub list (the far left-hand column of the table) and the column heads. Difficulty in identifying a suitable label is likely to indicate a problem in organization of the data.[18]
- Clearly indicate units of measurement.[16]
- Indicate totals, where applicable, to summarize the data in the table and to help reconcile the data with that in other tables and material in the text.[16]
- Show in which direction the percentages add to 100%. This informs the reader how the percentages in the table were derived.[16]
- Use tables when they promote a clearer summary of results than would prose.
- Avoid complex tables.

Carefully consider layout and organization[17]

- Provide a *visual focus* by giving averages for the rows and columns. (Often this is not possible for the types of data displayed in dietetics journals).
- Arrange the columns and rows in a logical order; facilitate comparisons when relevant.
- Round appropriately to improve ease of reading and recall.
- Use the text to lead the reader to important patterns and to exceptions.

Box 3
Categories of Information
Necessary for a Complete
Representation of Data in Tables

Category	Definitions	Examples (Comments)
Current source of the table	Author, publication date	From Smith, et al, 1990 (necessary only for data taken from sources apart from an original research effort, especially necessary in review articles)
Source of the data	Data collector and the period of data collection	Statewide Preschool Nutrition Survey, 1981–1982
Observer	Respondents: who reported the values?	Food intakes by preschoolers *as reported by their mothers and day care providers*
Matter	Entities involved in the event covered in the table	Preschoolers aged 3–5 years; milk consumption
Function	Nature of the event covered and factors that may influence it	Milk intake; race; income
Space	Location of the event	Large state, USA
Time	Period when the event occurred	1981–1982 (in studies examining past events—or exposures, as in case-control studies—this time may be much earlier than that given by the period of data collection)
Aspect	What was measured and to what topic does this point?	Mean intake in grams in a single 24-h period; (points to) weight of all forms of fluid milk
Domain	Range of values	0, . . . , 790 g

Compiled from Clark N.[18]

Figure 23.1
Example of undesirable and improved methods of depicting the same data. A is not a recommended method for several reasons: it appears to be a frequency polygon, but is not; it uses abbreviations that are not standard and may not be clear to all readers; there is no logical order to the arrangement of the data; and the actual frequencies are given on the graph (From Fiedler KM, Raguso A, Morgan G, Renker L.[12] Used by permission.) B is an improved version of the same graph. However, it would be even better if the order were changed so that positions (type of employment) appeared in descending order of frequency, if the shading reflected the relative frequency, and if the vertical axis displayed the percentage of graduates in each type of position, rather than absolute numbers.

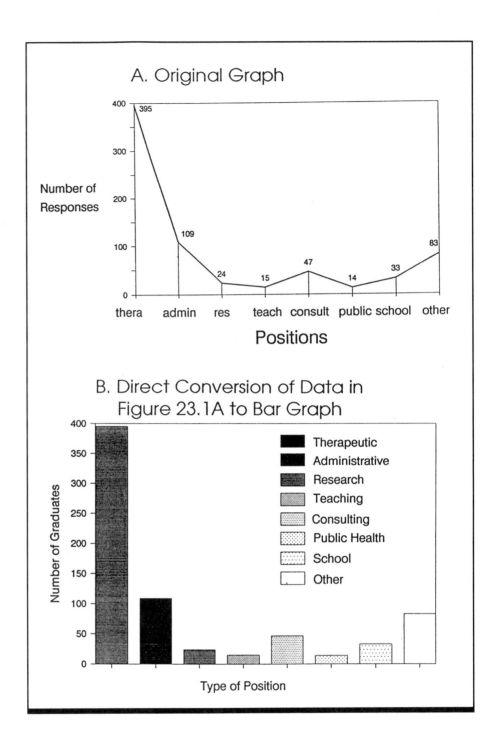

Presentation of Research Data

Figure 23.1 (continued)
C depicts some of these changes
and uses an alternative approach
for labeling. The names of the
positions have been changed
slightly to be more consistent in
style and more informative. D
shows how a vertical bar graph
can aid in labeling. This graph
was made with default settings. E
shows the same graph customized
by deleting vertical grid marks
and data labels, which cluttered
the graph and were therefore
considered undesirable.[13]

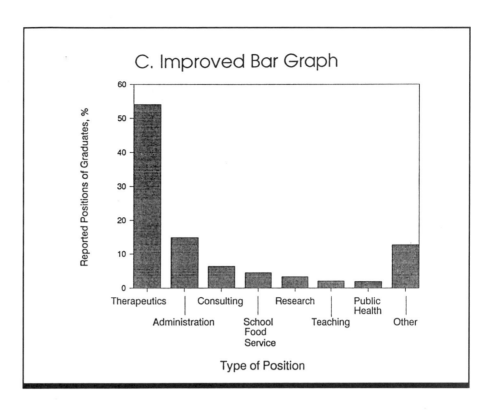

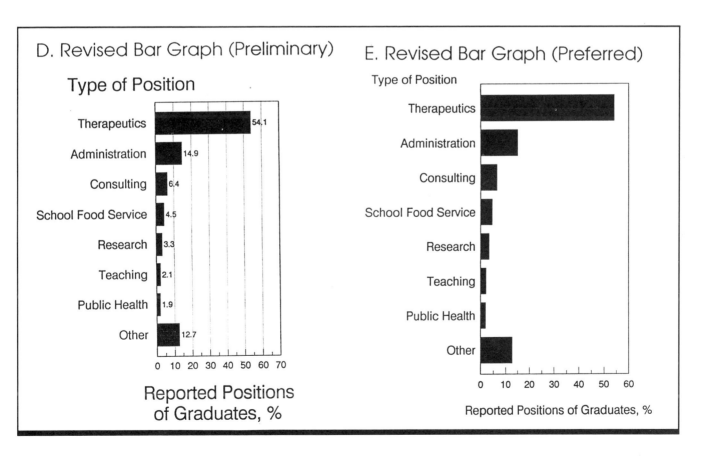

Stages of Table Reading

According to Clark,[18] there are three stages of table reading: the scanning stage, reading and primary comparisons, and second-level comparisons. In the scanning stage, the reader looks across the column heads and down the stub. Additional scanning practices appear to depend on the experience of the reader. In the reading stage, Clark asserts that readers read across the rows of data, and they assume that the column heads are the categories being presented for comparison, even if that was not the intent of the author. If this is true, it directly conflicts with Ehrenberg's advice to present the numbers to be compared in columns, rather than in rows.[17] No scientific basis was found for choosing one approach over the other. *Table 23.1* shows the effects of applying some of these recommendations, including the effect of transposing the rows and columns. The data in these tables are easy to transpose because the same units are used throughout.

Table 23.1
Series of Tables Containing the Same Data in Different Formats

A, reproduction of a table as it appeared in a journal article.

Comparison of Responses From Experimental (n = 22) and Control (n = 19) Groups to the Nutrition Knowledge Test (NKT) Prior to and Following the Nutrition Education Module*

Group	Percent Correct Mean ± SD Scores on NKT Pretest	Percent Correct Mean ± SD Scores on NKT Posttest	Percent Correct Adjusted Mean† Scores on NKT
Experimental (n = 22)	54.0 ± 14.4	65.3 ± 14.6	64.4[x]
Control (n = 19)	51.2 ± 11.4	53.3 ± 12.8	54.2[y]

* Values within a column with different letter superscripts are significantly different at the $P \leq 0.01$ level.

† Percent correct posttest scores in this column are adjusted based on percent correct pretest scores.

From Hart PC, Alford BB, Gorman MA.[19] Used by permission.

B, the same data displayed with simplified caption and column heads, deletion of redundancies, and the qualifier of missionaries. The organization facilitates comparison of pretest and posttest scores for those reading across rows.

Comparison of Pretest, Posttest, and Adjusted[a] Scores on the Nutrition Knowledge Test by Experimental and Control Groups of Missionaries

Group	Pretest Score	Posttest Score	Adjusted Mean Score[b]
	———Mean ± SD[c]———		
Experimental (no. = 22)	54.0 ± 14.4	65.3 ± 14.6	64.4[x]
Control (no. = 19)	51.2 ± 11.4	53.3 ± 12.8	54.2[y]

[a] Adjustments are based on pretest scores.

[b] Values within the column with different letter superscripts are significantly different at the $P \leq .01$ level.

[c] SD = standard deviation.

Adapted from Hart PC, Alford BB, Gorman MA.[19]

(Continued.)

C, the data arranged to favor comparison of controls with module participants when reading across the rows; this version also adds clarifying information about the experimental group.

Comparison of Control and Experimental[a] Group Scores Achieved by Missionaries on the Nutrition Knowledge Test

	Mean Test Score by Group	
Type of Test Score	Controls (no. = 19)	Module Participants (no. = 22)
Pretest	51.2 ± 11.4[b]	54.0 ± 14.4
Posttest	53.3 ± 12.8	65.3 ± 14.6
Adjusted mean score[c]	54.2	64.4*

[a] Experimental group members were required to attend a nutrition education module.

[b] Mean ± standard deviation.

[c] Posttest scores in this row are adjusted based on pretest scores.

* $P < 0.01$

Adapted from Hart PC, Alford BB, Gorman MA.[19]

One of the major advantages of placing the data to be compared in columns is that it often facilitates labeling. It is preferable to use consistent units of measurement for all items in a column. This sometimes is not done in the dietetic literature; listing nutrients down the stub may keep a table from becoming excessively wide and favors comparisons across the rows.

Sometimes it is possible and effective to set up a table to convey a strong visual message. For example, since incompatibility of vitamin-mineral preparations with enteral feeding mixtures can be of real concern, symbols might be used in a table to highlight this kind of problem. A visual approach is shown with a more standard approach in *Table 23.2.*

Table 23.2
*Alternate Approaches to
Presenting the Same
Information in Tabular Form*

A, slightly modified excerpt from a table by Burns PE, McCall L, Wirsching R.[20]

**Physical Compatibility of Vitamin/Mineral
Preparations With Products X, Y, and Z**

Medication	Degree of Compatibility[a]		
	Product X	Product Y	Product Z
Vitamin/mineral preparations			
Feosol®	4	4	C
Gevrabon liquid	4	4	C
KCl elixir	C	C	C
Fleets phosphosoda	1	4	C
Neocalglucon syrup	3	4	C
Theragran liquid	C	C	C
Zinc sulfate capsules	4	4	C

[a] C = Compatible. Incompatibility is measured on a scale of 1 to 4, with 4 being the most incompatible or hardest to unclog.

B, example of a more visual presentation of the same data.

**Physical Compatibility of Vitamin/Mineral
Preparations With Products X, Y, and Z**

Medication	Degree of Compatibility[a]		
	Product X	Product Y	Product Z
Vitamin/mineral preparations			
Feosol®	••••	••••	C
Gevrabon liquid	••••	••••	C
KCl elixir	C	C	C
Fleets phosphosoda	•	••••	C
Neocalglucon syrup	•••	••••	C
Theragran liquid	C	C	C
Zinc sulfate capsules	••••	••••	C

[a] C = Compatible. Incompatibility is measured on a scale of 1 to 4, with 4 dots (••••) being the most incompatible or hardest to unclog.

Adapted from Burns PE, McCall L, Wirsching R.[20]

GUIDELINES FOR PREPARING USEFUL GRAPHS

Many of the shortcomings of graphs published in the nutrition and dietetics literature appear to result from using computer graphics programs routinely, rather than taking the time to customize a graph for a particular application and carefully inspecting the result. Suggestions for avoiding unintentional misrepresentation of data or other common problems that may be associated with routine use of graphics software are incorporated in this section. Figure captions include additional tips.

When adding lettering to graphs, the use of initial capital letters only, rather than all upper case, is strongly urged. Words written in lower case are easier to read.[13,21,22]

Choice of Graph Type

Standard graph types include line graphs, scatter graphs, histograms, frequency polygons, bar graphs, stacked bar graphs, and pie charts. Readers are referred to works such as *Illustrating Science*[13] for information on the appropriate use of each type. Investigators need to take care not to let their decisions be driven by the choices offered by their graphics software package.

Presentation of Research Data

Graphs serve two general purposes: one is to examine data; the other is to communicate data to others. Stem and leaf diagrams and scatter plots are types of graphs useful for finding out if a few data points may be strongly influencing measures of effect. Such graphs are very useful for data interpretation, but are seldom used in communicating the results of studies. Box plots depict important aspects of the distribution of data.[23] (See *Figure 23.2* for a generic example of a box plot, and see articles by Hebert and Waternaux[24] and by Worthington-Roberts and associates[25] for examples of the use of this type of graph in reporting the results of nutrition research.)

Figure 23.2
Example of a single box plot. The elements define the mean, median (50th percentile), first and third quartiles (25th and 75th percentiles, respectively), 5th and 95th percentiles, and minimum and maximum values. Note that this plot depicts data that are skewed toward high values; the mean exceeds the median, there is considerable spread between the median and the 95th percentile, and there is at least one serious outlier. Several box plots may be presented on the same graph to allow comparison of the effects of three different treatments and to provide information about the distribution of data. Adapted from Worthington-Roberts BS, Breskin MW, Monsen ER.[25]

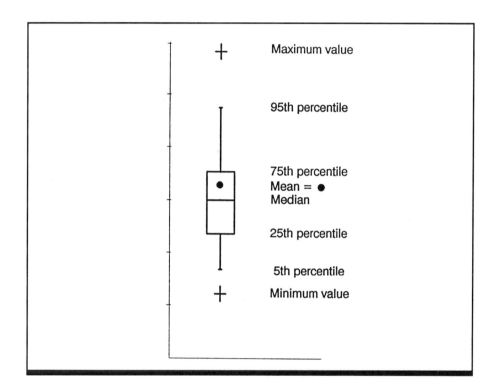

Important Characteristics of Graphs

According to Tufte,[22] "Graphical excellence is the well-designed presentation of interesting data—a matter of *substance*, of *statistics*, and of *design*." He demonstrates ways to achieve clear, precise, and efficient communication of complex ideas and emphasizes displaying truthful messages with the data. He objects to graphs that have a small ratio of data to ink (as is the case with many bar graphs, for example). Tufte compiled a useful list of qualities common to enhancing the visual quality of displays of statistical information:
* Choose proper format and design.
* Use words, numbers, and drawing together (eg, little messages that help explain the data).
* Produce a balanced, well-proportioned graph with a relevant scale.
* Display complex detail (the data) in a simple manner (avoiding abbreviations and elaborate codes).
* Tell a story with the data, if appropriate.
* Draw the graph in a professional manner.
* Avoid decorations and moire effects (as from hatched lines).

Colton[16] emphasizes three important characteristics of graphs:

- Graphs should aid the reader's comprehension of the material. They are unlikely to do this if they include a large number of variables, even with ingenious graph design.
- Their axes should be clearly labeled and include the units of measurement. A glance should suffice for alerting the reader to what is being illustrated and in what units. Cryptic labeling (eg, only the word *Percent*) of the vertical axis of graphs is common; more complete labeling (eg, "Percent of iron absorbed") helps convey the message.
- Graphs should be scaled to represent the data and their importance accurately.

Improper or misleading scaling often occurs unintentionally, especially if using graphics programs. Such programs include default settings—computer-selected settings for the range, the scales of the x and y axes, the typeface, and so forth—which are intended to make it easy to produce standard graphs that look good (at least to the casual observer). Default settings for the range of the vertical axis are based on the range of the data being displayed. Therefore, they minimize unused space—a desirable practice. However, the net result is that they often use an inappropriately high scale that makes minor changes appear major, as illustrated by *Figure 23.3*. The researcher should make sure that it is easy to tell if the scale does not start at zero and if the scales represent arithmetic or mathematical (eg, logarithmic) change; the investigator also should make sure that scales correspond exactly if graphs are to be compared (see below). Chapter 21 presents information about scale transformations. In all cases, the researcher needs to inspect all graphs visually for completeness, clarity, and accuracy before using them.

Figure 23.3
Inappropriate graph that overemphasizes the importance of the data. This graph was produced using default settings in a graphics program. The scaling of the Y axis is inappropriate, there is no break in the Y axis to show that the scale does not start at zero, and the lettering is too small to be reduced for publication.

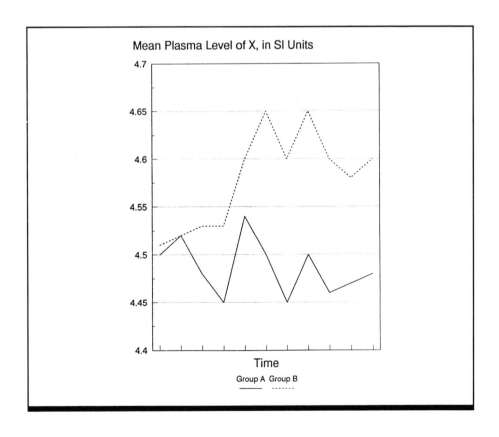

Presentation of Research Data

Figure 23.4
An example of lack of
consistency between figures. Note
that scale of the vertical axis of A
is slightly smaller than that of B
(probably because of inconsistent
size reduction, since the range
used is the same), that different
styles of lettering are used for
nutrient labels (those in B are
preferred), and that the intensity
of the fill is different for the bars
representing lower carbohydrate
diets. Hatching, as used for the
high carbohydrate group, is not
recommended.[22] The preferred
style for error bars on bar graphs
is illustrated on the bar for iron,
but the captions do not identify
whether the error bars represent
standard deviations or standard
errors. In these figures, the
message might be clearer if the
order used were low, moderate,
and high and if the intensity of
the shading corresponded to the
level of carbohydrate content.
From Alford BB, Blankenship
AC, Hagen RD.[26] Used by
permission.

Achieving Consistency

To achieve visual consistency, it is advisable to use the same computer software to prepare all graphs for a given paper. If two or more programs must be used, special steps may be required to achieve consistency in the use of symbols, fill, and lettering. Even if the same software is used to prepare all the graphs in a set, it is essential to achieve consistency of scale for those graphs that are likely to be compared; for example, the linear distance in millimeters between tick marks on graph A should be identical to that on graph B. To achieve this consistency, the preparer of the graphs must avoid the use of default settings for the vertical axis and be sure to specify the same range for all graphs to be compared (eg, 0% to 100% or 2.0 to 6.0 mmol). Some graphics software allows the user to change the size of the graph. If this is done for one, identical changes in size should be made in all graphs that are to be compared. Furthermore, the authors must specify that identical reductions be made in preparing the figure for printing. *Figure 23.4* shows two graphs that have the same range for the vertical axis, but slightly different scales. The figure caption points out other inconsistencies as well.

Illustrating Science: Standards for Publication[13] contains an outstanding set of guidelines for the preparation of graphs. Methods for improving the visual clarity of graphs are unusually detailed. The book advises those preparing graphs to choose symbols for data points that reproduce clearly and can be easily discerned. The recommended symbols are ●, ▲, ■; ○, △, □. The actual choice of symbols depends on what they represent and where they will appear in the graph. When only two symbols are required, black (filled) and white (open) circles are preferred; these might be used to represent black and white subjects, respectively. Similarly, white (open) symbols could be used to

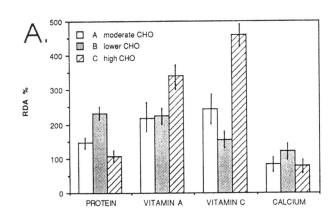

FIG. 3. *Average intakes of protein, vitamin A, vitamin C, and calcium of obese women on weight reduction diets*

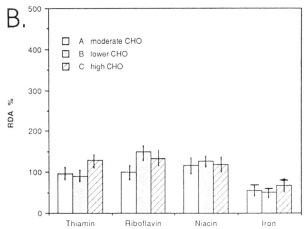

FIG. 4. *Average intakes of thiamin, riboflavin, niacin, and iron of obese women on weight reduction diets*

represent two groups before interventions and black symbols to represent them after the interventions (in this case, circles and triangles would be preferred). Although all the symbols shown above are acceptable, it is preferable if circles do not appear next to squares because these two shapes are difficult to distinguish, especially after reduction. If only one symbol is needed, black circles are recommended, since they are most like data points and are prominent.

Graphical Perception

Graphical perception involves the study of the way graphical information is visually decoded.[27] Since a graph is successful only if it is accurately and efficiently decoded, it may be helpful for researchers to be alert to new developments in this field of study. According to Cleveland and McGill,[28] the elementary tasks in graphical perception can be ranked from most to least accurate, as shown in *Box 4.*

These investigators provide experimental evidence that specific graph types are interpreted more accurately than are certain other types. In particular, they recommend dot or bar charts in place of pie charts, and dot or bar charts with grouping in place of stacked bars (*Figure 23.5*). Component (stacked) bar graphs merit special attention because they are widely used to depict the components of a whole and are easy to create with graphics software. A major problem with these graphs is that they require estimation of length along nonaligned scales. Thus, Figure 23.5B is clearly easier to interpret than Figure 23.5A. Cleveland and McGill further recommend direct display of the differences between two curves in place of the curves themselves (*Figure 23.6D*).

Box 4
Elementary Tasks in Graphical Perception in Decreasing Order of Accuracy

Elementary Estimation task	Examples
1. Position along a common scale	Height or length of a bar that is part of a bar graph
2. Position along nonaligned scales	Heights of segments in identical closed rectangles
3. Length, direction, angle	Comparison of line lengths without any point of reference; relative sizes of segments in a pie chart
4. Area	Difference in size of two circles
5. Volume, curvature	Difference in volume of two or more spheres
6. Shading, color saturation	Differences in shading on distribution maps

Compiled from Cleveland WS, McGill R.[28]

Presentation of Research Data

Figure 23.5
Stacked bar graph (A) compared with dot chart with grouping (B). B demonstrates improved ease of estimating the relative frequencies of the items within groups. The program used to produce the stacked bar graph used different kinds of hatching to denote the different groups; these were deleted to avoid a cluttered graph with moire effects. Adapted from Cleveland NS, McGill R.[28]

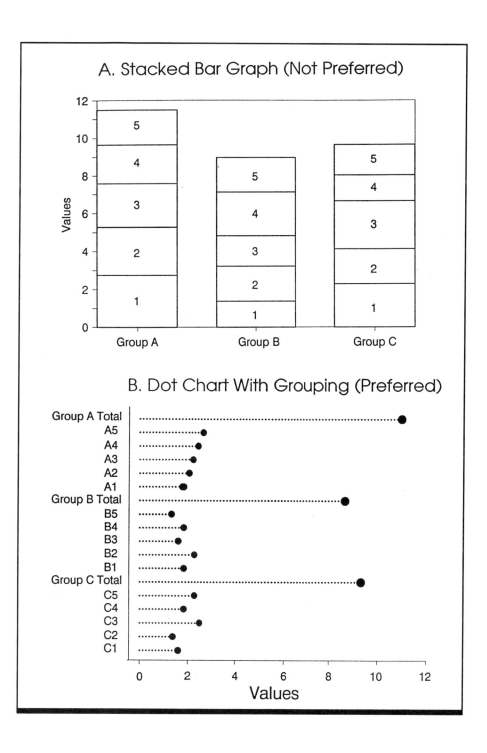

As can be seen in *Figure 23.6*, the messages conveyed by curve-difference graphs are greatly different from those conveyed by depicting the two curves separately. If the object is to show that one treatment consistently produces better results than another, it is more appropriate to use a graph like Figure 23.6A or B. On the other hand, if the difference between values at various time points is important, curve-difference graphs (Figure 23.6C and D) or a table of differences would be superior.

Figure 23.6
Curve difference graphs. A and B depict data for each treatment over time, whereas C and D depict the absolute difference between the treatments over time. Note the difference in message; the author should determine whether the difference between the curves warrants emphasis. Some readers who compare the two types of graphs suspect an error because of the great difficulty of visually perceiving absolute differences between two adjacent curves. Adapted from Cleveland WS, McGill R.[28]

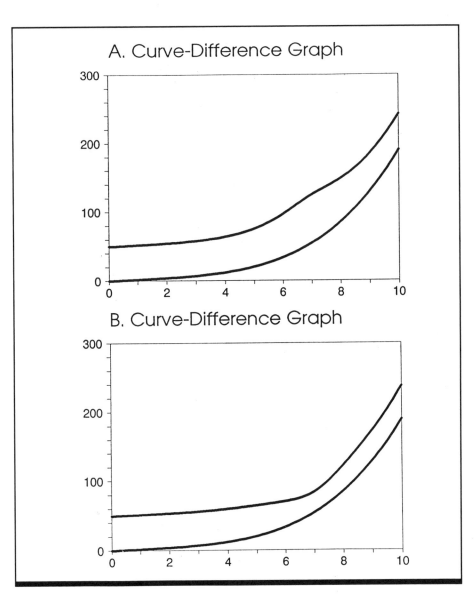

Presentation of Research Data

Figure 23.6 (continued)

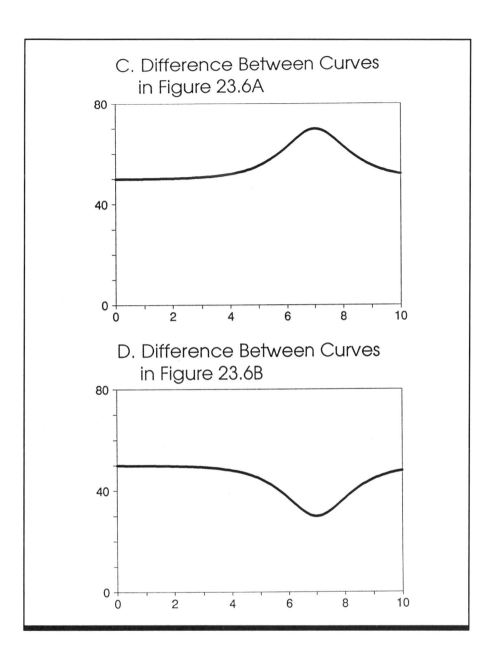

A few additional remarks may be useful to researchers trying to avoid some common pitfalls. Because histograms display frequency distributions, the area of the rectangles in the histogram must represent the frequency of the data. Thus, if intervals are unequal—representing different time periods, for example—the width of the rectangle should reflect this (ie, accurate scaling of the horizontal axis must be maintained). As shown earlier in Figure 23.1, graphics programs allow researchers to choose any one of many graph variations, not all of which are acceptable. Horizontal bar graphs (Figure 23.1E) make it possible to use complete labels rather than abbreviations or other sometimes awkward strategies.

Increased computer capabilities have resulted in rapid developments in the graphical display of results from multidimensional modeling. Although such displays are favorably described,[29] there is little information about how well these complex graphs convey messages to readers who are not specialists in the area.

OTHER FORMS OF ILLUSTRATIONS

Distribution Maps

Maps focus on the location of data and can be useful in depicting differences in rates, ratios, total amounts, or percentages by area. For example, a map of the United States in which states are grouped by census regions can be used to depict differences in breastfeeding rates in different parts of the country; a state map can be used to identify counties with unusually high or low prevalence of obesity, and a city map can be used to identify census tracts where members of an ethnic minority reside in large numbers. Shades from light to dark are often used to depict numerical values from low to high, as in *Figure 23.7A*. This practice has some serious drawbacks: regardless of the numerical value, large areas tend to appear more important, and there is a tendency to overestimate differences in the shades of gray and thus in the numerical values.[13] If such maps are used, seven is the maximum advisable number of intervals for the data.

Cleveland and McGill[28] suggest the use of framed rectangle (blocked rectangle) charts as replacements for distribution maps in which shading denotes quantitative information. Figure 23.7B is a framed rectangle chart that depicts the same data as that used for Figure 23.7A. Both figures were prepared with Freelance Plus* computer software.

Photographs

Photographs bring the element of reality to the reader. A photograph showing clinical signs of a rarely seen nutrient deficiency reinforces the author's statement that a specific treatment can lead to serious nutritional problems. Readers are referred to *Illustrating Science: Standards for Publication*,[13] *A Guide to Medical Photography*,[30] and *Halftone Reproduction Guide*[31] for detailed information on photography and points to consider concerning the reproduction of photographs .

*Lotus Development Corporation, Cambridge, MA 02142.

Presentation of Research Data

Figure 23.7
Distribution maps. A depicts the conventional approach of using different intensities of shading to denote different rates of X in various counties. The computer program automatically uses all upper case letters for the county names, and all upper case letters were used for the legend title for consistency. B depicts the framed (blocked) rectangle approach. In this approach, the area of the county has little or no effect on interpretation of the extent of the problem. Note the improved readability when only the initial letters are capitalized.

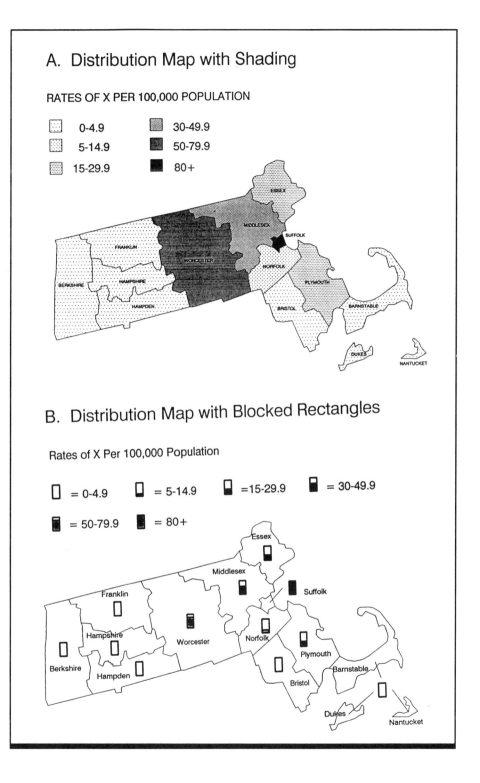

Algorithms and Flow Charts

Increasing numbers of algorithms and flow charts are appearing in the dietetic literature. Algorithms are used for clarifying complex decision-making processes; flow charts are used for organizing and presenting processes. *Figure 23.8* illustrates some features of a flow chart designed to highlight basic differences of two methods of dietary data collection. The major tasks involved are placed within carefully selected shapes and arranged logically. The shapes used are informative for those familiar with standard conventions, but knowledge of such conventions is not required for understanding the diagram. In the figure, the alignment of the steps makes it easy to identify where extra steps are required by the manual method of data collection. To make the diagram easy to read, active verbs are used, and the sentences are short and simple. Decision points are highlighted by question marks. Since the difference in time required by the two data collection methods was one of the reasons for the research, this information is included in the diagram in concise form.

If drawings are used as part of a flow chart, care should be taken to make them readily recognizable. If the purpose of the flow chart in *Figure 23.8* had been to provide a complete description of the methods, the diagram would include a much longer series of steps.

Care should be taken not to use the same symbol to represent two different variables. For example, if N is used in the legend to denote the number of an activity node, a different symbol, such as T, should be used to denote the time required for the activity. In Figure 23.8, which represents hypothetical data, different codes (eg, C1 and C2) were used to denote times at various steps so that the reader would realize that each time might be different.

Other Diagrams

Marcus[33] describes principles of visual organization and the limits of perception that can be useful in developing clear displays of complex relationships. Among his recommendations are use of sans serif typefaces (eg, sans serif rather than serif type), simplified imagery, open spaces, and consistency of design, including reliance on a grid of implied lines. Marcus recommends that similar things be arranged in similar ways and that they be positioned to make the visual hierarchy clear. He further recommends that lines and symbols in charts have a relationship to the information to which the chart refers (eg, relatively imprecise data should be represented by relatively thick, rather than thin lines) and that visual emphasis be achieved through use of heavier lines, larger type, and gray levels. These recommendations are more applicable to illustrations for posters or slides than for most published works.

Figure 23.8
Example of a flow chart. Adapted
from Fong AKH, Kretsch MJ. [32]

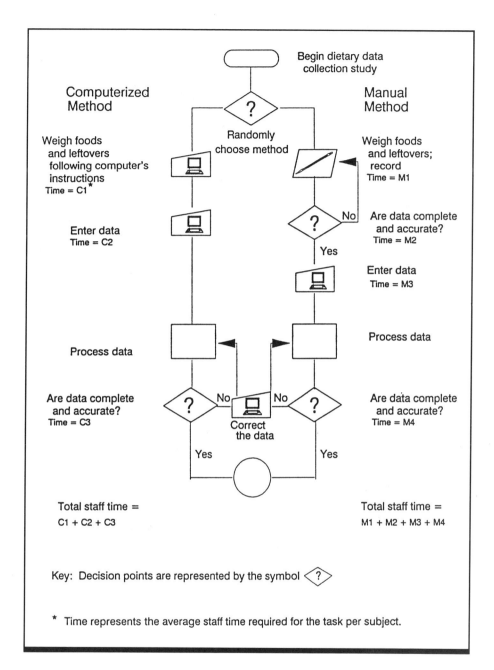

Begin dietary data
collection study

Computerized
Method

Manual
Method

Randomly
choose method

Weigh foods
and leftovers
following computer's
instructions
Time = C1 *

Weigh foods
and leftovers;
record
Time = M1

Enter data
Time = C2

No   Are data complete
and accurate?
Time = M2

Yes

Enter data
Time = M3

Process data

Process data

Are data complete
and accurate?
Time = C3

No   Correct
the data   No

Are data complete
and accurate?
Time = M4

Yes

Yes

Total staff time =
C1 + C2 + C3

Total staff time =
M1 + M2 + M3 + M4

Key: Decision points are represented by the symbol ⟨?⟩

* Time represents the average staff time required for the task per subject.

SUMMARY

When preparing illustrations for manuscripts, researchers need to select the proper type of illustrations to serve specific functions, identify the messages to be conveyed, and develop the illustrations as a compatible set. Special attention should be directed to conveying important messages with clarity, simplicity, consistency, and accuracy. Once the illustrations are prepared, the investigator is advised to examine the visual effect of those illustrations, both individually and as a set, and make adjustments as needed.

Acknowledgments

The author wishes to thank Marian M. F. Millstone, who used evenings and weekends to conduct the literature search and retrieve the articles. Without her assistance, the writing of this article would not have been possible.

References

1. Willows DM, Houghton HA. *The Psychology of Illustration, Volume 1, Basic Research.* New York, NY: Springer-Verlag; 1987.
2. Goldsmith E. *Research Into Illustration: An Approach and a Review.* Cambridge, England: Cambridge University Press; 1984.
3. Duchastel PC. Research on illustrations in text: Issues and perspectives. *Educ Commun Technol Journal.* 1980;28:283–287.
4. Levie WH, Lentz R. Effects of text illustrations: a review of research. *Educ Commun Technol Journ.* 1982;30:195–232.
5. Bailar JC III, Mosteller F. Guidelines for statistical reporting in articles for medical journals: Amplifications and explanations. *Ann Intern Med.* 1988; 108: 266–273.
6. Kroenke K. Poster sessions. *Am J Med.* 1987;83:1129-1130.
7. Warmuth JF. Perspectives on research. *J Nurs Staff Dev.* 1988;4:192-193.
8. Ryan NM. Developing and presenting a research poster. *Applied Nurs Res.* 1989;2:52-55.
9. Kroenke K. The 10-minute talk. *Am J Med.* 1987;83:329-330.
10. Garson A Jr, Gutgesell HP, Pinsky WW, McNamara DG. The 10-minute talk: organization, slides, writing, and delivery. *Am Heart J.* 1986;111:193-203.
11. Johnson V. Picture-perfect presentations. *Training Dev J.* May 1989;45-47.
12. Fiedler KM, Raguso A, Morgan G, Renker L. A retrospective study of graduates of a coordinated internship/master's degree program. *J Am Diet Assoc.* 1990; 90:591-596.
13. Scientific Illustration Committee of the Council of Biology Editors. *Illustrating Science: Standards for Publication.* Bethesda, Md: Council of Biology Editors; 1988.
14. *The Chicago Manual of Style.* 13th ed. Chicago, Ill: University of Chicago Press; 1982.
15. Day RA. *How to Write and Publish a Scientific Paper.* Philadelphia, Pa: ISI Press; 1979.
16. Colton T. *Statistics in Medicine.* Boston, Mass: Little Brown and Co; 1974.
17. Ehrenberg AC. The problem of numeracy. *Am Statistician.* 1981;35:67–71.
18. Clark N. Tables and graphs as a form of exposition. *Scholarly Publishing.* 1987;19:24–42.
19. Hart PC, Alford BB, Gorman MA. Evaluation of a nutrition education module as a component of the career orientation of foreign missionaries. *J Nutr Educ.* 1990;22:81–88.
20. Burns PE, McCall L, Wirsching R. Physical compatibility of enteral formulas with various common medications. *J Am Diet Assoc.* 1988;88:1094–1096.
21. Hartley J. Planning the typographical structure of instructional text. *Educational Psychologist.* 1986;21d:315–332.
22. Tufte ER. *The Visual Display of Quantitative Information.* Cheshire, Conn: Graphics Press; 1983.
23. Williamson DF, Parker RA, Kendrick JS. The box plot: a simple visual method to interpret data. *Ann Intern Med.* 1989;110:916–921.

24. Hebert JR, Waternaux C. Graphical displays of growth data. *Am J Clin Nutr.* 1983;38:145-147.
25. Worthington-Roberts BS, Breskin MW, Monsen ER. Iron status of premenopausal women in a university community and its relationship to habitual dietary sources of protein. *Am J Clin Nutr.* 1988;47:275-279.
26. Alford BB, Blankenship AC, Hagen RD. The effects of variations in carbohydrate, protein, and fat content of the diet upon weight loss, blood values, and nutrient intake of adult obese women. *J Am Diet Assoc.* 1990; 90:534–540.
27. Cleveland WS. Research in statistical graphics. *J Am Statis Assoc.* 1987; 82:419–423.
28. Cleveland WS, McGill R. Graphical perception: theory, experimentation, and application to the development of graphical methods. *J Am Statis Assoc.* 1984; 79:531–554.
29. Graedel TE, McGill R. Graphical presentation of results from scientific computer models. *Science.* 1982;215:1191–1198.
30. Hansell P, ed. *A Guide to Medical Photography.* Baltimore, Md: University Park Press; 1979.
31. Sternbach H. *Halftone Reproduction Guide.* Great Neck, NY: Halftone Reproduction Guide; 1965.
32. Fong AKH, Kretsch MJ. Nutrition evaluation scale system reduces time and labor in recording quantitative dietary intake. *J Am Diet Assoc.* 1990;90:664–670.
33. Marcus A. Computer-assisted chart making from the graphic designer's perspective. *Computer Graphics.* 1980;14:247–253.

24. RESEARCH PUBLICATIONS: THE PERSPECTIVES OF THE WRITER, THE REVIEWER AND THE READER

Judith A. Ernst, DMSc, RD

"I'm an expert in my area of research. I have something of value to contribute to the scientific community, and I want it published as soon as possible."—the Writer

"I assist the writer, the reader, and the editor. I volunteer my time to help assure the quality and clarity of research in the literature in as timely a fashion as possible."—the Reviewer

"I read in part to learn. I am not as familiar with some areas of research and have limited time to read. Therefore I expect articles to represent quality research and be communicated in simple, logical terms that I can understand and apply."—the Reader

Now is the time when the dietitian has the opportunity to assume major roles as writer, reviewer, and reader of research publications. Meaningful research that is original, well organized, meticulously conducted, and effectively communicated characterizes the ideal within the perspectives of all three roles. Guidelines have been developed that assist the writer, the reviewer, and the reader in the implementation, interpretation, and communication of meritorious research.

THE WRITER'S PERSPECTIVE

The writer is responsible for scrupulous behavior in the design and completion of research studies, intellectual honesty, and responsible coauthorship.[1]

The writer, as scientist, has an idea that emerges from an area of interest, from professional experience, or from the literature. He or she develops this idea into a research protocol and fosters it through the stages of implementation and data collection and interpretation. The author has an ethical obligation to society to design research that furthers the advancement of the science. Intellectual honesty, a responsibility of medical authors, is emphasized by Schiedermayer and Siegler[1] as essential for the continued professional and public trust of scientific research. Specific examples of scientific dishonesty, defined in 1830 by Babbage[2] as those of "trimming," "cooking," or "forging" data still apply to published literature today. Schiedermayer and Siegler also relate the three elements suggested by David Tracy to be essential for rational inquiry and intellectual honesty: Write only what you mean and mean what you write; provide all the evidence (including negative findings) honestly obtained and reason logically from the evidence; be aware of and discuss all substantive counter claims (based on evidence) to your claim (based on evidence).

Consultation with a statistician during the design phase and when results are analyzed is essential to prevent the collection of potentially worthless data that do not fit into an appropriate design for statistical analysis[3,4] (also see chapter 1). It may be necessary to establish a network within one's institution and create linkages to work with identified people who have statistical expertise. It is important to identify a statistician who meets the research needs; that is, a statistician who understands biomedical research if the research involves clinical subjects or who understands statistics related to epidemiology if the research involves that type of study. Chapter 1 authoritatively reviews methods for design, data analysis, and presentation of research methods in nutrition and dietetics, as well as a review and update for the researcher who already has background in basic statistics.

The 1988 edition of the Uniform Requirements for Manuscripts Submitted to Biomedical Journals[5] should be familiar to authors. It describes the format in which editors agree to receive articles and includes guidelines (*Table 24.1*) for presenting statistical aspects of scientific research in ways that are clear and helpful to readers.

Table 24.1
Guidelines for Statistical Reporting in Articles for Medical Journals[3,5]

1. Describe statistical methods with enough detail to enable a knowledgeable reader with access to the original data to verify the reported results.
2. When possible, quantify findings and present them with appropriate indicators of measurement error or uncertainty (such as confidence intervals).
3. Avoid sole reliance on statistical hypothesis testing, such as the use of P values, which fails to convey important quantitative information.
4. Discuss eligibility of experimental subjects.
5. Give details about randomization.
6. Describe the methods for, and success of, any blinding of observation.
7. Report treatment complications.
8. Give numbers of observations.
9. Report losses to observation (eg, dropouts from a clinical trial).
10. References for study design and statistical methods should be to standard works (textbooks or review papers with pages specified) when possible, rather than to papers in which designs or methods were originally reported.
11. Specify any general-use computer programs used.
12. Put general descriptions of statistical methods in the methods section. When data are summarized in the results section, specify the statistical methods used to analyze them.
13. Restrict tables and figures to those needed to explain the argument of the paper and to assess its support. Use graphs as an alternative to tables with many entries: do not duplicate data in graphs and tables.
14. Avoid nontechnical uses of technical terms in statistics, such as *random* (which implies a randomizing device), *normal, significant, correlation*, and *sample*.
15. Define statistical terms, abbreviations, and most symbols.

The writer, as communicator, needs to be logical, clear, and accurate in describing the methods and relating the results and conclusions of the research. He or she reads the literature and becomes knowledgeable about journals that would likely publish a particular topic, have a particular readership, and publish quality research. Tailoring the format of the manuscript to suit the chosen journal and following the set guidelines for authors[5,6-10] before submission, can expedite the reviewing process.[11]

Submitting a manuscript for peer review can be an invaluable educational experience for the author. Authors are entitled to expect a consistent response from the editor and prompt and courteous treatment of their articles, feel free to question why a paper has been turned down, and request reconsideration. Frequently, authors complain that the time spent in review of the paper delays the transmission of knowledge. The time spent refining an article, however, is well spent and relatively small, compared with the amount spent completing the research and writing.[12] The peer-review process is discussed more under The Reviewer's Perspective.

Irresponsible authorship and wasteful publication in scientific publishing is targeted by Huth[13] as offensive and perhaps far more damaging than fraud or plagiarism. He identifies irresponsible authorship as including as authors persons who make little or no contribution to the work reported and omitting persons who make major contributions. The responsible writer, as collaborator, acknowledges the complexity of modern medical research, which may require a variety of skills and techniques available only from the joint effort of several people. Principles that can be used for justification for multiple authorship are included in the Uniform Requirements for Manuscripts Submitted to Biomedical Journals (*Table 24.2*).

Table 24.2
Principles for Authorship

Principle 1
Each author should have participated sufficiently in the work represented by the article to take public responsibility for the content.

Principle 2
Participation must include three steps: (1) conception or design of the work represented by the article, or analysis and interpretation of the data, or both; (2) drafting the article or revising it for critically important content; and (3) final approval of the version to be published.

Principle 3
Participation solely in the collection of data (or other evidence) does not justify authorship.

Principle 4
Each part of the content of an article critical to its main conclusions and each step in the work that led to its publication (steps 1, 2, and 3 in Principle 2) must be attributable to at least one author.

Principle 5
Persons who have contributed intellectually to the article but whose contributions do not justify authorship may be named and their contribution described—for example, "advice," "critical review of study proposal," "data collection," "participation in clinical trial." Such persons must have given their permission to be named. Technical help must be acknowledged in a separate paragraph.

From International Committee of Medical Journal Editors.[5]

Wasteful publication includes reporting the results of a single study in two or more papers (or, as Huth puts it, "salami science") and republishing the same material in successive papers differing only in how the paper is formatted and the content discussed. Wasteful publication also includes blending data from one study with additional data that are insufficient to stand on their own to create another paper or, as Huth puts it, "meat extending."

The author is required to sign a copyright form stating that the article being submitted is exclusive and has not been published elsewhere. This procedure, it is hoped, prevents the problem of repetitive publication.[13]

THE REVIEWER'S PERSPECTIVE

Peer review plays a critical role in determining the nature and level of practice. About three quarters of major scientific journals use some sort of peer review.[12] A historical perspective of peer review and guidelines for the reviewer presented by Lock,[12] editor of the *British Medical Journal,* would be of interest to authors and critical readers as well as reviewers. In his guidelines for the reviewer, he emphasizes that the unpublished manuscript is a privileged document and should be protected from any form of exploitation. Reviewers are expected not to cite a manuscript or refer to the work it describes before it has been published, and to refrain from using the information it contains for the advancement of their own research. The reviewer, as confidant, must not plagiarize or use in any form the work that is being reviewed during the lengthy editorial process.[14] Therefore, the reviewer, as impartial referee, may be faced with important ethical questions because the author and reviewer often are competitors.[1] The reviewer, as protector of scientific integrity and excellence, may identify defects in a study design that, once corrected, permit the investigators to restructure their clinical experiment. Thus, the peer consultant plays a significant role in the improvement of research in progress.[14] In comments to the author, the reviewer should present criticism dispassionately and avoid abrasive remarks.[12] The reviewer looks for organization, originality, scientific reliability, clinical importance, clarity, correct and current referencing, and suitability for publication. *Table 24.3* presents the Guidelines for Manuscript Review, which reviewers for the *Journal of The American Dietetic Association* use when critiquing Perspectives in Practice articles, review articles, and Research and Professional Briefs, and when reviewing manuscripts presenting original research.

Table 24.3
***Guidelines for Manuscript Review:* Journal of The American Dietetic Association**

The following questions may guide you when critiquing Perspectives in Practice and review articles. Your comments will be most useful to the author if they are constructive and informative.

1. Does the *article,* in your opinion, make a valuable contribution to the field of dietetics?
2. Is that contribution clearly conveyed in the article?
3. Is the *title* clear and informative?
4. Is the *abstract* intelligible by itself? Does it summarize the purpose, content, and conclusions of the article?
5. Does the *introduction* state the intention of the article?
6. Is the *text* developed in logical order?
7. Is each *table/figure* intelligible by itself, concise, and necessary to the article? Are the legends understandable? Is the information in the text and *tables/figures* non-repetitive?
8. Are the *implications/applications/recommendations* logical, well-considered, and pertinent, yet far-sighted?
9. Are the *references* appropriate, current, and sufficient in number and scope?
10. Considering each of the *above sections,* is each presented concisely? Is the information relevant and non-repetitive?

(Continued.)

The following questions may guide you in critiquing Research and Professional Briefs. Criteria for a Research and Professional Brief are 1000 words or less (approximately three and one-half to four pages, double-spaced), plus one to two short tables/figures, and pertinent references from the scientific literature. Your comments will be most useful to the author if they are constructive and informative.

1. Does the *Research and Professional Brief,* in your opinion, make a valuable contribution to the field of dietetics?
2. Is the *title* clear and informative?
3. Does the *introduction* state the intention of the article?
4. Is the *text* developed in logical order?
5. If the *Research and Professional Brief* is research oriented, please consider the following two points:
   a. Are the *materials and methods* straightforward, well-conceived, and scientifically accurate? Is the research design appropriate to test the hypothesis? Is the sample selection appropriate? Is the sample size sufficient? Are suitable statistical tests applied?
   b. Are the *results* clear and appropriately analyzed? Do the *results* follow the same order presented under *methods?*
6. Is each *table/figure* intelligible by itself, concise, and necessary? Are the legends understandable? Is the information in the text and *tables/figures* non-repetitious?
7. Are the *implications/applications/recommendations* logical, well-considered, and pertinent, yet far-sighted?
8. Are the *references* appropriate, current, and sufficient in number and scope?
9. Considering each of the *above sections,* is each presented concisely? Is the information relevant and non-repetitious?

The following questions may guide you when reviewing manuscripts presenting original research. Your comments will be most useful to the author if they are constructive and informative.

1. Is the *article* of importance to the field of dietetics? Is that import clearly conveyed in the article?
2. Is the *title* clear and informative? Does it convey the major findings of the research?
3. Is the *abstract* intelligible by itself? Does it summarize the purpose, methods, sample, results, and conclusions of the article?
4. Does the *introduction* state the intention of the article?
5. Are the *materials and methods* straightforward, well-conceived, and scientifically accurate? Is the research design appropriate to test the hypothesis? Is the sample selection appropriate? Is the sample size sufficient? Are suitable statistical tests applied?
6. Are the *results* clear and appropriately analyzed? Do the *results* follow the same order presented under *methods?*
7. Is each *table/figure* intelligible by itself, concise, and necessary to the article? Are the legends understandable? Is the information in the text and *tables/figures* non-repetitious?
8. Is the *discussion* relevant to the findings? Are the results interpreted appropriately and compared with other published data of a similar nature?
9. Are the *implications/applications/recommendations* logical, well-considered, pertinent yet far-sighted?
10. Are the *references* appropriate, current, and sufficient in number and scope?
11. Considering each of the *above sections,* is each presented concisely? Is the information relevant and non-repetitious?

At the end of the process, the reviewer makes a recommendation to accept the paper for publication, accept it for publication after modification, or reject it for publication in a particular journal. The reviewer may recommend that the manuscript be submitted to another journal and may cite a particular journal.[14] Specific statements about the acceptability of a paper are directed to the editor in a confidential cover letter or on a form provided for that purpose. A reviewer's recommendations are gratefully received by the editor, but since editorial decisions are usually based on evaluations derived from several sources, a reviewer should not expect the editor to honor every recommendation.[13]

Robin and Burke[15] state that peer review not only influences the content of medical literature, but the process also directly affects medical education in the classroom and at the bedside, and influences the use or rejection of various medical innovations. They also comment that the peer review process benefits the readership by reducing the number of gross errors that appear in the literature, enforces some set of standards for practice, exerts a mechanism for quality control, and stimulates efforts to produce better work and better writing. Robin and Burke mention potential risks of peer review to include delay in transmission of helpful information, as well as the exclusion of new ideas or approaches that conflict with orthodoxy and thus retard progress.[15]

Soffer[14] in a proponent view to the statements of Robin and Burke, emphasizes that even though the current referee system may fail from time to time, it represents today's single greatest protection of scientific integrity and excellence. If the reviewer accepts the role of teacher by giving constructive criticism and remains open to feedback from the investigator, as in the case of a rebuttal, both investigator and reviewer are provided an educational experience. This effective communication within the editorial review process makes a good paper better and an excellent paper superb.[14] As Soffer states, nearly 50% of rejected manuscripts that had the benefit of additional peer review eventually have been accepted for publication. In an editorial in *JAMA*,[16] Rennie stated that the intent in medicine is to improve the peer review process. He referred to the International Congress on Peer Review in Biomedical Publications, which was sponsored by the American Medical Association and held in the spring of 1989. The goal of the Congress was to stress responsibility as it applies to authors and editors and the improvement of quality control over the entire process.

THE READER'S PERSPECTIVE

Research in the literature is read for a variety of reasons; two very good reasons are to keep abreast of professional news and to be titillated by the letters to the editor.[17] A group from the Department of Clinical Epidemiology and Biostatistics at McMaster University Health Sciences Centre stated in 1981 that more than 20 000 different biomedical journals were published. Furthermore, this group projected that the biomedical literature would double every 10 to 15 years and increase ten-fold every 35 to 50 years. The clinician, who has limited time available for reading, was estimated to need to read 200 articles and 70 editorials per month to keep up with the ten leading journals in internal medicine.[17]

The reader, as student and critic, reads the literature looking for scholarly articles that contribute to the scientific knowledge base, are clearly communicated, can be applied, and promote individual professional development. University-gained knowledge is significantly outdated after a few years; a professional must review and update knowledge regularly through journal publications. Students generally receive little exposure to any organized method for reading articles in the literature. Radack and Valanis[18] at University of Cincinnati School of Medicine taught critical evaluation of journal articles to medical students by presenting methodologic criteria for validity and usefulness of published data. They recommend that the critical evaluation of medical literature be incorporated into a course in biostatistics and clinical epidemiology in the second year of medical school. Robin and Burke[15] state that a reader who is trained to be more critical and skeptical of the printed word recognizes the limitations of individual papers as well as the limitations of the scientific method as applied to a given discipline. They feel that a critical readership would minimize the risks of peer review mentioned previously.

Scientific journals were identified as one of the most valuable resources for keeping current with the professional literature in a recent survey of dietitians.[19] Several of those who responded emphasized the need for a basic understanding of statistics to interpret the information presented in scientific journals adequately. Educators in dietetics are currently incorporating critical thinking into the dietetic internship experiences and at the undergraduate level. Likewise, dietetics students are encouraged to incorporate a course in statistics in their undergraduate curricula.

Stategies mentioned for keeping current with the literature included a journal club at work, allowing professional colleagues and students to share research articles. Another strategy was that reading be focused to only those articles specific to one's interest or area of expertise. A flow chart that guides the reader of clinical journals to critically select the best in the literature is proposed as follows (*Figure 24.1*).

- Look at the title and determine if the article is of interest or use to you. If not, go on to the next article.
- Review the list of authors and/or the institution where the research was completed. If the authors are well-known authorities in the subject area and have a good track record of careful and thoughtful work, read on.
- Determine the intent of the article as a Perspectives in Practice, review article, an original research article, or research or professional brief. If it tweaks your interest and meets your needs, read on.
- Read the abstract of a Perspectives in Practice, review article, or original research article and decide whether the brief description of the purpose, methods, and sample seem reasonable and the results and conclusions seem valid and useful. If further reading would be of value to you, read on.
- Read the text of a Perspectives in Practice or review article and check for clarity. Check also the references for appropriateness and sufficiency in number and scope.
- Read the materials and methods of a research article and critically review for scientific accuracy, research design, sample selection and suitability of applied statistical tests.
- Read the results and discussion and critically review them for clarity and appropriateness in interpretation. Check the references for appropriate incorporation into the discussion.
- Read the conclusions/implications/recommendations and critically review them for relevant application into practice.

Figure 24.1
A guide for the critical reader of
journal articles.

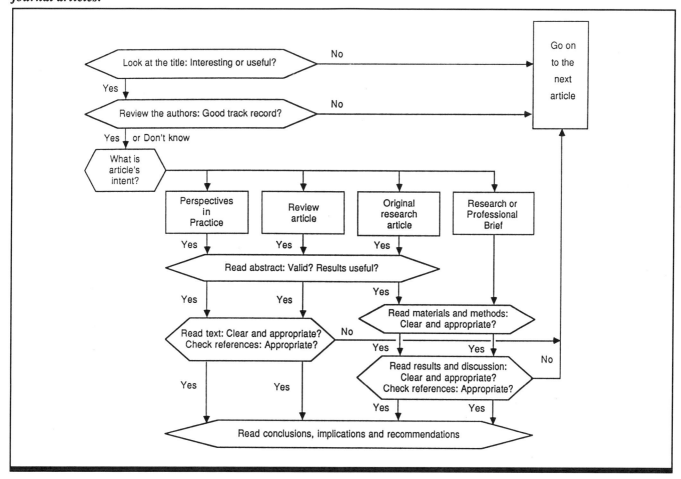

CONCLUSION

Dietitians have the opportunity to be viewed as the expert resources for nutrition knowledge and the primary communicators of that knowledge to their scientific and administrative colleagues as well as the lay public. The tools to achieve this challenging role lie in the development of a critical readership, a responsible authorship, and an invested group of peer reviewers. A critical readership will become critical reviewers of noteworthy information. Responsible authors will continue to be stimulated to research worthwhile ideas and effectively communicate the findings. Peer reviewers, through their efforts and expertise, guarantee quality and valid published knowledge. Journals are and will continue to be the most current source of nutrition knowledge; therefore, a personal commitment to develop and maintain skills in all aspects of the periodical arena is necessary to become the readers, writers, and reviewers that dietitians are called to be.

References

1. Schiedermayer DL, Siegler M. Believing what you read. Responsibilities of medical authors and editors. *Arch Intern Med.* 1986;146:2043.

2. Babbage C. *Reflections on the Decline of Science in England and on Some of its Causes.* London, England: Gregg International; 1969; reprint of 1830 ed.

3. Bailar JC, Mosteller F. Guidelines for statistical reporting in articles for medical journals. *Ann Intern Med.* 1988;108:266.

4. Gardner MJ, Machin D, Cambell MJ. Use of checklists in assessing the statistical content of medical studies. *Br Med J.* 1986;292:810.

5. International Committee of Medical Journal Editors. Uniform requirements for manuscripts submitted to biomedical journals. *Br Med J.* 1988;296:401. *Ann Intern Med.* 1988;108:258. *Med J Aust.* 1988;148:189.

6. Monsen ER. The Journal adopts SI units for clinical laboratory values. *J Am Diet Assoc.* 1987;87:356.

7. Now read this: the SI units are here. *JAMA.* 1986;255:2329. Editorial.

8. Chernoff R. Writing journal articles. In: Chernoff R, ed. *Communicating as Professionals.* Chicago, Ill: American Dietetic Association; 1986.

9. Perkin J. Developing tables, graphs, and figures. In: Chernoff R, ed. *Communicating as Professionals.* Chicago, Ill: American Dietetic Association; 1986.

10. Eichorn P, Yankauer A. Do authors check their references? A survey of accuracy of references in three public health journals. *Am J Public Health.* 1987;77:1011.

11. Mawyer G. Investigative grammar. *J Urol.* 1987;138:1340.

12. Lock S. *A Difficult Balance: Editorial Peer Review in Medicine.* Philadelphia, Pa: ISI Press; 1985.

13. Huth EJ. Irresponsible authorship and wasteful publication. *Ann Intern Med.* 1986;104:257.

14. Soffer A. Proponent view. *Chest.* 1987;91:255.

15. Robin ED, Burke CM. Peer review in medical journals. *Chest.* 1987;91:252.

16. Rennie D. Guarding the guardians: a conference on editorial peer review. *JAMA.* 1986;256:2391.

17. Sackett DL, Haynes RB, Tugwell P. *Clinical Epidemiology A Basic Science for Clinical Medicine.* Boston, Mass: Little Brown and Co; 1985.

18. Radack KL, Valanis B. Teaching critical appraisal and application of medical literature to clinical problem-solving. *J Med Educ.* 1986;61:329.

19. Wellman NS. The well-read dietitian. *J Am Diet Assoc.* 1990;90:996. President's page.

PART 8
APPLICATIONS OF RESEARCH TO PRACTICE

Research advances practice and allows effective decision making. Questions rising from practice provide practical focus for research. Quality of care may be improved and treatment modalities evaluated. Research may be extended and augmented through collaborative projects. The many techniques and guidelines presented in this volume can lead one toward successful research that will pleasurably enhance one's profession and practice.

Research opportunities exist in every facet of professional life. I hope that the following list will serve as a springboard to research projects that propel science forward and fascinate active investigators.

- Devise dietary intake methods for enhanced precision and validation through biochemical measurements (biological markers).
- Design and evaluate treatment modalities and dietary interventions appropriate in clinical practice; eg, in treating infants and children with HIV infection and cancer, elderly in ambulatory care settings, and adolescents with eating disorders.
- Conduct food composition research to supply data currently missing from existing databases; eg, trace minerals, engineered foods, therapeutically designed foods, culturally specific foods, individual fiber categories, phytochemicals, and food contaminants.
- Examine the role and effect of specific food components and nutrients in delaying onset of cardiovascular disease or in maintaining gut function through nutrition support.
- Evaluate the safety and suitability of medical foods.
- Assess bioavailability of nutrients, and estimate impact on specific populations.
- Estimate prevalence and interrelationships of health and nutrition characteristics through population surveys and record-based surveillance.
- Conduct sensory evaluation research to encompass intake, nutritional status, attitudinal, and psychosocial information; assess development, maintenance, and modification of sensory preferences.
- Examine gustatory, olfaction, texture, and other complex real food stimuli in controlled laboratory settings as well as realistic eating situations.
- In foodservice research, apply marketing techniques, devise effective training and retention techniques, incorporate robots, and address solid waste management.
- Examine service quality, evaluate decision support systems, and enhance computer applications, including use of artificial intelligence techniques.

- Document cost-effectiveness and cost-benefit of nutrition and dietetic services including the extent to which illness is prevented, its severity decreased, its duration curtailed, and the patient's rehabilitation facilitated and quality of life improved.
- Substantiate cost savings from nutrition and dietetic intervention; eg, recommending less costly products that have similar value in the healing process, improving life-style through patient education, establishing the number of visits appropriate for each diagnostic group, and evaluating cost-effectiveness of alternative foodservice production systems.
- Improve methods to manage confounding variables in attributing improved health status to nutrition care.
- Conduct marketing research to enhance one's competitive position; to evaluate audience readiness for new products and services, and to evaluate available avenues for promotion of services and products.
- In dietetic education research, devise cost effective curricula, identify factors that enhance the educational process, determine what motivates an individual's career choice, and devise and evaluate continuing education opportunities.
- Using meta-analysis research, address proposed hypotheses, observe the magnitude of an intervention, and determine the factors that influence an intervention.

A productive research environment encourages everyone to investigate, compare, document, validate, evaluate, refine, analyze, and design: that is, to study.

ERM, Editor

25. BRIDGING RESEARCH INTO PRACTICE

Margaret D. Simko, PhD, RD, and Judith A. Gilbride, PhD, RD

Research is the foundation and framework of a profession. The continuity and rigor of a well-planned research agenda help professionals develop and allow them to integrate findings into everyday practice. A vigorous plan of investigations is a challenge that may be difficult to achieve. True researchers may be absorbed in conducting studies for the sake of generating new knowledge, whereas practitioners may be so intent on meeting day-to-day job demands that research findings go unnoticed. Practitioners, in their eagerness to solve clinical problems, sometimes attempt to incorporate findings that have not been studied and tested adequately.[1] Monsen suggests that "stronger links must be built between research and practice to strengthen our profession because research is driven by practice, and practice is supported by research."[2]

Dietetics is at a stage in its development at which the link between practice and research is ready to grow and flourish. Research is necessary to advance professional practice.[3] Dietetic educators place high priority on research competence. A study of 79 dietetic internships and 46 coordinated undergraduate programs indicated a need for students to evaluate literature critically, have knowledge of research concepts, and make application of research findings to dietetic practice.[4] Rose stated in 1985 that: "Research is the fabric of effectiveness in operational management. And our professional responsibilities include reporting that research."[5]

FROM THE PERSPECTIVE OF THE PRACTICING DIETITIAN

Although "most problems in practice can be addressed through research" (chapter 1), job demands and time constraints may hamper investigators' efforts to solve practice problems. The practitioner is often so busy concentrating on meeting the routine responsibilities that he or she has little time to initiate research or even become involved in an ongoing study. This raises questions about recognizing the importance of research to the profession. The American Dietetic Association set a goal in 1987 to conduct research that will provide results that will be applicable to most dietetic practitioners, regardless of area of practice.[6]

WHY RESEARCH IS IMPORTANT TO THE PROFESSION

In the practice setting, the generation of scientific data keeps practitioners accurate and gives credibility to what they say.[6,7] Research results in solving problems that practitioners face every day.[7] Research is useful in monitoring ongoing activities in all areas of dietetics and provides feedback that serves as the basis for changing procedures to improve patient care. Well-designed studies can also provide data to assure quality care.

Studies are needed to document dietetic practice and to assess the effectiveness of nutrition intervention. Once effectiveness is determined, it is possible to evaluate the costs of intervention procedures and measure them against the efficacy of outcomes.

Another important need for outcome evaluation is that it keeps dietetics competitive as a profession. The National Science Foundation has expressed great concern over the fact that American industry has not allocated sufficient dollars for research and development, making businesses less competitive with foreign industries.[8] The profession of dietetics should heed this warning. In this era of shrinking financial resources, the evaluation of providing dietetic care delivery can demonstrate the value of nutrition services in competing for limited funds.

BASIC RESEARCH AND APPLIED RESEARCH: HOW THEY ARE USED

"Research encompasses facts that are not ends in themselves but merely are components in a total process whose ultimate aim is to reveal their significance in the quest for the discovery of truth."[9] Therefore, research studies do not always have immediate, practical application. To expect this is a narrow view of its value. The application of sound research principles can confirm impressions or observations about patient care. "Research is a systematic attempt to provide answers to questions. Such answers may be abstract and general as is often the case in *basic* research, or they may be highly concrete and specific as is often the case in *demonstration* or *applied* research. In both kinds of research, the investigator uncovers facts and then formulates a generalization based on the interpretations of those facts."[10]

WHAT IS RESEARCH AND HOW DOES IT RELATE TO PRACTICE?

Research, the discovery of new knowledge, pushes forward the frontiers of information. Research is almost always built on what was learned in previous studies. The analogy of the brick wall has been used to help conceptionalize research and place it in an appropriate context. The wall is methodically built, brick by brick. Each brick is a study that rests on the foundation of prior investigation, but provides a new block of information and advances the knowledge base. For the wall to endure, the bricks must be solid and correctly constructed, not only for their own integrity, but so that others can use this block as part of the base and build a firm foundation.

The application of research techniques in practice focuses on everyday operations and problem-solving. Data collection and its interpretation can provide insight and direction for doing collaborative projects with other colleagues and health care professionals. Rinke and Berry[11] presented a model that can serve as a guide to demonstrate the interactive relationship between practice and research (*Figure 25.1*). The model begins with questions generated by practice that lead to research projects designs that seek answers to unresolved problems in practice. Completion of the project produces new knowledge; however, incorporation of that new knowledge into practice usually requires teaching and disseminating findings to others who are involved in practice. Thus, the cycle is completed and starts again as other practice questions are raised and answers to new perplexing problems are sought.

Wylie-Rosett, Wheeler, Krueger, and Halford suggest that there are four levels of research for research-oriented dietitians.[12] Level 1 involves using a scientific approach in practice. This level would be illustrated in the Practice–Questions–Research steps in the proposed model (see Figure 25.1). Level 2 includes collaboration or translating the scientific approach into practice. This level would correspond to Education and Utilization of Knowledge in the model. Level 2 builds on Level 1 and includes publication of the findings. This is clearly a desirable outcome. Reaching Levels 3 and 4 involves participation and leadership. These levels can be achieved by following the model as the cycle is repeated and more knowledge, experience, and confidence are developed.

These authors[12] also suggest six useful steps to implement scientific principles in conducting research at level 1: (1) define the problem, (2) determine the probable causes, (3) develop the alternative solutions, (4) select the best solution, (5) test the solution, and (6) evaluate the solution. Practical examples are provided for each step in the process.

Figure 25.1
Bridging research into practice.
Adapted from Rinke WJ,
Berry MW.[11]

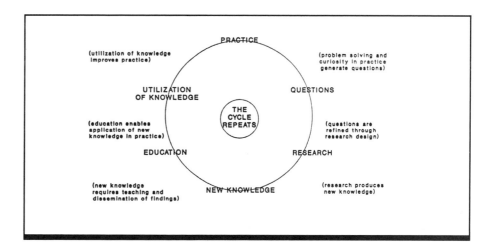

A study such as Wood's "Evaluation of a Hospital-Based Education Program for Patients with Diabetes"[13] can illustrate how the Rinke/Berry model can be facilitated.

The problem: Does nutrition education for patients with diabetes lead to improvement of control of the disease?

The questions: The investigator developed an inpatient diabetes education program that raised two questions: (1) Was the program effective in improving diabetes-related bahaviors and outcomes of the patients attending the program? (2) What were the effects of time on those behaviors and outcomes?

Method: Ninety-three hospitalized patients with diabetes were followed for a four-month period after discharge. Fifty-three had participated in a hospital-based diabetes education program. Participants were selected from hospitalized diabetic patients, 20 to 75 years of age, who had attended a two-session "Living with Diabetes" inpatient program. A control group consisted of 40 hospitalized diabetic patients who had equal opportunity to attend the program but had not participated. Descriptive statistics compared the two groups and no significant differences were found. Patients identified as medically unstable were not included in the study. Pre-established outcome measures included lower fasting blood glucose levels, decrease in insulin requirements, fewer hospitalizations, and fewer emergency room visitations. Results of the study indicated that blood glucose levels and emergency room visits were significantly lower in the experimental group.

Education: The diabetes education program had been conducted for 53 patients. Clearly, it appears to have merits that warrant expansion to other diabetic patients. Expanding the program requires education of other dietetic staff and administrators. Informing other hospital professionals of the existence of the program and its outcome may generate additional resources and support.

READING RESEARCH LITERATURE

Utilization of knowledge: Continuation and expansion of the diabetes education program as resources permit is indicated by these findings. A case for additional resources and program continuance and expansion could be supported by data generated by this study.

Practice: As the research findings are incorporated into clinical practice, further questions arise that would warrant additional study. In this case, the investigator raised two questions: Is there a direct relationship between the program and adherence to diabetes self-care behaviors, and does adherence positively affect outcomes? Thus, new research questions are devised and the practice-research-practice model continues in its cycle.

As dietitians read research studies in the literature, they should look for ways to integrate findings into practice. When reading and examining reports, questions should come to mind: "Are there practical applications for these investigative findings?" "Can I apply this information to my setting?"

Critical analysis is useful when reading investigative report articles to determine if the purpose and need of the study are supported, the methods are appropriate, the conclusions indicate accurate interpretation of the data, and if the references are well-chosen and up to date. Some published research studies may contain limitations. Practitioners should evaluate the quality of each report and determine if the study has weaknesses that limit its application to a particular health care setting.

Example 1. A study was designed to examine three different methods of estimating phosphorus and calcium content and to compare each method with the chemical analysis of 20 daily diets.[14] The rationale for the study was established because low intakes of calcium and high intakes of phosphorus in the diet have been considered risk factors for the development of osteoporosis and hypertension. The methods for analyzing calcium and phosphorus incorporated the use of two computer programs and a handbook providing chemical analysis. Results showed an insignificant trend toward underestimation of calcium content in the diets; however, phosphorus intakes were significantly underestimated by 15% to 25% of the actual level determined by chemical analysis.

Application: Based on these findings, the estimation of calcium intake from available composition tables suggests an acceptable margin of error, while phosphorus estimates cannot be relied upon as sufficiently accurate. Therefore, estimates of patients' calcium intake may be reasonably accurate, but phosphorus estimates may not be as reliable. Further exploration of other nutrient databases could provide the practitioner with greater confidence in estimating calcium and phosphorus in the diet.

Example 2. A study was conducted to determine parameters of operating costs in conventional, cook-chill, and cook-freeze systems and to compare the costs for the three foodservice systems.[15] Data were collected for 33 conventional, 22 cook-chill, and 11 cook-freeze hospital foodservice systems. Results indicated few differences among the three systems for most operational and financial variables. The number of full-time equivalents (FTEs) was found to be the strongest predictor of operating costs in all three systems.

Application: Based on these findings, installation of a ready-food system may not lead to cost savings. The authors suggested that, when seeking reduction of expenditures, it may be more appropriate to study labor costs than install a ready-food system.

SOME USES OF RESEARCH IN THE PRACTICE SETTING

Research to Assess and Analyze the Setting

To develop a framework for investigation of nutrition care delivery research, grounded research theory (see chapter 2) can be employed to collect data about the patient population, the institution, and/or the community. This information is vital in planning and testing the most efficient and effective delivery of nutrition services. Questions such as the following can be asked: What is the population serviced by this institution or agency? (Numbers, age, sex, economic status.) What are their nutrition needs? (Diagnosis, health status, mobility.) What resources are available to help deliver nutrition services? (Time, funds, personnel, other health care professionals.) An instrument can be developed to collect pertinent information, or a model may be found in the literature[16] and adapted to a specific setting. This kind of investigation can precede a research design and assists in formulating appropriate, practical research questions such as: How are resources organized to meet the needs of the population? Starting with a needs assessment can be very useful because the problem selected for study depends on the needs in the practice setting as well as funding sources, constraints of time and personnel, and answers to the question: Will method X or method Y be more effective in solving problems relating to this population?

Research to Measure Practice

Documentation and measurement of practice standards can provide evidence of the effectiveness of nutrition care being delivered. If effectiveness is not demonstrated, the findings can provide a framework for further study that changes practice and produces more positive outcomes.

Example 1. A study was conducted to examine whether cystic fibrosis patients who received nutrition counseling had higher caloric intakes and body mass index values.[17] Thirty-seven patients were followed on a nonrestricted nutrition program for four years. Bandura's self-management principles were applied in teaching patients to meet their nutrition needs. The results showed significant increases in energy intake and body mass index. Based on these findings, the nutrition education and counseling had a positive effect on patient outcome.

Example 2. The eating habits of 683 persons were studied by means of the 24-hour dietary recall.[18] At the beginning of the study there were no differences in food recall scores among the entire group. From this group, 355 research subjects were randomly selected for participation in a specialized nutrition education program for a six-month period. After the instruction, there was a significant increase in food recall scores for the research group and no change in the control group. Based on these findings it was concluded that the specialized nutrition education program was effective in producing significant changes in the eating habits of the subjects.

Example 3. A fiber-supplemented dietary regimen was started to alleviate constipation problems among 300 elderly residents in a nursing home.[19] Bran was added to the hot breakfast cereal, increasing the crude fiber content of the diet to 6 to 8 g, compared with the former 4 to 6 g. The bran was effective in reducing or preventing constipation in 60% of the residents, even though many of them had previously required laxatives. In the year following initiation of the program, the use of laxatives was almost eliminated in the research group with a reported saving of $44 000 in expenditures for laxative medications. This study, which involved a change in practice by the dietary department, demonstrated a positive health outcome as well as a cost savings.

Research to Change Practice

Research is useful to monitor activities or procedures, solve problems, and change practice by finding a better way to deliver nutrition services.

Example 1. A monitoring system of tray assembly rates was designed to evaluate patient tray accuracy and to identify types of assembly errors.[20] Errors were classified according to type: omission, addition, or substitution, as well as by severity. The methodology used in this study serves as the basis for quality improvement and as a motivational factor to stimulate enhanced performance by tray employees.

Example 2. A computer-assisted management information system for nutrition services was created to facilitate effective management of clinical nutrition services and labor resources in a teaching and research hospital.[21] Standards were developed for quality and quantity of nutrition care, time required to provide nutrition care, and utilization of dietitians' time. Data were evaluated to determine whether services were consistent with standards and to calculate a recommended number of clinical dietitian FTEs for the hospital. The management information system was instrumental in developing a fee-for-service structure, for evenly distributing workloads among dietitians, and for monitoring adherence to standards of care. The system provided a better way to deliver nutrition care.

Example 3. A study was designed to develop and validate a nutrient adequacy score to be used by nutrition programs for women and children.[22] A dietary score was developed to be limited if certain targeted subgroups of major food groups were not included. The population of 1431 was divided into nine different segments. The score correctly classified 69% to 98% of the persons in each population segment. The score was simple to implement, requiring just three steps, from assessing the food frequency to determining risk. Development of the nutrient adequacy score provided a more efficient method to assess client's nutrition needs.

UTILIZING RESEARCH REPORTS TO HELP SOLVE PROBLEMS

The earlier discussion of the Rinke and Berry model[11] drew on the study of Wood[13] to illustrate implications of the model. An examination of the other steps to developing a research project helps to clarify further the process of incorporating research into practice.

Planning the Project

When confronting a practice problem, some steps may serve to facilitate planning the project and moving it along. Among them are: appointing a committee or work group, defining the problem and subproblems, making assignments to committee members, setting a time frame, and organizing ongoing committee meetings to discuss progress, refocus if necessary, and keep the project progressing toward completion.

Applications to Practice

Example. Collaborative teamwork is illustrated in the development of a nutrition priority system by the New York State Department of Mental Health (NYSDMH).[23] Although this would not be defined as research per se, the organizational steps followed illustrate those recommendations made above.

The problem was to devise a nutrition screening system that would set priorities for nutrition needs and ensure individualized nutrition care for all patients. The existing system focused on the diet order, rather than the needs of the patient. Dietitians felt uncomfortable that some patients in need of care were being excluded.

The first step was to *establish a committee* of dietitians from the NYSDMH facilities. The committee met and *defined their goal:* to "identify objective or quantifiable indicators to categorize patients at the greatest nutritional risk and to establish classifications based on those categories according to the level of nutrition care needed." The first phase included a literature search by committee members to learn what systems had been reported. The committee members also conducted a telephone survey of other health care facilities to determine whether priority systems were in use. Finally, *each committee member received a section of the NYSDMH proposed priority system* and, after establishing a subcommittee, fully developed that section. The project was *completed in one year* with *committee meetings held at intervals* during that time.

Defining the Problem

Research begins with a problem or question: what one wants to know about one's practice that would be useful. The question should be clearly defined at the outset with an answer that is measurable. After putting the question in writing, the practitioner should work on refining and improving it. With further thought, the question usually expands and evolves into a broader statement; however, an effort should be made to tighten and focus the problem and allow measurement of very specific variables.

Twomey[24] provides a good example of the stages of evolution of a research question in a practice setting:
Beginning question: "It sure seems like we have a lot of malnourished patients on our surgical service."
Question becoming more specific: "What is the rate of wound infections in our malnourished patients undergoing cholecystectomy?"
Introducing definitions to be used for this research: "What is the rate of wound infection (= discharge of pus) in our cholecystectomy patients who are malnourished (albumin less than 3.0)?"
Best question, providing comparison or controls; making the problem measurable: "What is the rate of wound infection in our cholecystectomy patients who are malnourished (albumin less than 3.0) compared with those who are well nourished (albumin 3.0 or above)?"

The Literature Search

Literature related to the selected problem provides the foundation or "bricks" for the planned study. A review of the literature provides ideas for methodology and shows how other researchers have handled a similar question. It can disclose sources of information that may not be known. It can assist in evaluating the proposed project and comparing it with other studies. Monsen and Cheny provide an in-depth discussion of this topic in chapter 1.

In reviewing the literature, it may be useful to pose some questions to clarify the problem and develop the study:

- Can this information help solve the problem? A literature review sometimes provides the information that answers the question without further study. This is an efficient use of existing research.
- Is there a model that can be used to study the problem? Some studies may provide such a model and eliminate some steps in the research process.
- Can the information in the literature be modified or adapted for the case in question? Other models, findings, methodology, or instruments may be discovered through the literature review and discussion with peers—especially peers with research experience—that would be appropriate for the study under consideration.

Implementing the Plan

After developing the question and conducting the literature search, a design for the study is selected. Preparation of a proposal or research protocol is necessary to delineate clearly the procedures and processes that will be utilized for data collection. A pilot study is useful to test for any problems in the methodology and provide an opportunity to make adaptions prior to undertaking the larger investigation.

Analysis of Results

The procedures for analysis of data need to be planned at the beginning of the study, not after the data are collected. In conducting research in the practice setting, resources for collection, analysis, and interpretation of data may be limited. The process may need to be simplified to complete the project with the resources available in the health care setting and within a specific time frame.

OTHER EXAMPLES OF NUTRITION CARE DELIVERY RESEARCH

Clinical example 1. One hundred eighty-five Medicare patients were assessed for malnutrition.[25] Patients were classified as malnourished if they fell below at least two of four parameters: percentage ideal body weight, percentage weight loss, total lymphocyte count, and serum albumin concentration. Based on those criteria, 8.6% of the subjects were classified as malnourished. Submitting ICD-9-CM codes for a potential enhancement of Medicare reimbursement was not possible, since for all patients in this study in whom malnutrition was diagnosed, additional comorbidity and complication (CC) factors existed.

Application: If malnutrition had been the only CC factor, hospital reimbursement may have been increased. However, patients who are classified as malnourished require intensive nutrition intervention, and it is essential to identify malnutrition and treatment for this population.

Clinical example 2. Dietetic technicians screened 225 patients to identify those at nutritional risk during a three-month period.[26] Results indicated that, based on the parameters established, one-third were at nutritional risk. A standardized screening protocol was developed from those data.

Application: Standardization of a screening tool and utilization of support personnel can simplify the process of meeting the needs of a patient population.

Administrative example 1. To assess productivity, data were collected from observations of foodservice workers' activities during three days in each of three senior centers utilizing cook-serve food production systems.[27] Productivity ratios were calculated as average labor minutes in each activity per meal served. Although productivity varied with the number of meals served, labor time was consistent within the three centers.

Application: This study provides a model from which a similar study can be developed to compare productivity within other foodservice operations.

Administrative example 2. A study was conducted to determine the feasibility of a centralized choice menu plan with the "offer versus serve" self-serve lunch program.[28] The same menu was offered to children in two elementary school districts during a one-week period. The two schools selected had similar total enrollment and foodservice. Once school was in a high-poverty area and the other school enrolled more middle-income children. Students were able to choose the minimal number of three foods required by the USDA. The portions chosen and the amount of plate waste were recorded and a nutrition analysis was completed for all foods chosen and consumed. Sixty-six percent of the food choices were similar at the two schools. Except for pyridoxine and ascorbic acid, three-fourths of the students at both schools selected more than 75% of one-third of the RDA. Overall plate waste was 12.9%. The conclusions from this study indicated that a centralized menu within the serving options of a self-service, choice menu was feasible for this school district.

Application: This study demonstrates the use of research to explore a more efficient system of food production for a school district while maintaining quality in the lunch served and consumed by the children.

NOW WHAT? WHERE DO WE GO FROM HERE?

Getting started with research in the practice setting is the first giant step. Aside from one's own curiosity, reading the research literature helps to generate ideas. Identifying possible questions to address is a good starting point. Assessment of the needs of the population and the resources available to implement investigations are crucial to productive planning.

Creativity and imagination are useful tools to assist with conducting research and managing the barriers that may impede implementation of practice-related research projects. Barriers include:

Time. Time must be found to conduct practice-related research. Sufficient time generally needs to be carved out of an already full schedule. An evaluation of existing responsibilities to determine if some can be simplified, delegated, or eliminated may open up some blocks of time. Reading articles on time management may help with this task. First, an attempt should be made to conduct the study within the working day. Structuring professional reading time into the working day is positive time management and not only helps keep the practitioner current about professional development, but also helps generate research ideas. However, a willingness to devote some personal time to early development of research investigation is usually necessary.

Staffing. Usually additional staff members are not available for beginning projects. Enlisting other staff members to collaborate in at least some part of the project is crucial. It may be easier to motivate staff members if the investigation has the potential to make their jobs easier or more efficient. Other health care personnel within an institution may be interested in the project, and volunteers or students sometimes may be eager to participate.

Money. A practitioner must be realistic and recognize that funds generally are not allocated for beginning research. This dictates a simple design. Selecting data that are readily available would be desirable; for example: What laboratory values are already collected that could be used for end points? Are data analysis systems in place in the institution? Working through a pilot study may be an excellent method of learning how to utilize an existing data analysis program. The project should be planned to keep within the resources available. If data analysis must be done with a hand calculator, the study design should be in keeping with this limitation.

Permissions. Implementing any research necessitates permission from supervisors or superiors. Reorganization of duties or staffing must be authorized. Cooperation and permission are needed to make use of facilities such as computer time. Permissions from physicians and patients are necessary for human subject research. The practitioner must go through the appropriate channels to organize the project, or the barriers could lead to frustration. Potential benefits of study to patients, potential higher productivity, or both will encourage cooperation.

Knowledge. Learning how to conduct research is essential for success. Taking a course or courses is a good way to learn. However, reading research literature and talking with researchers is also very helpful. Many people are afraid to initiate investigations, but involvement usually builds confidence. Coulston explains how to develop "a good, clear research question" in her article, "Nutrition Research in the Clinical Setting: Getting Started."[29] These guidelines are very useful for developing a research project. Leontos and colleagues[30] shared their experiences in developing and conducting a study in the hope that by knowing some of the problems in advance, practitioners would avoid some of the pitfalls and be encouraged to develop successful projects.

Resources need to be skillfully mobilized and managed to integrate research into practice. The profession of dietetics desperately needs a much broader practical research base. This chapter—and indeed, this book—has been designed to provide background and technical information that will assist in this effort. It is the authors' hope that it will motivate and inspire practitioners to approach research questions in practice with new vigor and self-confidence.

SUGGESTIONS FOR FUTURE RESEARCH

There are a vast array of topics that could be studied by the practitioner to improve practice and open up new vistas for the profession. The following suggestions would be most useful in expanding the dietetics database:
1. Documentation of clinical practice and assessment of the effectiveness of nutrition intervention.
2. Investigation of the team approach as to what aspect of care provided by the dietitian contributed to improved patient outcome.
3. Comparison of different prevention and treatment models of dietary intervention and patient outcomes.
4. Expansion and extension of some of the studies presented in this chapter.

References

1. Angier N. Cultures in conflict: M.D.'s and Ph.D.'s. *New York Times.* April 24, 1990.
2. Monsen ER. New practices and research in dietetics. The 1988 Journal. *J Am Diet Assoc.* 1988;88:15.

3. Sims LS, Simko MD. Applying research methods in nutrition and dietetics: embodiment of the profession's backbone. *J Am Diet Assoc.* 1988;88:1045–1046.

4. Fitz P, Winkler MF. Education, research, and practice: bridging the gap. *J Am Diet Assoc.* 1989;89:116–117.

5. Rose JC. Research or practice? *J Am Diet Assoc.* 1985;85:797.

6. Smitherman AL, Wyse BW. The backbone of our profession. *J Am Diet Assoc.* 1987;87:1394–1396. President's page.

7. Satter E. Relating research to practice. *Nutr News.* 1987;50:1.

8. A corporate lag in research is causing worry. *New York Times.* Jan 1, 1990.

9. Leedy PD. *Practical Research.* New York, NY: Macmillan Publishing Co Inc; 1974:5.

10. Tuckman BW. *Conducting Educational Research.* 2nd ed. New York, NY: Harcourt Brace Jovanovich Inc; 1978.

11. Rinke WJ, Berry MW. Integrating research into clinical practice: a model and call for action. *J Am Diet Assoc.* 1987;87:159–161.

12. Wylie-Rosett J, Wheeler M, Krueger K, Halford B. Opportunities for research-oriented dietitians. *J Am Diet Assoc.* 1990;90:1531.

13. Wood ER. Evaluation of a hospital-based education program for patients with diabetes. *J Am Diet Assoc.* 1989;89:354.

14. Oenning LL, Vogel J, Calvo MS. Accuracy of methods estimating calcium and phosphorus intake in daily diets. *J Am Diet Assoc.* 1988;88:1076.

15. Greathouse KR, Gregoire MB, Spears MC, Richards V, Nassar RF. Comparison of conventional, cook-chill, and cook-freeze foodservice systems. *J Am Diet Assoc.* 1989;89:1606.

16. Cowell C, Simko MD, Gilbride JA. The nutrition profile as a tool for identifying who needs nutritional care. In: Simko MD, Cowell C, Gilbride JA, eds. *Nutrition Assessment: A Comprehensive Guide for Planning Intervention.* Rockville, Md: Aspen Publishers Inc; 1984; chap 4.

17. Luder E, Gilbride JA. Teaching self-management skills to cystic fibrosis patients and its effect on their caloric intake. *J Am Diet Assoc.* 1989;89:359.

18. Del Tredici AM, Omelich CL, Laughlin SG. Evaluation study of the California expanded food and nutrition education program: 24-hour food recall data. *J Am Diet Assoc.* 1988;88:185.

19. Hull C, Greco RS, Brooks DL. Alleviation of constipation in the elderly by dietary fiber supplementation. *J Am Ger Soc.* 1980;28:410.

20. Dowling RA, Cotner CG. Monitor of tray error rates for quality control. *J Am Diet Assoc.* 1988;88:450.

21. Duffy KM, Fromm BA, Sorensen DA. A computer-assisted management information system for nutrition services. *J Am Diet Assoc.* 1989;89:1296.

22. Krebs-Smith SM, Clark LD. Validation of a nutrient adequacy score for use with women and children. *J Am Diet Assoc.* 1989;89:775.

23. McClusky KW, Fishel L, Stover-May R. Nutrition priority system: a model for patient care. *J Am Diet Assoc.* 1987;87:200.

24. Twomey P. *Getting Started in Clinical Nutrition Research.* Washington, DC: American Society for Parenteral and Enteral Nutrition; 1981.

25. Delhey DM, Anderson EJ, Laramee SH. Implications of malnutrition and diagnosis-related groups (DRGs). *J Am Diet Assoc.* 1989;89:1448.

26. Hedberg AM, Garcia N, Trejus IJ, Weinmann-Winkler S, Gabriel ML, Lutz AL. Nutritional risk screening: development of a standardized protocol using dietetic technicians. *J Am Diet Assoc.* 1988;88:1553.

27. Lieus EM, Winkler LL. Assessing productivity of foodservice systems in nutrition programs for the elderly. *J Am Diet Assoc.* 1989;89:826.

28. Dillon MS, Lane HW. Evaluation of the offer vs. serve option within self-serve, choice menu lunch programs at the elementary school level. *J Am Diet Assoc.* 1989;89:1780.

29. Coulston AM. Nutrition research in the clinical setting: getting started. *Clin Nutr Management.* 1991;10:1.

30. Leontos CJ, Harveywebster MJ, Palmer-Lynch CB. Research: an attainable goal for the successful practitioner? *Top Clin Nutr.* 1990;5:69.

INDEX

INDEX

factors to consider when analyzing survey data, 213–215
  health and nutrition examination surveys, 212
  Nationwide Food Consumption Surveys, 208, 212
  Ten-State Nutrition Survey, 212
reason for development of, 204
record-based surveillance systems, 205
  Pediatric Nutrition Surveillance System (PedNSS), 205–206
  Pregnancy Nutrition Surveillance System (PNSS), 206

Nationwide Food Consumption Surveys, 208, 212
Natural context, and qualitative research, 79–80
Negligence, 39
Neonatal mortality rate, 105
Nested case-control design, 141
Networking, in obtaining funding, 61
NIH grant application, 6
Nominal data, 348
Nominal response, 116
Noncoverage error, 39, 41–42
Nonparametric methods, 351
Nonparametric tests, 29
Nonprofit organizations, obtaining research funding from, 66
Nonresponse biases, 300–301
Nonresponse error, 39, 42–43
Nonsampling bias, in analyzing national nutrition survey data, 214
Null hypothesis, 28–29, 144, 354
  in sample size calculation, 337
Nuremberg Code, 39
Nutrient Data Bank Directory, 196
Nutrient Database for Standard Reference, 196, 197
Nutrition care delivery research, examples of, 428–429

O

Objectivity, 301
  continuous, 352
  discrete, 352
  of qualitative research, 78
Observation
  in dietetic education research, 317–318
Observational studies, 15, 131
  case-control studies, 137
    analysis and interpretation in, 139
    design of, 137–139
    strengths and limitations, 139
  cohort studies, 140
    analysis and interpretation in, 141–142
    design of, 141
    strengths and limitations, 142
    types of, 140–141
Observation forms, pilot-testing of, 86

Observer subjectivity, 13
Occurrence sampling, in human resource management research, 267
Odds ratio, 134, 139, 356
Odor classification, 222
Olfaction, 222
Olfactory detection threshold testing, 226
One-sided test, 29, 351
Open-ended questions, 115
Operational costs, 279
Oral presentations, 379
  developing visual materials for, 380
    handout materials, 382–383
    oration techniques, 383–384
    overhead projectors and transparencies, 380–381
    slides, 381–382
    videotape and film, 382
  organization of, 379–380
  planning and preparation of, 380
Oration techniques, 383–384
Ordinal data, 301, 348
Ordinal response categories, 116–117
Outcome event, 356–357
Outliers, 31, 196
Overgeneralization, 39, 46
Overhead projectors and transparencies, 380

P

Paired observations, in sample size determination, 340–341, 344–345
Paired *t* test, 340–341, 349
Paranetric tests, 350
Partially controlled quasi-experimental designs, 3, 23
Participant observation, 82
Path analysis, 32
Pearson correlation coefficient, in assessing validity, 187
Pediatric Nutrition Surveillance System (PedNSS), 205–206
Peer review
  and ethics, 45–46
  submitting manuscript for, 387, 411–412, 413
  value of, 387
Per capita intakes, 173
  correlation of, with incidence or mortality rates, 174
Perceived intensity, 227–229
Personal interviews, in collecting primary data, 309
Personnel, budgeting for, 59
Photographs, 404
Pie charts, 396, 400
Pilot study, 12
  for clinical trial, 167–168
  conducting, 6
  of interview scripts, 86

Quality control
  procedures in, 195
  and selection of food analysis
    laboratory, 162
Quantitative models, in information
  systems, 254
Quantitative research
  application of, to management
    practice, 264–265
  meta-analysis in, 321
  similarities to qualitative
    research, 74, 75
Quasi-experimental design, 278
Question length, in questionnaire, 117
Questionnaire, 111
  administration, 120
    interviews, 121
    mailed questionnaires, 120–121
  analysis and reporting of results
    validity reliability, 122
  computer administration of, 113
  conceptualization in, 111–112
  design and construction, 13
    considerations, 118–119
    language and readability, 113
    mode of administration, 112–113
    question construction, 114–115
    questionnaire length, 117
    question placement, 117
    response formats, 115–117
    role of computers in, 118
    visualization, 113
  in dietetic education research, 317
  pretesting, 119–120
  as research instruments, 72
  utilization of results, 122
Question order, in questionnaire, 113
Question placement, in
  questionnaire, 117
Questions, construction of, in
  questionnaire, 114–115

R
Random assignment, 146
Random-digit dialing, 309
Randomization, and bias, 145
Randomized clinical trial, 157
  assignment to treatment
    groups, 18–19
  choice of intervention or
    treatment, 17–18
  end points and data
    collection, 19–21
  factorial design, 22
  features, 16–17
  selection of subjects, 17
  size of the sample, 19
  statistical analysis and
    interpretation, 21–22
  uses of, 16
Random misclassification, 139, 142
Ratings, in data collection, 318
Ratio response, 116

Readability, in questionnaire, 113
Readers' Guide to Periodical
  Literature, 302
Reader's perspective, on research
  publications, 415–416
Recency principle, 112
Recognition threshold testing, 226
Record-based surveillance sys-
  tems, 205, 491
  factors to consider when analyzing
    data from surveillance
    systems, 206–208
  Pediatric Nutrition Surveillance Sys-
    tem (PedNSS), 205–206
  Pregnancy Nutrition Surveillance Sys-
    tem (PNSS), 206
Record volume, as factor in national
  nutrition monitoring
  system, 207–208
Recruitment, of study subjects for
  clinical study, 153–154
Reference groups, 298
Regression analysis, 31–32, 357
Regression coefficients, in
  meta-analysis, 324
Rejection of research proposal
  coping with
    asking for list of reviewers, 67
    asking for pink slip, 67, 68
    avoiding discouragement, 66–67
    obtaining list of funded
      research, 67
Relational research question, 347–348
Relative rate, 134
Relative risk, 134, 356
  formula for estimating, 135
"Relative-to-ideal" ratings, 234
Relative validity, 187
Release time, 59
Reliability
  definition of, 13
  in descriptive research, 71
  and experimental errors, 301
  of food frequency
    questionnaire, 123–124
  in meta-analysis, 326–330
  in questionnaire design, 122
  and sample size determination, 343
  of screening tests, 105
Repetition, and statistical
  analysis, 30–31
Replicate measurements, 349
Replicate samples, 10
Replication, and statistical
  analysis, 30–31
Representativeness of sample, assessment of, 146
Reproducibility, of dietary intake methodology studies, 188–189
Research
  bridging into practice, 421–430
  definition of, 422
  ethics in, 7

Vote counting, in meta-analysis, 326

W

Walker-Duncan procedure, 31
Weight, 277
Weighted average, and
  meta-analysis, 329–330
White House Conference on Food,
  Nutrition, and Health, 212

Working hypothesis, 354
Writer's perspective, on research
  publications, 410–413

Z

Zeroes, handling of, in magnitude
  estimation, 230–231
Z test, 361